Online Resources

Included with your purchase are multiple online resources. This includes the practice tests in an interactive format and a convenient study timer to help you manage your time.

Instructions for accessing these resources can be found on the last page of this book.

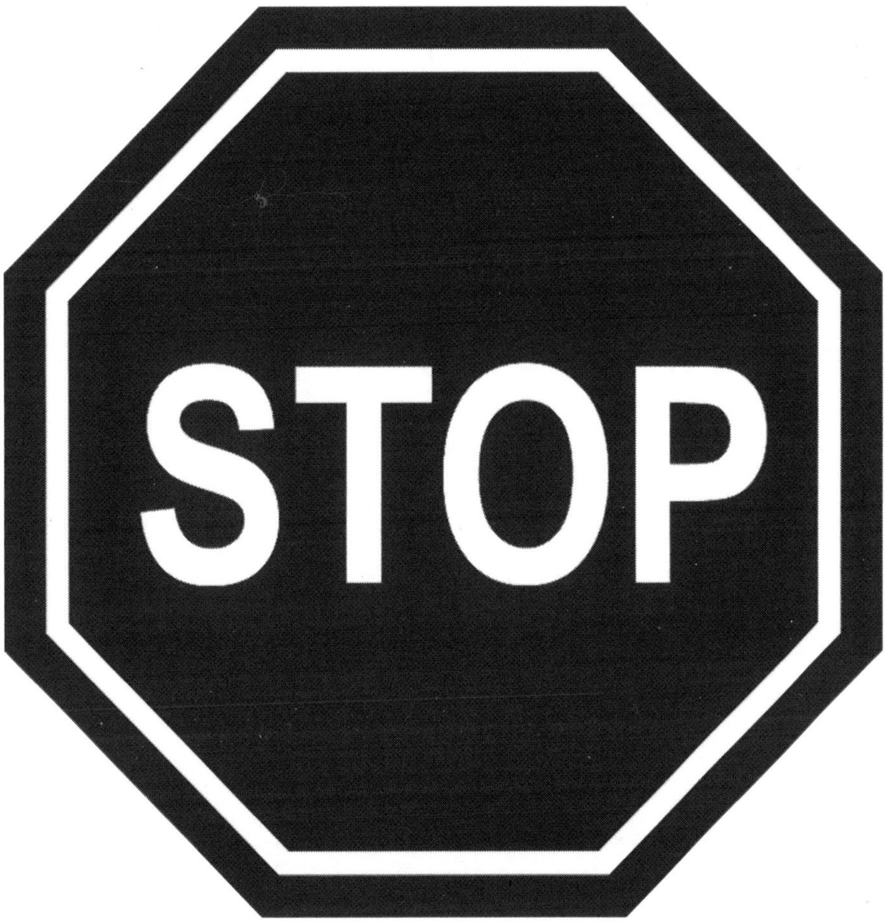

Adult CCRN® Exam Prep 2026 and 2027

15 Full-Length Practice Tests + Online Exam Simulator + CCRN Study Guide Review Book + Audiobook Access [8th Edition]

Lydia Morrison

Written and edited by TPB Publishing.

ISBN 13: 9781637751282

Table of Contents

Welcome

Dear Reader,

Welcome to your new Test Prep Books study guide! We are pleased that you chose us to help you prepare for your exam. There are many study options to choose from, and we appreciate you choosing us. Studying can be a daunting task, but we have designed a smart, effective study guide to help prepare you for what lies ahead.

Whether you're a parent helping your child learn and grow, a high school student working hard to get into your dream college, or a nursing student studying for a complex exam, we want to help give you the tools you need to succeed. We hope this study guide gives you the skills and the confidence to thrive, and we can't thank you enough for allowing us to be part of your journey.

In an effort to continue to improve our products, we welcome feedback from our customers. We look forward to hearing from you. Suggestions, success stories, and criticisms can all be communicated by emailing us at support@testprepbooks.com.

Sincerely,

Test Prep Books Team

Quick Overview

As you draw closer to taking your exam, effective preparation becomes more and more important. Thankfully, you have this study guide to help you get ready. Use this guide to help keep your studying on track and refer to it often.

This study guide contains several key sections that will help you be successful on your exam. The guide contains tips for what you should do the night before and the day of the test. Also included are test-taking tips. Knowing the right information is not always enough. Many well-prepared test takers struggle with exams. These tips will help equip you to accurately read, assess, and answer test questions.

A large part of the guide is devoted to showing you what content to expect on the exam and to helping you better understand that content. In this guide are practice test questions so that you can see how well you have grasped the content. Then, answer explanations are provided so that you can understand why you missed certain questions.

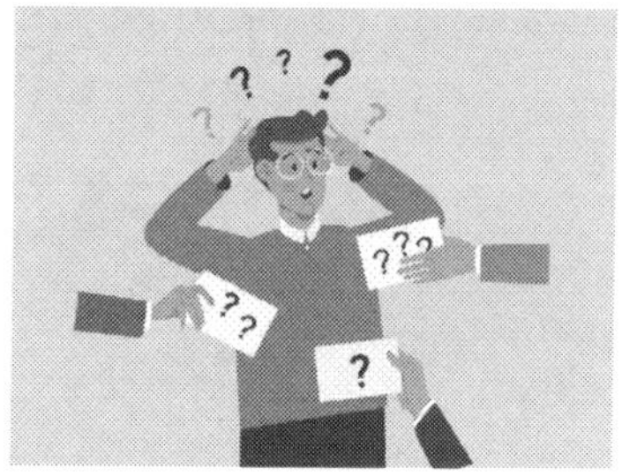

Don't try to cram the night before you take your exam. This is not a wise strategy for a few reasons. First, your retention of the information will be low. Your time would be better used by reviewing information you already know rather than trying to learn a lot of new information. Second, you will likely become stressed as you try to gain a large amount of knowledge in a short amount of time. Third, you will be depriving yourself of sleep. So be sure to go to bed at a reasonable time the night before. Being well-rested helps you focus and remain calm.

Be sure to eat a substantial breakfast the morning of the exam. If you are taking the exam in the afternoon, be sure to have a good lunch as well. Being hungry is distracting and can make it difficult to focus. You have hopefully spent lots of time preparing for the exam. Don't let an empty stomach get in the way of success!

When travelling to the testing center, leave earlier than needed. That way, you have a buffer in case you experience any delays. This will help you remain calm and will keep you from missing your appointment time at the testing center.

Be sure to pace yourself during the exam. Don't try to rush through the exam. There is no need to risk performing poorly on the exam just so you can leave the testing center early. Allow yourself to use all of the allotted time if needed.

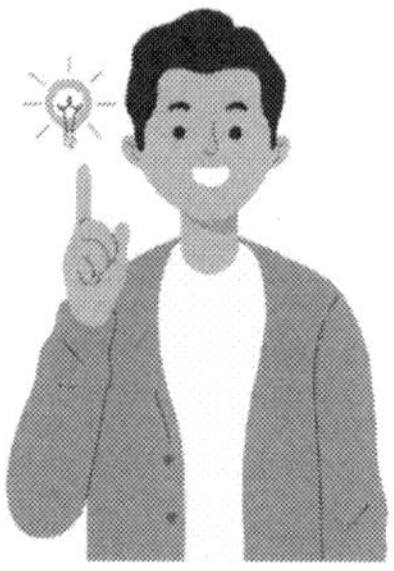

Remain positive while taking the exam even if you feel like you are performing poorly. Thinking about the content you should have mastered will not help you perform better on the exam.

Once the exam is complete, take some time to relax. Even if you feel that you need to take the exam again, you will be well served by some down time before you begin studying again. It's often easier to convince yourself to study if you know that it will come with a reward!

Test-Taking Strategies

1. Predicting the Answer

When you feel confident in your preparation for a multiple-choice test, try predicting the answer before reading the answer choices. This is especially useful on questions that test objective factual knowledge. By predicting the answer before reading the available choices, you eliminate the possibility that you will be distracted or led astray by an incorrect answer choice. You will feel more confident in your selection if you read the question, predict the answer, and then find your prediction among the answer choices. After using this strategy, be sure to still read all of the answer choices carefully and completely. If you feel unprepared, you should not attempt to predict the answers. This would be a waste of time and an opportunity for your mind to wander in the wrong direction.

2. Reading the Whole Question

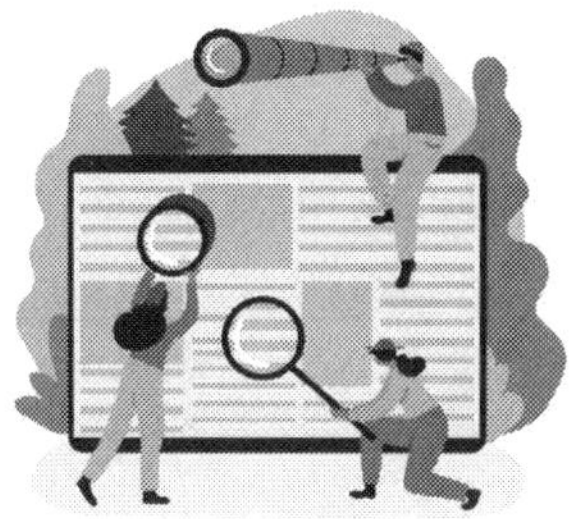

Too often, test takers scan a multiple-choice question, recognize a few familiar words, and immediately jump to the answer choices. Test authors are aware of this common impatience, and they will sometimes prey upon it. For instance, a test author might subtly turn the question into a negative, or he or she might redirect the focus of the question right at the end. The only way to avoid falling into these traps is to read the entirety of the question carefully before reading the answer choices.

3. Looking for Wrong Answers

Long and complicated multiple-choice questions can be intimidating. One way to simplify a difficult multiple-choice question is to eliminate all of the answer choices that are clearly wrong. In most sets of answers, there will be at least one selection that can be dismissed right away. If the test is administered on paper, the test taker could draw a line through it to indicate that it may be ignored; otherwise, the test taker will have to perform this operation mentally or on scratch paper. In either case, once the obviously incorrect answers have been eliminated, the remaining choices may be considered. Sometimes identifying the clearly wrong answers will give the test taker some information about the correct answer. For instance, if one of the remaining answer choices is a direct opposite of one of the eliminated answer choices, it may well be the correct answer. The opposite of obviously wrong is obviously right! Of course, this is not always the case. Some answers are obviously incorrect simply because they are irrelevant to the question being asked. Still, identifying and eliminating some incorrect answer choices is a good way to simplify a multiple-choice question.

4. Don't Overanalyze

Anxious test takers often overanalyze questions. When you are nervous, your brain will often run wild, causing you to make associations and discover clues that don't actually exist. If you feel that this may be a problem for you, do whatever you can to slow down during the test. Try taking a deep breath or counting to ten. As you read and consider the question, restrict yourself to the particular words used by the author. Avoid thought tangents about what the author *really* meant, or what he or she was *trying* to say. The only things that matter on a multiple-choice test are the words that are actually in the question. You must avoid reading too much into a multiple-choice question, or supposing that the writer meant something other than what he or she wrote.

5. No Need for Panic

It is wise to learn as many strategies as possible before taking a multiple-choice test, but it is likely that you will come across a few questions for which you simply don't know the answer. In this situation, avoid panicking. Because most multiple-choice tests include dozens of questions, the relative value of a single wrong answer is small. As much as possible, you should compartmentalize each question on a multiple-choice test. In other words, you should not allow your feelings about one question to affect your success on the others. When you find a question that you either don't understand or don't know how to answer, just take a deep breath and do your best. Read the entire question slowly and carefully. Try rephrasing the question a couple of different ways. Then, read all of the answer choices carefully. After eliminating obviously wrong answers, make a selection and move on to the next question.

6. Confusing Answer Choices

When working on a difficult multiple-choice question, there may be a tendency to focus on the answer choices that are the easiest to understand. Many people, whether consciously or not, gravitate to the answer choices that require the least concentration, knowledge, and memory. This is a mistake. When you come across an answer choice that is confusing, you should give it extra attention. A question might be confusing because you do not know the subject matter to which it refers. If this is the case, don't eliminate the answer before you have affirmatively settled on another. When you come across an answer choice of this type, set it aside as you look at the remaining choices. If you can confidently assert that one of the other choices is correct, you can leave the confusing answer aside. Otherwise, you will need to take a moment to try to better understand the confusing answer choice. Rephrasing is one way to tease out the sense of a confusing answer choice.

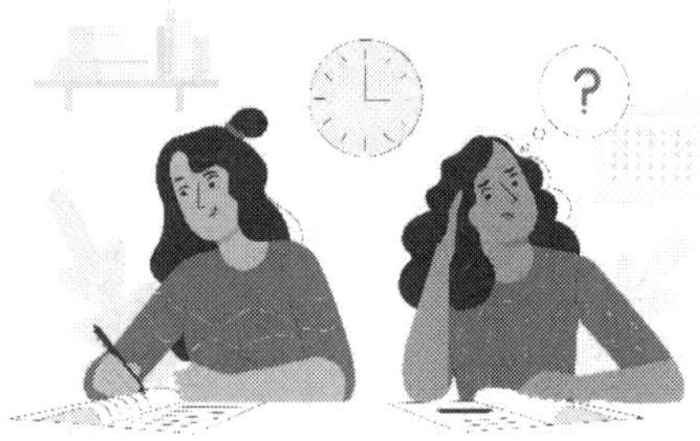

7. Your First Instinct

Many people struggle with multiple-choice tests because they overthink the questions. If you have studied sufficiently for the test, you should be prepared to trust your first instinct once you have carefully and completely read the question and all of the answer choices. There is a great deal of research suggesting that the mind can come to the correct conclusion very quickly once it has obtained all of the relevant information. At times, it may seem to you as if your intuition is working faster even than your reasoning mind. This may in fact be true. The knowledge you obtain while studying may be retrieved from your subconscious before you have a chance to work out the associations that support it. Verify your instinct by working out the reasons that it should be trusted.

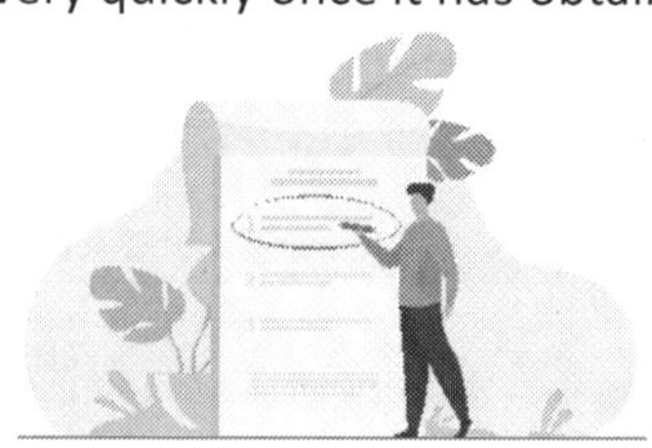

8. Key Words

Many test takers struggle with multiple-choice questions because they have poor reading comprehension skills. Quickly reading and understanding a multiple-choice question requires a mixture of skill and experience. To help with this, try jotting down a few key words and phrases on a piece of scrap paper. Doing this concentrates the process of reading and forces the mind to weigh the relative importance of the question's parts. In selecting words and phrases to write down, the test taker thinks about the question more deeply and carefully. This is especially true for multiple-choice questions that are preceded by a long prompt.

9. Subtle Negatives

One of the oldest tricks in the multiple-choice test writer's book is to subtly reverse the meaning of a question with a word like *not* or *except*. If you are not paying attention to each word in the question, you can easily be led astray by this trick. For instance, a common question format is, "Which of the following is...?" Obviously, if the question instead is, "Which of the following is not...?," then the answer will be quite different. Even worse, the test makers are aware of the potential for this mistake and will include one answer choice that would be correct if the question were not negated or reversed. A test taker who misses the reversal will find what he or she believes to be a correct answer and will be so confident that he or she will fail to reread the question and discover the original error. The only way to avoid this is to practice a wide variety of multiple-choice questions and to pay close attention to each and every word.

10. Reading Every Answer Choice

It may seem obvious, but you should always read every one of the answer choices! Too many test takers fall into the habit of scanning the question and assuming that they understand the question because they recognize a few key words. From there, they pick the first answer choice that answers the question they believe they have read. Test takers who read all of the answer choices might discover that one of the latter answer choices is actually *more* correct. Moreover, reading all of the answer choices can remind you of facts related to the question that can help you arrive at the correct answer. Sometimes, a misstatement or incorrect detail in one of the latter answer choices will trigger your memory of the subject and will enable you to find the right answer. Failing to read all of the answer choices is like not reading all of the items on a restaurant menu: you might miss out on the perfect choice.

11. Spot the Hedges

One of the keys to success on multiple-choice tests is paying close attention to every word. This is never truer than with words like *almost*, *most*, *some*, and *sometimes*. These words are called "hedges" because they indicate that a statement is not totally true or not true in every place and time. An absolute statement will contain no hedges, but in many subjects, the answers are not always straightforward or absolute. There are always exceptions to the rules in these subjects. For this reason, you should favor those multiple-choice questions that contain hedging language. The presence of qualifying words indicates that the author is taking special care with his or her words, which is certainly important when composing the right answer. After all, there are many ways to be wrong, but there is only one way to be right! For this reason, it is wise to avoid answers that are absolute when taking a multiple-choice test. An absolute answer is one that says things are either all one way or all another. They often include words like *every*, *always*, *best*, and *never*. If you are taking a multiple-choice test in a subject that doesn't lend itself to absolute answers, be on your guard if you see any of these words.

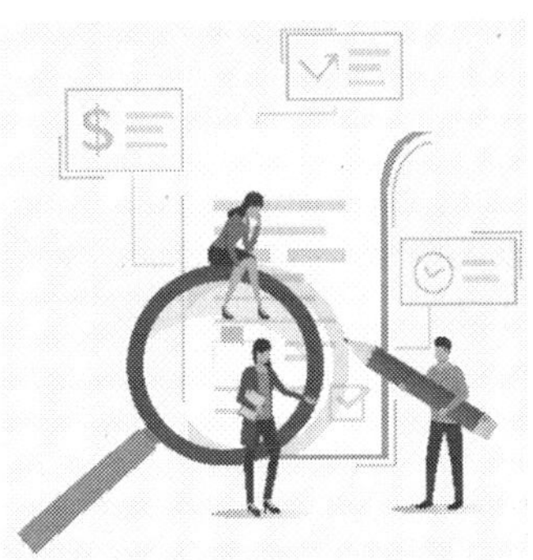

12. Long Answers

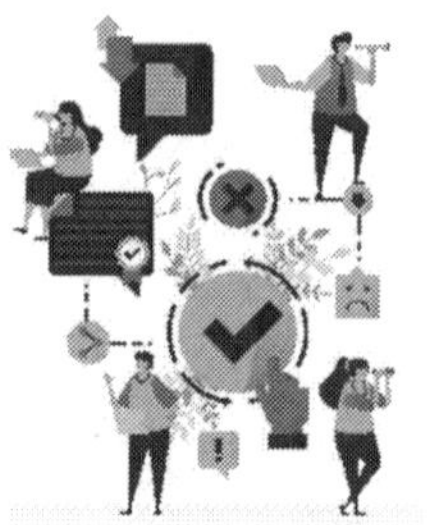

In many subject areas, the answers are not simple. As already mentioned, the right answer often requires hedges. Another common feature of the answers to a complex or subjective question are qualifying clauses, which are groups of words that subtly modify the meaning of the sentence. If the question or answer choice describes a rule to which there are exceptions or the subject matter is complicated, ambiguous, or confusing, the correct answer will require many words in order to be expressed clearly and accurately. In essence, you should not be deterred by answer choices that seem excessively long. Oftentimes, the author of the text will not be able to write the correct answer without offering some qualifications and modifications. Your job is to read the answer choices thoroughly and completely and to select the one that most accurately and precisely answers the question.

13. Restating to Understand

Sometimes, a question on a multiple-choice test is difficult not because of what it asks but because of how it is written. If this is the case, restate the question or answer choice in different words. This process serves a couple of important purposes. First, it forces you to concentrate on the core of the question. In order to rephrase the question accurately, you have to understand it well. Rephrasing the question will concentrate your mind on the key words and ideas. Second, it will present the information to your mind in a fresh way. This process may trigger your memory and render some useful scrap of information picked up while studying.

14. True Statements

Sometimes an answer choice will be true in itself, but it does not answer the question. This is one of the main reasons why it is essential to read the question carefully and completely before proceeding to the answer choices. Too often, test takers skip ahead to the answer choices and look for true statements. Having found one of these, they are content to select it without reference to the question above. The savvy test taker will always read the entire question before turning to the answer choices. Then, having settled on a correct answer choice, he or she will refer to the original question and ensure that the selected answer is relevant. The mistake of choosing a correct-but-irrelevant answer choice is especially common on questions related to specific pieces of objective knowledge.

15. No Patterns

One of the more dangerous ideas that circulates about multiple-choice tests is that the correct answers tend to fall into patterns. These erroneous ideas range from a belief that B and C are the most common right answers, to the idea that an unprepared test-taker should answer "A-B-A-C-A-D-A-B-A." It cannot be emphasized enough that pattern-seeking of this type is exactly the WRONG way to approach a multiple-choice test. To begin with, it is highly unlikely that the test maker will plot the correct answers according to some predetermined pattern. The questions are scrambled and delivered in a random order. Furthermore, even if the test maker was following a pattern in the assignation of correct answers, there is no reason why the test taker would know which pattern he or she was using. Any attempt to discern a pattern in the answer choices is a waste of time and a distraction from the real work of taking the test. A test taker would be much better served by extra preparation before the test than by reliance on a pattern in the answers.

Introduction to the Adult CCRN Exam

Function of the Exam

The Adult Acute/Critical Care Nursing Certification (CCRN®) exam is required to obtain the CCRN specialty certification, which is one of several specialty certifications offered to nurses by the AACN Certification Corporation. Nurses who work in settings where they provide direct care to adult, pediatric, or neonatal patients needing acute or critical care can seek CCRN® certification, which demonstrates competency in the knowledge and skills needed for their job, as well as professional recognition of their commitment to the field, their careers, and the care of acutely/critically ill patients. Accordingly, CCRN® test takers are nurses who typically work in intensive care units, combined ICU/CCUs, trauma units, cardiac care units, medical/surgical ICUs, or in critical care transport. CCRN® nurses need to deliver high-intensity, specialized care to their patients with a high degree of vigilance. Care may be focused on a specific system, such as renal, cardiac, or pulmonary, or it may be more generalized, geared toward multisystem, systemic issues.

The CCRN® exams are designed based on a job analysis, which examines the practice and skills of registered nurses (RNs) or advanced practice registered nurses (APRNs) who provide direct care to adult, pediatric, or neonatal patients who are acutely/critically ill. This process occurs at least every five years and helps determine and validate the abilities, skills, and knowledge needed to work with one of these patient populations in situations where the patients are acutely/critically ill. An expert CCRN® panel then works to ensure the exams are designed to reflect the findings of the job analysis and clinical practice. There is a separate exam for each patient population—adult, pediatric, and neonatal—and candidates should select the exam that best reflects the primary patient population for whom they provide direct care.

Exam candidates must have a current, unencumbered RN or APRN license from the United States. Additionally, one of the following two clinical practice requirements must be met prior to sitting for the exam:

- At least 1,750 hours providing direct care to acutely ill adult patients over the previous two years as an RN or APRN, with at least 875 of those hours obtained in the most recent year
- At least 2,000 hours providing direct care to acutely ill adult patients over the previous five years as an RN or APRN, with at least 144 of those hours obtained in the most recent year

It should be noted that orientation hours do not count towards minimum hour requirements unless the candidate was the assigned nurse who was providing direct care to patients with acute/critical illnesses during those hours.

Test Administration

Candidates can register online or via a paper application for the exam. After receiving an approval-to-test email, they can schedule their exam administration. The email will include a specific 90-day period during which the candidate must schedule and take the exam. The exam is offered twice daily, Monday through Friday, and some Saturdays, at more than 300 PSI/AMP testing locations around the United States. The exam is offered in a computer and paper-and-pencil format. Scores are provided immediately after submitting the computer-based version, and are received three to four weeks after sitting for the paper version. The exam may be retaken for an additional fee.

Test Format

The Adult CCRN® exam, like the pediatric and neonatal versions, contains 150 multiple-choice questions, of which, 125 are scored. The remaining 25, which are randomly scattered throughout the exam, are used to gauge their worth for inclusion in future versions. Test takers are given three hours to complete the exam. Clinical Judgment comprises 80% of the questions, while Professional Caring and Ethical Practice topics contribute 20% of the questions. It should be noted that the Clinical Judgment questions pertain only to adult patients, while the Professional Caring and Ethical Practice questions will address patients across the lifespan. The following table provides the domains of the adult version of the exam and the breakdown of their approximate percentage contributions to the total:

Domain	**Percentage of Exam***
Clinical Judgment	80%
Cardiovascular	13%
Respiratory	12%
Endocrine/Hematology/Gastrointestinal/Renal/Integumentary	21%
Musculoskeletal/Neurological/Psychosocial	18%
Multisystem	16%
Professional Caring and Ethical Practice	20%

*Note that the percentage of questions from the Clinical Judgement and Professional Caring and Ethical Practice domains are fairly firm at 80% and 20%, respectively. However, the percent contribution of questions pertaining to the specific body systems are approximated and therefore, do not necessarily sum to exactly 80%.

Scoring

A panel of subject matter and exam experts establish the passing score of the Adult CCRN® exam. The passing score is established via the modified Angoff, a criterion-referenced process for setting standards. Each test taker's CCRN® exam performance is compared to the predetermined standard to determine their passing status. The difficulty rating of each question also impacts the value of answering a question correctly. The passing score is said to be established to identify those candidates who possess an acceptable level of knowledge and skill in providing care to acutely ill adult patients. Candidates who successfully pass the exam receive a certificate denoting their specialty certification within three to four weeks after passing the test.

Study Prep Plan for the Adult CCRN Exam

1. **Schedule** - Use one of our study schedules below or come up with one of your own.

2. **Relax** - Test anxiety can hurt even the best students. There are many ways to reduce stress. Find the one that works best for you.

3. **Execute** - Once you have a good plan in place, be sure to stick to it.

One Week Study Schedule

Day 1	Clinical Judgment
Day 2	Respiratory
Day 3	Endocrine/Hematology/Gastrointestinal/ Renal/ Integumentary
Day 4	Practice Test #1
Day 5	Practice Test #2
Day 6	Practice Test #3
Day 7	Take Your Exam!

Two Week Study Schedule

Day 1	Clinical Judgment	Day 8	Practice Test #1
Day 2	Cardiac Surgery	Day 9	Answer Explanations #1
Day 3	Respiratory	Day 10	Practice Test #2
Day 4	Endocrine/Hematology/ Gastrointestinal/Renal/ Integumentary	Day 11	Answer Explanations #2
Day 5	Musculoskeletal/ Neurological/ Psychosocial	Day 12	Practice Test #3
Day 6	Professional Caring & Ethical Practice	Day 13	Answer Explanations #3
Day 7	The American Hospital Associations Patient...	Day 14	Take Your Exam!

One Month Study Schedule

Day 1	Clinical Judgment	Day 11	Transfusion-Related Acute Lung Injury (TRALI)	Day 21	The American Hospital Associations Patient Care Partnership Document
Day 2	Acute Peripheral Vascular Insufficiency	Day 12	Endocrine/Hematology/ Gastrointestinal/Renal/ Integumentary	Day 22	Facilitation of Learning
Day 3	Acute Pulmonary Edema	Day 13	Hematology/ Immunology	Day 23	Systems Thinking
Day 4	Cardiac Surgery	Day 14	Renal/Genitourinary	Day 24	Practice Test #1
Day 5	Cardiac/Vascular Catheterization	Day 15	Musculoskeletal/ Neurological/ Psychosocial	Day 25	Answer Explanations #1
Day 6	Heart Failure	Day 16	Behavioral and Psychosocial	Day 26	Practice Test #2
Day 7	Structural Heart Defects	Day 17	Multisystem	Day 27	Answer Explanations #2
Day 8	Respiratory	Day 18	Professional Caring & Ethical Practice	Day 28	Practice Test #3
Day 9	Acute Respiratory Infections	Day 19	Caring Practices	Day 29	Answer Explanations #3
Day 10	Status Asthmaticus	Day 20	The Needs of the Critical Care Family (Molter, 1997)	Day 30	Take Your Exam!

Build your own prep plan by visiting the Online Resources page.

Instructions and a QR code can be found on the last page of this guide.

As you study for your test, we'd like to take the opportunity to remind you that you are capable of great things! With the right tools and dedication, you truly can do anything you set your mind to. The fact that you are holding this book right now shows how committed you are. In case no one has told you lately, you've got this! Our intention behind including this coloring page is to give you the chance to take some time to engage your creative side when you need a little brain-break from studying. As a company, we want to encourage people like you to achieve their dreams by providing good quality study materials for the tests and certifications that improve careers and change lives. As individuals, many of us have taken such tests in our careers, and we know how challenging this process can be. While we can't come alongside you and cheer you on personally, we can offer you the space to recall your purpose, reconnect with your passion, and refresh your brain through an artistic practice. We wish you every success, and happy studying!

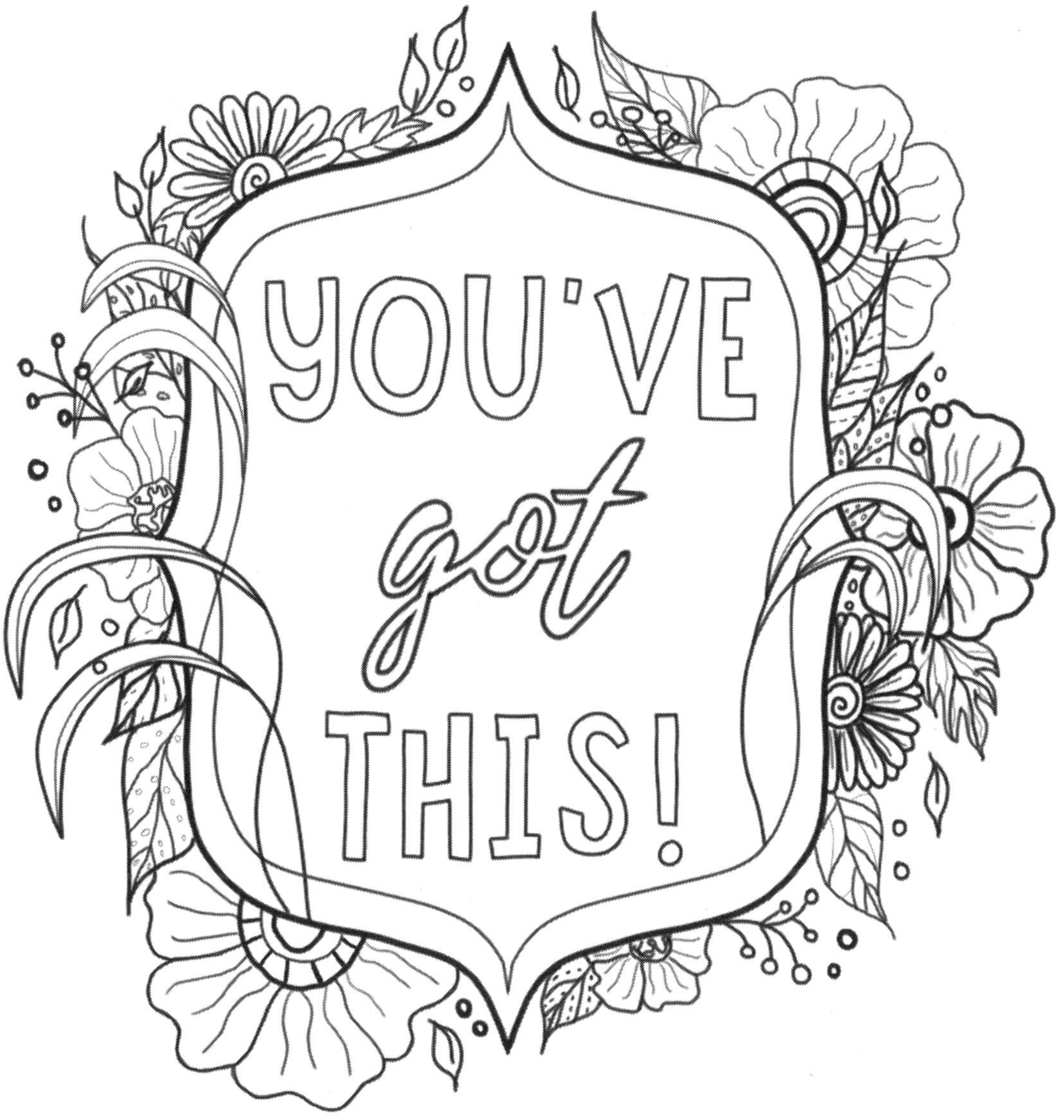

Clinical Judgment

In the world of patient care, the nurse is the vigilante, always watching and guarding the patient. A continuous series of clinical judgments are made based upon patient assessment, tests, lab work, procedure results, data analysis, and team collaboration. The critical care registered nurse (CCRN) is highly adept at putting together all these pieces of the patient puzzle, making informed clinical judgments that will greatly benefit the patient's care. The following is a review of cardiovascular and pulmonary maladies. The nurse pursuing CCRN certification must be familiar with these conditions, causes, signs and symptoms, and course of treatment to make appropriate clinical judgments regarding the patient's care.

Cardiovascular

The critical care nurse is an expert at recognizing a cardiovascular illness, from the crushing weight felt by a patient with angina, to the classic shooting pain up and down the left arm of a patient experiencing a heart attack, to the pooling of blood in the legs when one's circulatory system has weakened. Savvy knowledge of the cardiovascular system and the different ways it can malfunction is a key factor in a critical care nurse's ability to make sound clinical judgments. The following is a review of acute cardiovascular diseases in critical care settings.

Acute Coronary Syndrome

An **acute coronary syndrome** is any instance in which the coronary arteries of the heart are blocked, causing an interrupted flow in crucial oxygen delivery to the heart muscle. This causes immediate damage to the areas affected, and if left untreated, tissue death. A more common term for the syndrome, though less precise, is a **heart attack**.

There are three distinct types of acute coronary syndromes: Non-ST-Segment Elevation Myocardial Infarction (NSTEMI), STEMI, and unstable angina. The first two refer to what most people know as "heart attacks," differing only by the amount of the heart wall that is damaged. **Angina**, a term for chest pain, can occur without heart tissue damage. All three categories can occur because of increased oxygen demand in the heart tissue or the body at large, such as during exercise and emotional distress.

In any of the three cases, major determining factors for tissue damage include the severity of the arterial blockage, the length of time the arteries are blocked, the percentage of the heart that is affected, the magnitude of the demand for oxygen in the heart, and the extent to which the heart can compensate for the oxygen loss.

A patient may be experiencing a different condition than acute coronary syndrome, such as an anxiety attack or acid reflux, that may mimic the same signs and symptoms. The clinician must be aware of this possibility when making a clinical judgment. An accurate assessment will be made based on patient history, clinical presentation, and events leading up to the current symptoms.

The most common symptom that signals acute coronary syndrome is chest pain. The chest pain of a heart attack has been described as "crushing pressure," "heavy weight," "tightness," and/or "fullness" in the chest area above the heart. Other accompanying symptoms include a shooting pain radiating down one or both arms, along the jawline, or even in the back or abdomen. The patient may present with complaint of "not being able to catch their breath," breathing rapidly, or shallow breathing. Dizziness, lightheadedness, nausea, and profuse drops of sweat may be part of the patient's presentation.

It is important to note that gender plays a role in how patients may present with a heart attack. Considering that heart disease is the leading cause of death for women in the United States, the critical care nurse should be aware that women may not exhibit the classic signs of a heart attack. A woman is more likely to have non-chest-related symptoms, such as nausea, anxiety, and radiating pain in the upper or lower back and jaw region. These symptoms may occur weeks before the actual attack, making correct diagnosis even more difficult to pinpoint. That being said, knowing that there may be a different presentation will help the critical care nurse make the correct clinical judgment regarding the situation, considering all involved factors.

Diagnosis of MI is made by electrocardiogram (ECG) reading as well as serological markers such as elevated troponin.

Diagram illustrating normal ECG, ST elevation, ST depression, and T inversion

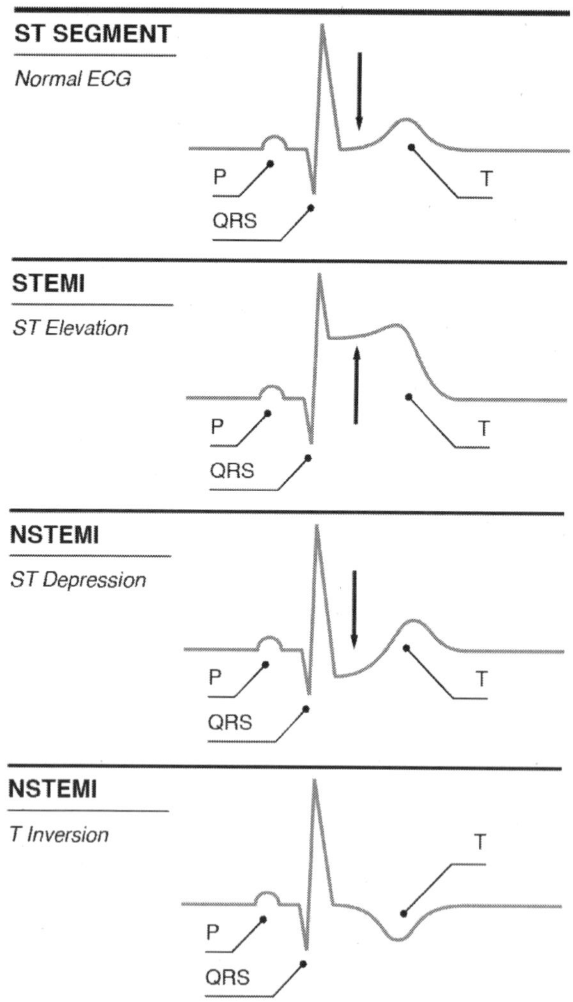

An **NSTEMI** is an MI in which the ST segment of the ECG is not elevated. This important distinction arises from the amount of heart muscle damaged. In an NSTEMI, not enough heart tissue is damaged to make the ST segment rise on the ECG, whereas a **STEMI** does just that.

Serological markers such as an elevated troponin level indicate cardiac muscle damage. When the muscle is injured, it releases muscle cell contents into the bloodstream; the greater the damage, the higher the muscle cell contents, such as troponin, in the bloodstream. Other serological markers indicating heart muscle damage include the cardiac enzymes CK-MB and muscle cell component myoglobin.

After the ECG has been checked and the blood has been sent to the lab to evaluate for elevated serological markers of a heart attack, the patient will likely be whisked away for a cardiac catheterization. This standard procedure includes accessing the patient's femoral artery, threading a thin tube, or catheter, up through the abdominothoracic blood vessels directly into the heart to assess for blockages and damage. During the test, dye is released into the heart, and x-ray images are obtained for better visualization. The patient will often be given medication to relax, but they will still be awake for the procedure. This procedure can allow the cardiologist to open up coronary vessels that have been occluded with atherosclerotic plaques using a tiny balloon and place tiny metal scaffolds called **stents**, if necessary, and determine if further interventions such as cardiac surgery are needed to repair valves or bypass severely blocked arteries.

Illustration of the thickness of heart muscle affected in the heart wall in NSTEMI vs. STEMI

Transverse section of the heart

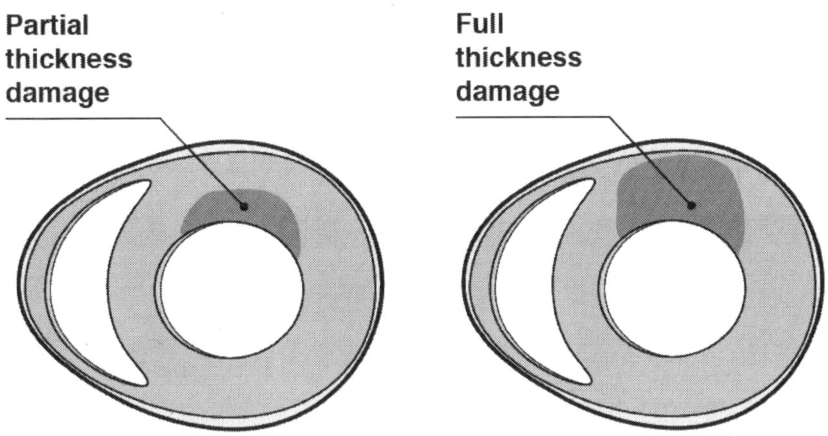

Aortic Aneurysm

A patient experiencing a sudden onset of tearing chest pain may be experiencing a rupture or dissection of an aortic aneurysm. Aortic aneurysms may occur at the top of the aorta, right after exiting the heart, termed **thoracic aortic aneurysms**. Aortic aneurysms may also occur farther down the aorta, then called either **thoracoabdominal aortic aneurysms** or **abdominal aortic aneurysms**. An **aneurysm** is any ballooning or enlargement of a blood vessel, often caused by atherosclerosis. When an aneurysm suddenly tears apart, massive amounts of the patient's blood start surging out with each and every heartbeat, making it an immediate medical emergency. A patient experiencing an aortic aneurysm dissection needs immediate surgical repair followed by intensive cardiac and hemodynamic monitoring until stabilized.

Patients with unruptured aortic aneurysms may be completely asymptomatic. Detection of an aortic aneurysm occurs through ultrasonography, abdominal CT, echocardiography, and/or transesophageal echocardiography. Treatment for aortic aneurysms that have not ruptured includes elective surgical repair along with encouragement to quit smoking, a major cause of atherosclerosis, and drug therapy including antilipids and BP control.

Illustration showing the difference between an abdominal and thoracic aortic aneurysm

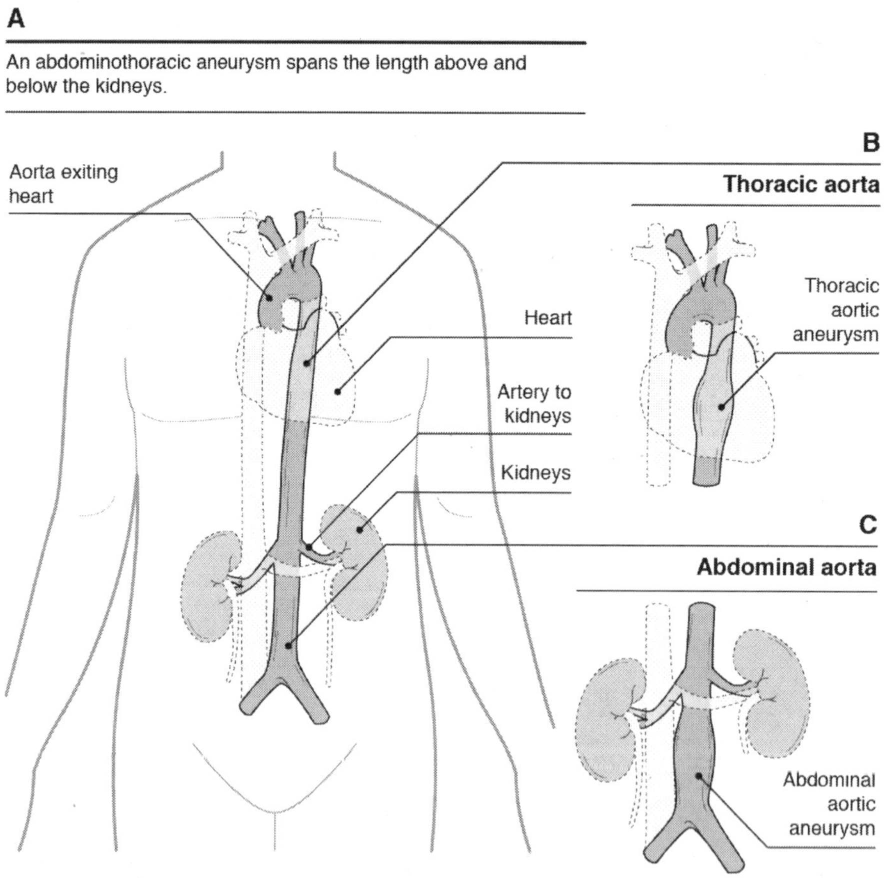

Aortic Dissection

Aortic dissection is a condition in which the layers of the arterial wall become separated and blood leaks in between the layers of the vessel. A dissection represents damage through at least the first layer of an artery. It is a more serious form of aneurysm because all of the layers are compromised.

A dissection is different from a rupture. With a dissection, blood leaks in and through the layers of an artery, but the artery remains structurally intact, albeit weakened. Blood is still contained within the vessel. When a rupture occurs, it is similar to the popping of a balloon. The integrity of the artery is disrupted, and blood leaks out of the artery. Dissections increase the risk of rupture. Medical management with beta-blockers is the treatment of choice for stable aortic dissections.

Aortic Rupture

The aorta is the main artery in the body and provides oxygenated blood to all other arteries in the cardiovascular system. An **aortic rupture** is damage to the aorta in which it breaks or bursts. The primary symptom is sharp pain in the torso, back, or groin. Other signs may include visible bruising, low blood pressure, confusion, and blue-tinged skin; however, patients typically lose consciousness quickly when the aorta ruptures. Aortic ruptures are extremely serious events with a high mortality rate (up to 90%); emergency surgery is required to repair the aorta and most patients are simply not able to receive adequate care before fatal hemorrhage occurs.

Aortic ruptures are classified based on cause, either due to traumatic or aneurysm event. Traumatic aortic ruptures result when the aorta is hit, punctured, or otherwise wounded through blunt force or penetration. This most commonly occurs in motor vehicle accidents in which a person's chest takes impact or in assault victims who have been shot or stabbed in the chest. Aortic aneurysms are typically triggered by aortic swelling, which then causes the artery to balloon and burst. Aortic aneurysms are usually symptomless until a rupture occurs. Risk factors for aortic aneurysms include coronary artery disease, hypertension, heavy smoking or alcohol use, or vascular diseases. These factors result in a weakening of the arterial walls, therefore making the artery more vulnerable to breaking down.

As aortic aneurysms cause more cases of aortic ruptures than traumatic events, patients with risk factors should undergo regular screenings. Chest ultrasounds and imaging scans are the only methods with which to know whether a patient is at risk of experiencing an aortic aneurysm. Preventive treatments in high-risk patients include smoking cessation, stress reduction, and long-term medication to ensure that blood pressure remains in a moderate range.

Cardiac Infection and Inflammatory Diseases

Endocarditis

By definition, **endocarditis** is the inflammation of the endocardium, or innermost lining of the heart chambers and valves. It is also called infective endocarditis, or bacterial endocarditis.

To review, there are three layers of tissue that comprise the heart. A double-layer serous membrane, known as the **pericardium**, is the outermost layer. The pericardium forms the pericardial sac that surrounds the heart. The middle and largest layer is the **myocardium**. Since an MI occurs when the heart muscle is deprived of oxygen, the myocardial layer of the heart is where the damage due to lack of oxygen occurs. The innermost layer that lines the heart chambers and also the heart valves is called the **endocardium**. Endocarditis occurs when the endocardial layer and heart valves become infected and inflamed.

The most common cause of endocarditis is a bloodstream invasion of bacteria. Staphylococci and Streptococci account for the majority of infective endocarditis occurrences. During medical or dental procedures—such as a colonoscopy, cystoscopy, or professional teeth cleaning—bacteria may enter the bloodstream and travel to the heart. Inflammatory bowel disease and sexually transmitted diseases also foster bacterial transmission to the bloodstream and, ultimately, the heart.

Risk factors for the development of endocarditis include valve and septal defects of the heart, an artificial heart valve, a history of endocarditis, an indwelling long-term dialysis catheter, parenteral nutrition or central lines in the right atrium, IV drug use, and body piercings. Patients taking steroids or immunosuppressive medications are susceptible to fungal endocarditis. Regardless of the source, the bacteria infect the inside of the heart chambers and valves. Clumps of infective bacteria, or vegetation, develop within the heart at the site of infection. The heart valves are a common infection site, which often results in incomplete closure of the valves.

The classic symptoms of endocarditis are fever, cardiac murmur, and petechial lesions of the skin, conjunctiva, and oral mucosa. However, symptoms can range in severity. Flu-like symptoms, weight loss, and back pain may be present. Dyspnea and swelling of the feet and ankles may be evident. Endocarditis caused by Staphylococcus has a rapid onset, whereas Streptococcus occurs more slowly with a prolonged course.

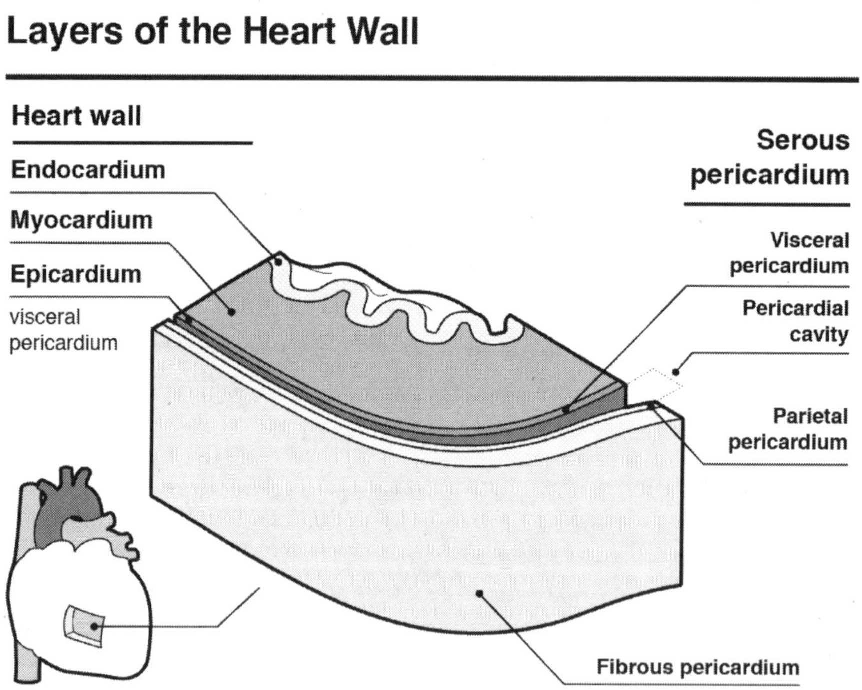

Antimicrobial treatment for four to six weeks is the standard of care. In some cases, two antimicrobials are used to treat the infection and prevent drug resistance. The objective of treatment is to eradicate the infection and treat complications. Surgery may be required for persistent recurring infections, one or more embolic occurrences, or if heart failure develops.

Left untreated, endocarditis can result in stroke or organ damage, as the vegetation breaks off, travels through the bloodstream, and blocks circulation. The spread of infection and subsequent formation of abscesses throughout the body may also occur. Heart failure may develop when the infection hampers the heart's ability to pump effectively or with perforation of a valve.

A complete history and physical that includes inquiry about medications, recent surgeries, screening, and diagnostic testing may provide the crucial piece of information that identifies endocarditis in the face of otherwise vague symptom presentation. The nurse should anticipate the order for blood cultures, an erythrocyte sedimentation rate (ESR), a CBC, an ECG, a chest x-ray, and a transthoracic or transesophageal echocardiogram to identify the location of the infected area.

An in-depth patient interview and assessment by the nurse are essential. Diagnostic and laboratory results coupled with data from the patient interview will aid in early recognition and treatment of endocarditis. Because an incident of endocarditis places one at a higher risk for future infections, patient teaching should include informing all providers and dentists prior to treatment. Antibiotic prophylaxis may be indicated.

Myocarditis

Myocarditis is inflammation of the myocardium, or the central muscle tissue that forms the heart. This inflammation can be caused by reactions of the immune system, such as infections (usually viral, but may also be bacterial or fungal) or autoimmune conditions, such as lupus. Myocarditis can also be caused by medications, including chemotherapy as well as some antidepressants and antipsychotics. Finally, myocarditis can be caused by drug use (e.g., cocaine) and exposure to toxins, such as spider or snake bites. Regardless of the cause, myocarditis can lead to both acute and chronic cardiac conditions, making its identification and prompt treatment vital to improving patient outcomes.

A patient with myocarditis may present with the following symptoms:

- Chest pain
- Shortness of breath
- Increased fatigue
- Syncope
- Tachycardia or other arrhythmias
- Signs of poor peripheral perfusion (e.g., cool extremities or peripheral edema)
- Signs of infection (e.g., fever)

As with most patients presenting with these signs and symptoms, initial diagnosis will likely start with laboratory testing, an electrocardiogram (ECG), and imaging. Laboratory tests will likely include the following:

- Complete blood count (CBC) to check for signs of infection or anemia
- Metabolic panel (CMP) to check for electrolyte abnormalities
- Cardiac enzymes (e.g., troponin) to look for stress on the cardiac muscle
- B-type natriuretic peptide (BNP) to check for signs of heart failure
- Potentially other samples to find a source of suspected infection (e.g., viral panels, streptococcus testing, or blood cultures).

ECG results will generally show tachycardia and/or T wave changes but may also reveal prolonged QT or other abnormalities, depending on the location of the inflammation and the progression of the disease process. Initial imaging will likely be x-ray, which may show an enlarged heart in the patient with myocarditis. Additional imaging may include a cardiac computed tomography (CT) scan to rule out blocked arteries, magnetic resonance imaging (MRI) to show a more detailed image of the cardiac inflammation, and an echocardiogram to evaluate the heart's ability to pump efficiently and to find any possible abnormalities in valves or heart chambers. These diagnostics will allow the treatment team to identify the presence of myocarditis, find a potential cause, and help determine necessary treatment.

Treatment of myocarditis depends on its cause, severity, and any other resulting sequelae of the condition. If myocarditis is found to be caused by an infection, initial treatment will likely involve administration of antivirals, antibacterials, or antifungals. If the cause is determined to be medication, the treatment team may have to determine the risks and benefits of holding, changing, or decreasing the medication. For example, it may not be possible to stop a specific chemotherapy drug; however, other medications such as steroids may be added to decrease inflammation. If the cause is recreational drug use, the patient will likely be given resources and education on drug cessation. If the cause is some other toxin, treatment will vary based on the specific toxin and what resources are available to either counter the toxin (e.g., antivenom) or symptomatically treat the patient.

If the myocarditis progresses into other heart conditions, those will also need to be treated. For example, myocarditis can lead to heart failure and valve abnormalities. These may require blood pressure medications, rate control medications, diuretics, and potentially surgical intervention. Arrythmias may need to be treated depending on the rhythm and stability of the patient. If the arrythmias become chronic, the patient may also require placement of a pacemaker or implantable cardioverter-defibrillator device (ICD). In the most severe cases of myocarditis, the patient may even require **extracorporeal membrane oxygenation (ECMO)**.

Nursing management of patients with myocarditis involves continued assessment of the patient for signs of worsening cardiovascular symptoms. These may include the following: worsening chest pain or shortness of breath; changes in mental status; changes to peripheral vascular perfusion (e.g., edema or decreased perfusion); changes in cardiac monitoring (e.g., life-threatening arrhythmias); and changes in monitoring of laboratory values. Nursing management also requires providing patient education throughout the disease process. The nurse should educate patients on ways to prevent myocarditis, such as taking antibiotics when they have strep throat or cessation of recreational drugs. For those who have been diagnosed, the nature of the condition should be thoroughly explained, including potential complications and treatment expectations depending on the patient's individual needs. For example, if the patient's myocarditis progresses into heart failure, the patient should be educated on diuretic and cardiac medication usage as well as what signs and symptoms may imply an exacerbation of their condition that requires further treatment (e.g., worsening extremity swelling, shortness of breath, and/or chest pain).

Pericarditis

Pericarditis is inflammation of the pericardium, which forms the pericardial sac that surrounds the heart.

Look at this graphic again for reference:

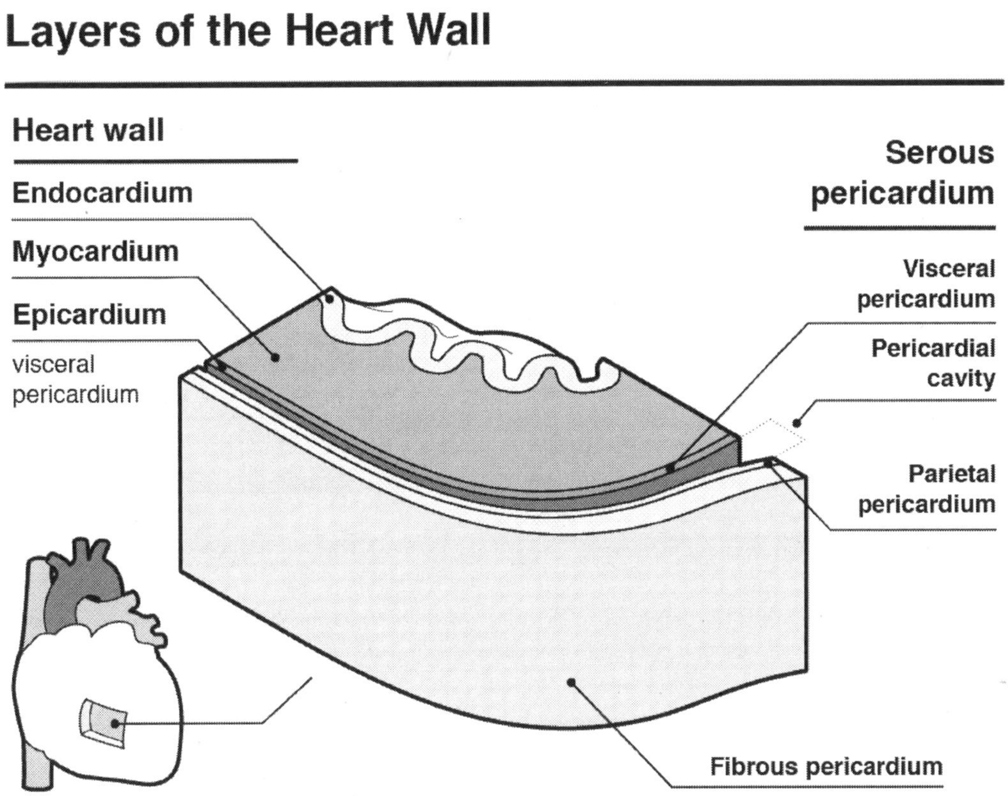

The fibrous attachments between the pericardium the mid-diaphragm and to the back of the sternum keep the heart in place during acceleration or deceleration. The fibrous nature of the parietal layer prevents cardiac distention into the mediastinal region of the chest. It separates the heart from the surrounding structures, and it protects the heart against infection and inflammation from the lungs. The pericardium contains pain receptors and mechanoreceptors, both of which prompt reflex changes in the BP and HR.

Pericarditis can be either acute or chronic in presentation. Causes are varied and include an acute MI; bacterial, fungal, and viral infections; certain medications; chest trauma; connective tissue disorders such as lupus or rheumatic fever; metastatic lesions from lung or breast tumors; and a history of radiation therapy of the chest and upper torso. Frequent or prolonged episodes of pericarditis can lead to thickening and scarring of the pericardium and loss of elasticity. These conditions limit the heart's ability to fill with blood, and therefore limit the amount of blood being pumped out to the body. The result is a decrease in cardiac output (CO). Pericarditis can also cause fluid to accumulate in the pericardial cavity, known as pericardial effusion.

A characteristic symptom of pericarditis is chest pain. The pain is persistent, sharp, pleuritic, felt in the mid-chest, and aggravated by deep inhalation. Pericarditis may also cause ST elevation, thereby mimicking an acute MI, or it may be asymptomatic.

A **pericardial friction rub** is diagnostic of pericarditis and characterized by a creaky or scratchy sound heard at the end of exhalation. The rub is best heard when the patient is sitting and leaning forward. Stethoscope placement should be at the left lower sternal border in the fourth intercostal space. The rub is audible on auscultation and synchronous to the heartbeat. A pericardial friction rub is differentiated from a pleural friction rub by having patients hold their breath. The pericardial friction rub will remain constant with the heartbeat. Other presenting symptoms include a mild fever, cough, and dyspnea. Common laboratory findings are elevated white blood cell (WBC), ESR, or CRP levels.

The diagnosis of pericarditis is based on history, signs, and symptoms. Treatment goals are to determine the cause, administer therapy for treatment and symptom relief, and detect signs of complications. A thorough medical and surgical history will identify patients at risk for developing pericarditis. The physical assessment should evaluate the reported pain level during position changes, inspiration, expiration, coughing, swallowing, and breath holding. In addition, flexion, extension, and rotation of the neck and spine should be assessed for their influence on reported pain.

In patients not showing signs of any specific etiology or a poor prognosis, a one-week trial of NSAIDs with follow-up is recommended for patients with acute pericarditis. Physical activity in non-athletic patients should be restricted to regular daily activity until symptoms resolve, and a three-month minimal restriction on activity for athletes. In patients with moderate risk not responding ideally to NSAIDs, an etiological search is advised to diagnose and manage the specific form of pericarditis.

Cardiac Surgery

Cardiac surgery refers to any surgery of the heart itself, as well as the adjacent large vessels that carry blood to or from the heart. Cardiac surgery is most commonly performed to treat heart defects, heart damage, decreased function, or trauma. Cardiac surgery may be needed for congenital reasons, lifestyle factors, or acute injury. Cardiac surgery may be performed by physically cutting through the chest wall and rib cage to operate on the heart or cardiac region. This is known as open-heart surgery. In the last decade, minimally invasive cardiac surgeries have become more common for many cardiac procedures. These types of surgeries utilize endoscopic cameras and catheters to conduct surgical procedures through small incisions in less risky parts of the body. Clinicians are able to use imaging techniques and catheters to guide medical instruments into the cardiac regions, rather than making a large incision to the chest and directly entering the cardiothoracic cavity. This reduces the risk of surgical complications and post-surgical infections while reducing overall recovery time for the patient.

A **coronary artery bypass graft** (**CABG**) is a surgical procedure for patients with coronary heart disease, in which the left or right coronary arteries become narrow and are susceptible to clogs. These two arteries are the main supply of oxygenated blood to the heart to support its tissues and functions; when they are diseased, it often causes angina in the patient. Angina is severe chest pain caused by a decrease in oxygen supply to the heart. Diseased coronary arteries and angina significantly increase the patient's risk for heart attack, so a CABG is often recommended to reduce the risk.

During a CABG, a healthier blood vessel from another part of the body is removed and attached to the coronary artery. Blood flow is redirected through the grafted vessel, which then supplies the heart. Recovery after this procedure is significant. Most people require a minimum of inpatient recovery, and three months for a full recovery. Complications can include infections at the surgical site. If the graft is not successful, patients can still experience a heart attack. Finally, if patients do not make lifestyle decisions that support their artery health, they may require repeat CABGs.

Valve repairs and replacements may be needed in patients with congenital heart conditions (such as heart murmurs or congenital valve anomalies) or in patients who have worn heart valves due to age. Patients may also choose poor lifestyle behaviors, such as a sedentary lifestyle, unhealthy diet, or habitual smoking, which can narrow and harden the valve (valve stenosis). Patients whose valves do not open or close effectively are unable to efficiently circulate blood through the body and may feel fatigue, dizziness, and chest pain; they may also have difficulty carrying out physical activities. Patients are also at increased risk of heart failure.

Valves may be repaired or replaced through open-heart surgery but are increasingly remedied through minimally invasive endoscopic procedures. Repair procedures include patching worn valves, reconnecting loose valves, or loosening valves that have adhesions or scarring. Narrow valves may be treated with a temporary or permanent stent. As a last resort, the entire affected valve will be replaced with a valve manufactured from pig or cow cardiac tissue.

Cardiac Tamponade

Cardiac tamponade, or pericardial tamponade, is a syndrome caused by the excessive accumulation of blood or fluid in the pericardial sac, resulting in the compression of the myocardium and reduced ventricular filling. It is a medical emergency with complications of pulmonary edema, shock, and death, if left untreated.

The pericardium, or outer layer of the heart wall, is a two-layer membrane that forms the pericardial sac, which envelops the heart. The parietal (outer) layer of the pericardium is made of tough, thickened fibrous tissue. This layer is attached to the mid-diaphragm and to the back of the sternum. These attachments keep the heart in place during acceleration or deceleration. The fibrous nature of the parietal layer prevents cardiac distention into the mediastinal region of the chest.

The visceral (inner) layer of the pericardium is a double-layered membrane. One layer is affixed to the heart. The second layer lines the inside of the parietal (outer) layer. The small space between the parietal and visceral layers is the pericardial space. The space normally contains between 15 and 50 milliliters of pericardial fluid. The pericardial fluid lubricates the membranes and allows the two layers to slide over one another as the heart beats.

Symptoms of a pericardial tamponade are dyspnea, chest tightness, dizziness, tachycardia, muffled heart sounds, and restlessness. **Pulsus paradoxus** is an important clinical finding in tamponade; it represents an abnormal BP variation during the respiration cycle and is evidenced by a decrease of 10 mmHg or more in systolic BP during inspiration. Pulsus paradoxus represents decreased diastolic ventricular filling and reduced volume in all four chambers of the heart. The clinical signs associated with tamponade are distended neck veins, muffled heart sounds, and hypotension. These clustered symptoms are known as **Beck's triad**.

Removal of the pericardial fluid via **pericardiocentesis** is the definitive therapy. A pericardiectomy or pericardial window may be performed to remove part of the pericardium. Fluid removed during the procedure is analyzed to determine the cause of the effusion. Malignancies, metastatic disease, and trauma are major causes of the development of pericardial effusions.

Identification and treatment of a tamponade requires emergent medical intervention. A rapid focused assessment of heart sounds and BP, including assessing for pulsus paradoxus, is a critical first step. An in-depth medical and surgical history can aid in identifying the etiology.

Cardiac Trauma

Cardiac trauma cases are categorized into those that occurred from blunt impact or penetrating force. **Blunt cardiac trauma** results from high force contact upon a person's chest, which can occur suddenly and last moments, or from prolonged compression. Common causes of blunt cardiac trauma include motor vehicle accidents, falls, and impact that occurs during recreational activities. **Penetrating cardiac trauma** occurs when an object is able to pierce the skin and tissues over the cardiac region, as well as cardiac tissue itself. This results in an open wound. Penetrating cardiac trauma is most commonly caused by knife and bullet impact but can also occur from impalements.

Since the organs and vascular networks in the cardiac region are so vital to life, cardiac trauma should be assessed comprehensively, with Advanced Trauma Life Support measures in mind. This clinical system includes a **primary survey**, which entails airway management, spinal support, breathing and ventilation support, and bleeding control. The primary survey aims to stabilize the patient's vital functions and ensure that the patient's heart, lungs, and spinal section deep to the thoracic cavity are supported. A secondary survey by clinicians is used to assess other health outcomes of cardiac trauma that are not directly threatening the patient's life.

A **secondary survey** may include physical examination of other body parts, addressing other aspects of the patient's medical history, and continuously monitoring vital signs such as temperature, pulse rate, and respiration. Sudden changes to these vital signs can indicate deterioration in the patient. In cardiac trauma patients, clinicians should note dysrhythmias, myocardial contusions, cardiac ruptures, and damage to coronary arteries. Blunt cardiac trauma typically requires prolonged monitoring of heart function, heartbeat rhythm, and electrical activity. Penetrating cardiac trauma typically requires emergency surgery to repair any lacerations and open wounds. Patients with penetrating cardiac trauma are more vulnerable to the presence of foreign bodies and infections.

Cardiac/Vascular Catheterization

A critical care nurse is well-acquainted with the **cardiac catheterization** procedure, as it is such a powerful and common tool to determine if a patient has cardiac disease. The test involves the threading of a small, thin catheter through peripheral arteries or veins up to the heart, obtaining information about the chambers, valves, and structures therein, as well as about the pulmonary artery, the coronary arteries, and the veins.

There are two different approaches to cardiac catheterization: left heart and right heart. If the cardiologist wishes to access the left heart, commonly to determine anatomy of the heart, BP in the aorta, or to assess aortic or mitral valve function, they will access the femoral artery and enter the heart through the aorta on the left side. For left heart catheterization, the subclavian, radial, or brachial arteries may also be accessed, but less commonly.

For right heart catheterization, the venous system is accessed. The heart is approached from the right side, entering through the right atrium where venous blood is returning. Right heart cardiac catheterization is used to determine the pressures in the right atria, right ventricle, and pulmonary arteries, as well as the pulmonary artery occlusion pressure (PAOP). Common venous access sites used for right heart catheterization are the femoral, subclavian, internal jugular, or antecubital veins.

The method of visualization used in cardiac catheterization is through the injection of radiopaque contrast into the heart chambers and surrounding structures while x-ray images are taken to produce images. This is called **angiography**. Another visualization technique uses tiny ultrasound transducers placed at the end of the catheter to produce images. Angiography and ultrasonography can be used at the same time.

Patients with kidney disease may not be good candidates for undergoing a cardiac catheterization due to the contrast that is used. When this dye is shot into the heart, it must be metabolized by the kidneys, which in a damaged kidney, could lead to further damage. Patients with active infections, fever, heart failure, heart arrhythmias, and coagulopathies may also be poor candidates for cardiac catheterizations, at the discretion of the physician.

To prepare for a cardiac catheterization, the patient will be kept nil per os (NPO) for 4 to 6 hours pre-catheterization. During the procedure, the patient will be given medication to help them relax but will not be put under general anesthesia.

Diagnostic

There are two uses for cardiac catheterization: diagnostic and interventional. The diagnostic approach means the cardiologist is looking to assess the anatomy of the heart, determine its functioning ability, and evaluate disease states. Common diagnostic uses of cardiac catheterization include angiography, intravascular ultrasonography, measuring of cardiac output, biopsy of tissues within the heart, shunt detection, and measurement of the heart's metabolic function.

Interventional

The second approach to cardiac catheterization is interventional, often occurring during a diagnostic procedure. A problem is seen, and action is taken to correct it. Common interventions during cardiac catheterization are percutaneous transluminal coronary angioplasty and stent insertion.

The tip of the cardiac catheter is a tiny balloon that can be inflated to open occluded arteries, a procedure termed **angioplasty.** After balloon inflation, the cardiologist may choose to insert a stent into the reopened artery to maintain patency of the vessel. Stent placement is used often in the case of acute MI. This intervention helps restore blood flow to areas of ischemia in the heart following a coronary artery occlusion.

Illustration of catheter insertion, balloon inflation, and stent placement during cardiac catheterization

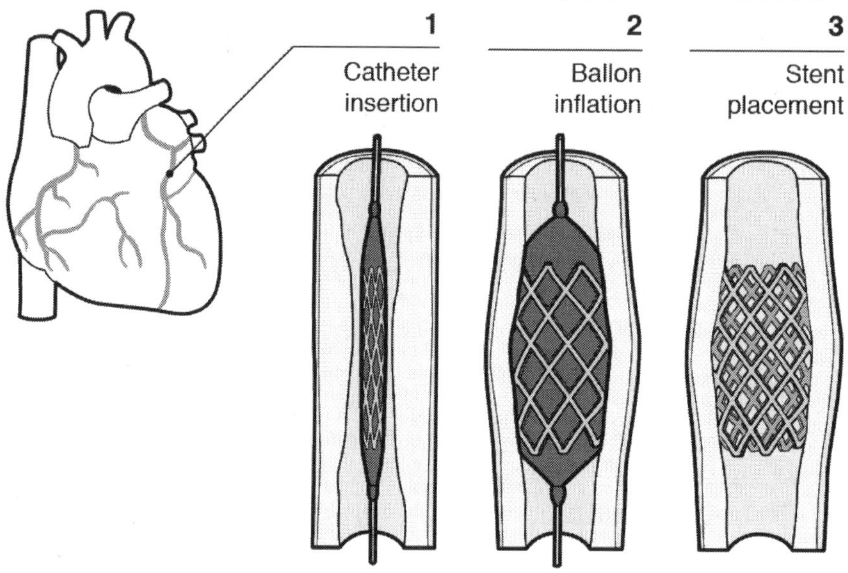

Cardiogenic Shock

The critical care nurse should be familiar with a dangerous condition known as **cardiogenic shock**. **Cardiogenic** means originating in the heart. **Shock** is a state in which blood flow in the body has dramatically decreased, and tissues are not getting adequate oxygen to perform their metabolic functions. Cardiogenic shock is when the heart has stopped pumping blood adequately through the body, characterized by critically low cardiac output, marked hypotension without volume loss, and signs of poor tissue perfusion such as cyanosis, oliguria, coolness of the extremities, and decreased level of consciousness. The nurse may see mottling of the skin in the legs and arms of the patient, detect a rapid and faint pulse, and auscultate distant-sounding heart sounds with a possible third and fourth heart sound present.

Cardiogenic shock often occurs following an acute MI. The ischemia that results from this condition causes the heart to fail in its ability to adequately circulate blood in the body. Mortality rates for cardiogenic shock are high if swift, aggressive intervention does not occur as soon as possible.

Cardiogenic shock is an emergency, and the patient must be treated immediately to prevent death. Admission to an ICU is likely, where the patient may have a central line put in to ensure rapid volume replacement and allow for multiple infusions of medicines to help maintain BP and cardiac output. The patient may have an arterial line placed to monitor BP continuously while BP is treated. Pharmacologic therapy will likely include drugs to improve cardiac contractility, such as dopamine, and diuretics to maintain volume and prevent volume overload during fluid resuscitation. If dopamine does not do an adequate job of maintaining BP, a stronger option would be norepinephrine, a potent vasoconstrictor. Any electrolyte abnormalities, such as acidosis, hypokalemia, or hypomagnesemia, should also be corrected.

Some patients will have an **intra-aortic balloon pump** inserted in the aorta to assist the heart's function. When the heart pumps, during systole, the balloon is deflated. When the heart rests, during diastole, the balloon inflates. This inflation helps push blood into the coronary arteries, reperfusing them. The deflation allows for more space in the aorta and thus more blood to flow out to the body and the tissues needing oxygen.

Patients in cardiogenic shock are likely candidates for a percutaneous intervention (PCI) or coronary artery bypass graft (CABG) surgery to immediately correct the issue. Research has shown that a PCI is most effective within 90 minutes of patient presentation to prevent mortality and long-term damage.

Cardiomyopathies

A **cardiomyopathy** is any condition in which the heart muscle is diseased. There are four categories of cardiomyopathy that will be discussed here: dilated, hypertrophic, idiopathic, and restrictive cardiomyopathy.

Dilated

Dilated cardiomyopathy is a primary myocardial disorder, meaning it occurs on its own without any coronary artery disease or anything else. Usually both ventricles will be affected, and will be dilating, thinning, becoming hypertrophic, and causing systolic dysfunction. Mitral and tricuspid regurgitation often develop because of the dilation. When the left ventricle is affected, the patient will have exertional dyspnea and fatigue because the left ventricle diastolic pressure rises and cardiac output is reduced. When the right ventricle is affected, the patient may present with edema of the legs and arms along with jugular vein distention. The symptoms of dilated cardiomyopathy typically develop slowly over time, except for acute cases such as takotsubo.

Takotsubo cardiomyopathy, also known as **acute apical ballooning cardiomyopathy** or **broken heart syndrome**, is triggered by a sudden and extreme amount of emotional distress. The patient may have experienced the loss of a loved one or some other catastrophic life event, which set in motion a hyperadrenergic state in the body. *Takotsubo* is a Japanese word for a fishing pot used for capturing octopuses, which is what the left ventricle has been said to look like during this type of cardiomyopathy. Patients typically present in a similar manner to those experiencing an ischemic event, with dyspnea, chest pain, nausea, and vomiting, among other symptoms. This type of heart failure is typically reversible, requiring acute hemodynamic support and similar treatment to patients with acute coronary syndrome.

Typical dilated cardiomyopathy has several different potential causes, including chronic tachycardia, connective tissue disorders such as rheumatoid arthritis, drugs and toxins such as alcohol and cocaine, inherited genetic factors, infections, and metabolic disorders such as diabetes mellitus. Viral infections are a well-known cause of dilated cardiomyopathy, with over twenty different viruses identified, such as human immunodeficiency virus (HIV) infection.

A patient with dilated cardiomyopathy will be diagnosed using a chest x-ray, which will show the enlargement of the heart, called **cardiomegaly**. The chest film may also show pleural effusions, a result of ventricular failure. Serological markers such as troponin may be elevated in dilated cardiomyopathy. Tissue samples from the heart muscle may be obtained for biopsy in some cases. ECG and imaging studies, such as echocardiography and cardiac magnetic resonance imaging (MRI), will also be used to make a diagnosis of dilated cardiomyopathy.

Patients with dilated cardiomyopathy will be treated with angiotensin-converting enzyme (ACE) inhibitors, beta blockers, angiotensin-receptor blockers (ARBs), diuretics, and digoxin, among other pharmacologic therapies. These drugs are often used in heart failure with a lowered ejection fraction. **Ejection fraction** is a term of measurement used to quantify the percentage of blood leaving the heart with each beat. A patient with heart failure, as is the case with dilated cardiomyopathy, will have a much lower ejection fraction than normal. A normal ejection fraction is around 55 to 70 percent.

Hypertrophic

Hypertrophic cardiomyopathy is an inherited condition due to a genetic mutation. In very rare cases, this type of cardiomyopathy may be acquired, as is the case in patients with acromegaly. **Hypertrophy** refers to a thickening of the cardiac muscle, often becoming stiff and noncompliant. Ejection fraction in patients with hypertrophic cardiomyopathy may be elevated as the smaller heart chamber empties completely with each beat to maintain cardiac output.

This type of cardiomyopathy often occurs in athletes, frequently causing sudden death and the official diagnosis being made upon autopsy. Symptoms are like acute coronary artery occlusion, such as chest pain, dyspnea, and syncope. Patients will be diagnosed using echocardiography or cardiac MRI, where the heart structures are visualized and the severity of the hypertrophy is analyzed.

Family history of sudden death or patient history of unexplained syncope are clues that the patient may have this type of cardiomyopathy.

The treatment plan for a patient diagnosed with hypertrophic cardiomyopathy usually includes beta-blockers, such as metoprolol, and calcium channel blockers, such as verapamil. Beta-blockers and calcium channel blockers help with this type of cardiomyopathy because they slow the heart rate, decrease contractility, and prolong the time that the heart chambers can fill between beats. Nitrates, diuretics, and ACE inhibitors should be avoided because they reduce preload, which worsens the condition. Implantable cardioverter defibrillator (ICD) is recommended to prevent death in patients with a history of cardiac arrest and syncope.

Idiopathic

When the cause of the cardiomyopathy is unknown, it is called **idiopathic**. This type of cardiomyopathy is responsible for up to half of the occurrences of heart failure. Patients with this type of cardiomyopathy are typically between twenty and sixty years of age. Their clinical presentation will be like other patients experiencing cardiomyopathy, with fatigue and dyspnea on exertion being a primary symptom if the left ventricle is affected. If the right ventricle is affected, jugular vein distention and edema may be present.

Like the other types of cardiomyopathies, **idiopathic cardiomyopathy** is believed to be the result of a viral infection, immune dysfunction, genetic factors, toxins, metabolism, and/or tachycardia-induced conditions. Alcohol and chemotherapeutic drugs are believed to be toxins that may cause cardiomyopathy.

The role of viruses must be investigated when determining the cause of idiopathic cardiomyopathy, as this root cause starts the chain reaction of inflammation and autoimmune dysfunction leading to cardiomyopathy. Viruses that have been associated with this type of cardiomyopathy include herpes, adenovirus, and enterovirus.

Treatment for the patient with idiopathic cardiomyopathy may include lifestyle modification of risk factors such as alcohol abuse; drug therapy with ACE inhibitors, beta-blockers, diuretics, and digitalis; and possible resynchronization therapy in patients experiencing dysrhythmias. Patients experiencing cardiomyopathy in the absence of a viral cause may be good candidates for immunosuppressive therapies such as prednisone, per the discretion of the physician.

Restrictive

A cardiomyopathy characterized by noncompliant heart walls that are resistant to filling during the diastolic period is termed **restrictive cardiomyopathy**. There are two categories of restrictive cardiomyopathy: obliterative and nonobliterative. Obliterative means that there is fibrosis within the endocardium and subendocardium, while nonobliterative entails that the myocardium has been infiltrated by an abnormal substance. One or both ventricles of the heart may be affected. Restrictive cardiomyopathy is much less common than dilated, idiopathic, and hypertrophic cardiomyopathies.

A patient with restrictive cardiomyopathy may present with fatigue and exertional dyspnea, like the other cardiomyopathic presentations. This is due to decreased cardiac output and oxygen delivery to the tissues and organs of the body.

Restrictive cardiomyopathy may arise because of genetic factors. The resistance to diastolic filling results in an increased filling pressure, followed by pulmonary venous hypertension.

A patient will be diagnosed with restrictive cardiomyopathy using echocardiography to visualize the ventricles and other structures of the heart. Cardiac MRI, heart catheterization, and biopsy may also be used to confirm the diagnosis.

A patient diagnosed with restrictive cardiomyopathy has a poor prognosis, unfortunately, as diagnosis is often made in the later stages of the disease. The cause will be treated if possible along with supportive treatment for symptoms. Diuretics will be used to relieve pulmonary vascular congestion if appropriate.

Illustration comparing a normal heart muscle with dilated, hypertrophic, and restrictive cardiomyopathies

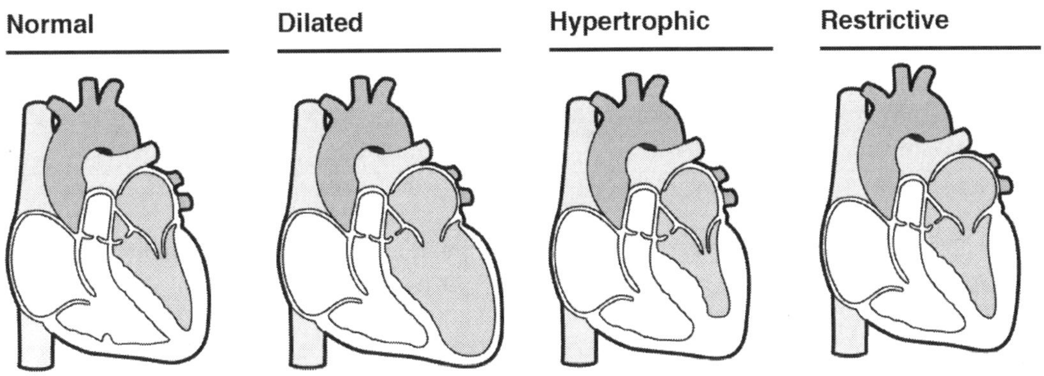

Dysrhythmias

A normal, healthy heart is a muscular pump powered by an electrical current that passes throughout its myocytes with every beat. The electrical impulse that triggers heart contractions can be measured using an ECG. In a disease state, abnormalities in electrical activity and conduction arise leading to irregular contractions of the chambers of the heart, called **dysrhythmias**.

Normal or **sinus rhythm** involves regular contraction of the atria followed by contraction of the ventricles. Atrial contraction fills the ventricles, and ventricle contraction pushes the blood to the lungs to be oxygenated or to the body to distribute the blood. Normal heart rate in an adult is 60 to 100 beats per minute. Slower rates are called **bradycardia,** while faster rates are called **tachycardia**.

Fibrillation is a movement of the heart best described as a flutter or a quiver. It is an ineffectual contraction of a chamber of the heart, in which inadequate blood flow is produced. **Atrial fibrillation**, often shortened to "AFib," is an abnormal but constant and rapid rhythm of the atria. AFib puts the patient at risk for the formation of clots in the atrial chambers. These clots, formed in pooling blood that is not adequately pumped out of the heart, may dislodge and travel to other parts of the body, such as the heart and brain, causing ischemic syndromes.

While a patient can live with AFib for some time without knowing it or needing much treatment, **ventricular fibrillation** is a different story. When the ventricles fibrillate and fail to adequately pump blood out of the body, it is a medical emergency requiring immediate intervention. Cardiopulmonary resuscitation with defibrillation is necessary, the pumping action of chest compressions making up for the ventricular failure in perfusing vital organs. Ventricular failure is the presenting rhythm for most patients experiencing cardiac arrest, often being the ultimate cause of death if resuscitation is unsuccessful.

Other common heart dysrhythmias include atrial flutter, atrioventricular block, bundle branch block (BBB), long QT syndrome, Torsades de pointes, and ventricular tachycardia.

Heart Failure

In a normal heart, when preload increases, the heart rises to meet the demand, pumping harder and faster to maintain perfusion of vital body organs. In **heart failure**, the heart no longer is able to meet the demands of the body, with weakened contractions and less cardiac output.

The **Frank-Starling Law of the Heart** describes the relationship between preload, heart contractility, and heart failure. In heart failure, the heart can no longer meet the demands of preload, and decreased contractility and cardiac output result.

Heart failure can arise from many different causes, including myocardial damage from an MI, disorders of the heart valves such as aortic stenosis, arrhythmias (both bradycardia and tachycardia), defects in the conduction system such as a left BBB, or even systemic disorders such as anemia, hyperthyroidism, and hypertension.

Treatment is available and can help with overall quality of life, but no cure is currently available. Drug therapy will target symptoms with diuretics, nitrates, or digoxin with long-term management in the form of ACE inhibitors, beta-blockers, and ARBs. Some patients may have an ICD placed to help with dysrhythmias and to resuscitate them should they go into cardiac arrest. Surgeries such as valve repairs, CABG, and even heart transplantation may be considered.

Hypertensive Crisis

A patient may present to the urgent care center or emergency room with uncontrolled hypertension, resulting in a systolic reading greater than 200 and a diastolic reading greater than 120. Blood pressure (BP) readings that are this high, rightly-called **malignant hypertension**, can cause damage to the organs supplied by the blood vessels, such as the heart, kidneys, brain, and lungs. A **hypertensive crisis** may arise if the patient forgets to take their BP medication, they've experienced a heart attack or stroke, their kidneys are failing, and many other scenarios.

Symptoms of hypertension include a severe headache, severe chest pain, nausea and vomiting, anxiety, shortness of breath, seizures, and unresponsiveness.

Upon presentation with malignant hypertension, the doctor may decide to infuse intravenous (IV) medications to reduce the BP. Such medications include sodium nitroprusside and esmolol, a beta-blocker. The clinician will be very careful not to lower the BP too quickly, as a dramatic drop in BP could cause further damage to end organs.

Possible comorbidities of a hypertensive crisis include the organs that such a hypertension could damage: cerebral vascular accident, myocardial ischemia or infarction, bleeding in the brain such as subarachnoid hemorrhage, pulmonary edema, aortic dissection, and acute renal failure.

Severe hypertension in pregnancy is called **preeclampsia** or **eclampsia**. Women experiencing this condition may be given hydralazine to lower their pressure, which presents not only a danger to them but to the forming fetus in the uterus. Magnesium sulfate is also given to pregnant women to prevent them from experiencing a seizure while hypertensive.

Myocardial Conduction System Abnormalities

Myocardial conduction refers to the movement of an electrical impulse across the myocytes, or muscle cells, that causes contractions. Common conduction disorders include bundle branch block (BBBs), heart block, long QT syndrome, and Wolf-Parkinson-White Syndrome.

Bundle Branch Block

Bundle branch block (BBBs) occurs when there is a block in either the right, left, or both branches of the heart's conduction system, traveling the length of the ventricles. A patient with BBB may be asymptomatic, as the heart compensates by having the electrical impulse travel down a different path than the blocked branch to stimulate ventricular contraction. The ventricle affected will then beat just a fraction of a second slower than the other one, not producing any noticeable symptoms. BBB will likely be found when diagnosing some other heart condition, but it is good to know it is there. No treatment is usually required if the patient is asymptomatic.

Heart Block

A **heart block** is any instance in which the electrical impulse of the heart does not travel correctly from the atria to the ventricles, occurring in varying degrees from first degree to third degree. First-degree heart blocks are defined by a slower movement of the electrical signal, while second-degree heart blocks are defined by missed beats caused by electrical impulses that never reach the ventricles. In third-degree, or complete heart block, the electrical impulse is not passing to the lower chambers at all, resulting in ineffective blood pumping and a very slow heart rate. Patients with third-degree heart block will likely need a pacemaker implanted.

Prolonged QT Interval

Long QT syndrome occurs when the QT segment of the ECG wave form is prolonged, representing the electrical activity in the ventricles. This hereditary and rare disorder usually occurs in healthy adults and children and is characterized by fainting episodes, feelings of "fluttering" in the chest, and abnormal heart rate or rhythm. Diagnosis occurs with ECG and stress testing. Long QT syndrome may be fatal, as it could potentially cause sudden cardiac arrest. A treatment plan for long QT syndrome may include beta-blockers, avoiding drugs that aggravate the syndrome, and possibly implantation of an ICD or pacemaker.

Wolff-Parkinson-White Syndrome

Wolff-Parkinson-White (WPW) Syndrome is a congenital cardiac syndrome characterized by an additional accessory electric pathway that can lead to abnormal conduction and tachyarrhythmias. The addition of an accessory pathway in WPW can result in electrical impulses that skip the AV node and go directly to the bundle of His and Purkinje fibers. Many patients with WPW will remain asymptomatic with a normal ECG, although there are cases of concealed bypass grafts in patients with a history of normal ECGs who develop tachyarrhythmia. Patients with no present arrhythmia are typically asymptomatic. Patients with tachyarrhythmia from WPW typically present with dizziness, syncope, palpitations, dyspnea, chest pain, and even death. Symptoms may be ongoing or episodic, depending on the nature of the arrhythmia. Diagnosis follows a complete history and physical, abnormal vital signs including tachycardia, and a remarkable 12-lead ECG with a short PR interval less than 120ms and long QRS complex over 120ms with an abnormal delta wave. Additional studies such as CBC, BMP, cardiac enzymes, and chest radiography may be needed to confirm diagnosis. Treatment is typically not necessary for asymptomatic patients but may involve a referral to cardiology. Accessory pathway catheter ablation is the first-line treatment for symptomatic WPW patients, although surgical ablation may also be performed with a high success rate. Medications such as propafenone and flecainide may be utilized in patients with ischemic heart disease who are not candidates for ablation therapy.

Structural Heart Defects

Congenital Heart Defects

The most common types of heart defects occur in developing fetuses and are often diagnosed prenatally or shortly after the child is born. Some common types of congenital defects are **atrial septal defects** (ASDs), **patent foramen ovale** (PFO), patent ductus arteriosus (PDA), coarctation of the aorta, and tetralogy of Fallot.

ASD and PFO are similar in that there is a hole between the two atria of the heart, and oxygen-rich blood leaks from the left chamber to the right. In ASD, the tissue never forms, and in PFO, the hole that is normally there does not close after birth as it should. An ASD hole is generally larger than a PFO.

Patent ductus arteriosus occurs when the **ductus arteriosus**, the vessel that connects the pulmonary artery and the aorta, does not close as it should after birth. The ductus arteriosus is vital for fetal development; however, if it remains open after birth, the oxygen-rich blood of the aorta that is meant for body circulation gets mixed with the oxygen-poor blood of the pulmonary artery. This results in increased pulmonary pressures and stress on the heart.

A narrowing of the aorta in a baby is called **coarctation of the aorta** and results in hypertension and heart damage.

Tetralogy of Fallot is a complex congenital heart defect involving four defects: a hole between the two ventricles, called a **ventricular septal defect** (VSD); pulmonary valve stenosis; an aorta that is located between the two ventricles and above the VSD; and hypertrophy, or a thickening of the right ventricle that results from the increased workload of pulmonary valve stenosis. Patients with Tetralogy of Fallot must have open heart surgery to repair the defects.

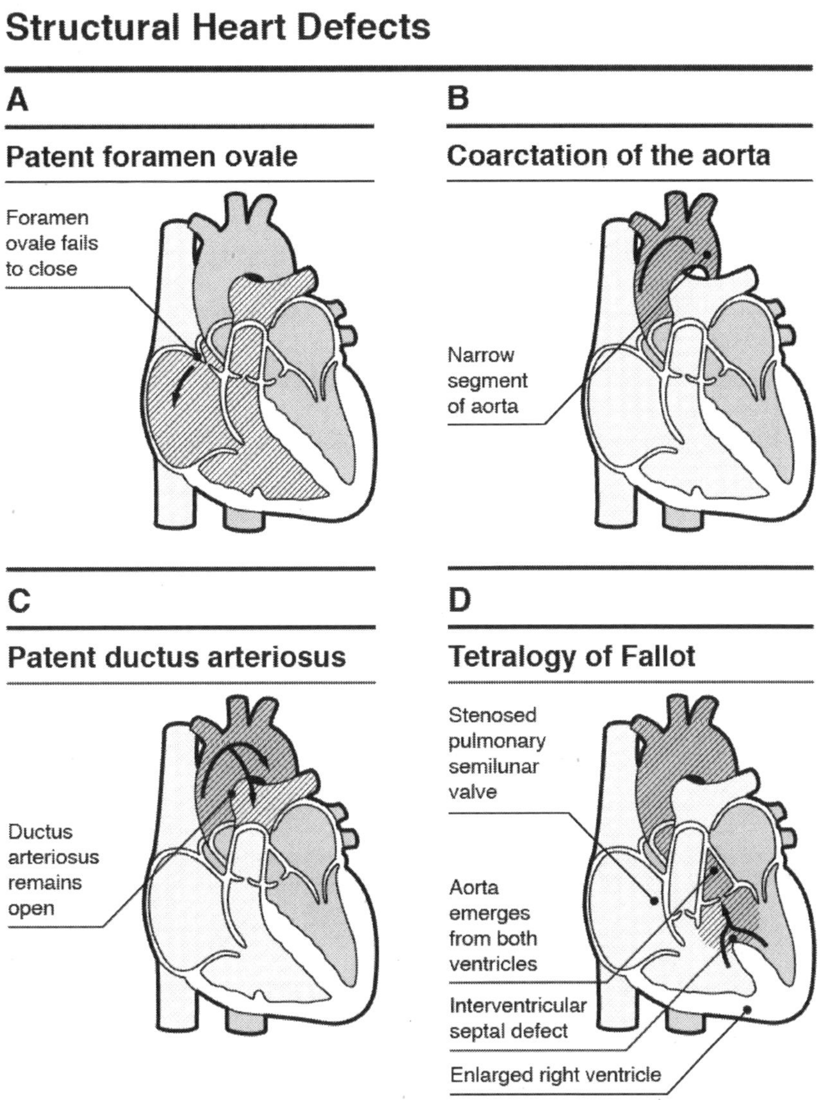

Acquired Heart Defects

Structural heart defects occurring in adulthood include **valvular disease**. There are four valves in the heart: mitral, tricuspid, aortic, and pulmonary. These valves control the flow of blood between the chambers of the heart, the lungs for oxygenation, and the body for circulation. Valvular defects occur because of normal aging and degeneration, infections, hypertension, atherosclerosis, ischemic conditions such as heart attack, tumors, radiation, and even some medications. Valve dysfunctions can include stiffening, in which blood is forced backward rather than forward, or weakening, in which blood leaks inappropriately between chambers. The severity of the valve dysfunction determines the number of symptoms and the amount and type of treatment needed. Patients with valvular disease may experience palpitations, fatigue, dizziness, and/or chest pain. Diagnosis is made with an ECG, stress tests, chest x-rays, echocardiograms, and/or cardiac catheterization. Management and treatment options can include encouragement of smoking cessation, antithrombotics or anticoagulants, and possible surgery to repair the valves.

Vascular Disorders

Acute Peripheral Vascular Insufficiency

Some patients may suffer with chronic insufficiencies of the peripheral vascular system, both arterial and venous. In either case, insufficiency predominantly occurs in the legs rather than the arms because of gravity on the lower portion of the body. This is not to say that arms cannot be affected by vascular insufficiency, but it occurs there more rarely.

Arterial insufficiency can be acute or chronic, and it varies in severity. The more severe the narrowing of the arteries in the extremity, the more profound the symptoms will be. Caused by sclerosis in the arteries of the lower extremities, arterial insufficiency causes pain in the legs, due to a decreased blood flow and thus a decreased delivery of oxygen to the muscle tissue. Other manifestations of an atherosclerotic arterial system are loss of hair; bluish tint, or cyanosis, of the skin; gangrene; and ischemic ulcers.

Treatment for arterial insufficiency includes diet modification, risk factor reduction, exercise, and medications targeted at preventing clots and treating symptoms such as pain. Arterial insufficiency can occur acutely because of a clot.

Diagnosis for peripheral arterial insufficiency is obtained through a comparison of the ankle BP and the brachial BP, called the **ankle-brachial BP index**. Blood vessels will be visualized using ultrasonography as well as angiography if the patient will be going for surgery to correct the issue.

Venous insufficiency occurs when the valves and walls of the venous system weaken and malfunction. The result is pooling of blood in the extremities that would have normally returned to the heart for recirculation. This can be an acute occurrence in the case of volume overload, such as in pregnancy.

Edema caused by venous insufficiency may be accompanied by throbbing, cramping pain along with aches, heaviness, and fatigue of the legs. Risk factors include having a clot in the leg called a **deep vein thrombosis (DVT)**, which is the most common cause, as well as obesity, older age, and a direct trauma to the venous vasculature.

Peripheral arterial disease (PAD) is a chronic condition in which the arteries of the extremities—almost always lower extremities—are narrowed and sometimes blocked by atherosclerotic plaques. This causes **ischemia**, in which vital oxygen delivery is interrupted and tissue damage and death occurs. Symptoms of PAD include claudication, wounds or ulcers that will not heal, cyanosis of the extremity, loss of hair in the extremity, and atrophy of the skin. Treatment usually involves lifestyle modifications (e.g., smoking cessation) and drug therapy with antiplatelets such as aspirin or cilostazol.

Chronic venous insufficiencies occur when the veins' ability to return blood to the heart is impaired. This disease also occurs more frequently in the lower extremities because of gravity. The cause of this insufficiency usually arises from immobility, in which lack of muscle contraction surrounding the veins leads to vein weakness and dysfunction. Another cause is venous hypertension, which usually occurs after a DVT. Symptoms of chronic venous insufficiencies include a feeling of fullness or heaviness in the legs, aching, cramping, and fluid accumulation, or edema. Treatment includes elevation of the affected limb(s), compression to encourage flow, and treatment of a secondary infection, if present.

Patients with chronic venous insufficiency are at high risk for developing venous stasis ulcers. Areas where blood has pooled are vulnerable to injury, followed by wounds that will not heal due to poor circulation.

Both patients with venous and arterial insufficiencies are prone to these types of nonhealing ulcers. A differentiating factor between venous and arterial ulcers is that venous are usually superficial and arterial are deeper, eventually exposing deep fascia such as tendons and bones. Adequate care of lower extremities in both cases of venous and arterial insufficiencies is vital to prevent secondary infections.

Carotid Artery Stenosis

Carotid artery stenosis is a subcategory of peripheral vascular insufficiency involving the arteries of the neck that supply the brain with nutrient-filled blood. This condition may exist long before symptoms occur, as the narrowing may not be severe enough to significantly reduce blood flow to the brain. Stenosis, the narrowing of a blood vessel, in this case is most often caused by **atherosclerosis**. This entails a building up of a fatty substance called **plaque** inside the artery walls, which leads to reduced blood flow.

An acute condition involving carotid artery stenosis is when a clot occurs at the site of the stenosis, interrupting blood flow completely. This leads to a **transient ischemic attack (TIA)**, or worse, a cerebrovascular accident (CVA), commonly referred to as a **stroke**. A TIA is an episode that mimics stroke symptoms, such as slurring of speech, drooping of face, and other neurologic deficits, and lasts for less than an hour but longer than five minutes. There is no long-term damage, as the episode is transient enough that no brain tissue is injured. A TIA may be the first clue to signal that the patient has carotid artery stenosis, as there may be few to no symptoms beforehand.

Risk factors for developing carotid artery stenosis include alcohol abuse, hypertension, smoking, high cholesterol, diabetes, obesity, stress, heart disease, drug abuse (especially cocaine and amphetamines), vascular inflammation, history of stroke, and old age. Smoking cessation information should be given to the patient to encourage them to quit.

Carotid artery stenosis is diagnosed most commonly with carotid ultrasound, using sonography to visualize the arterial structures in the neck. Other tests that may be ordered include carotid angiography, magnetic resonance angiography, and computerized tomography angiography (CAT).

The arteries may be stented or partially removed to correct the stenosis. Antiplatelet and anticoagulant therapies will be used to prevent future blood clots.

Arterial/Venous Occlusion

When an artery or vein is blocked by a clot, this occlusion is termed a **thrombosis**. Clot formation is a normal hemostatic adjustment that occurs in a healthy individual to prevent excessive bleeding and promote wound healing. Inappropriate clotting, however, can interrupt critical blood flow, and thus oxygen delivery to the tissues of the body. Interruption in oxygen delivery, if not corrected, will lead to tissue damage and death.

Occlusion of an artery may sometimes occur because of atherosclerosis, in which fatty deposits called plaques build up over time, sticking to the walls of the vessels. These fatty deposits are composed of lipids, inflamed smooth muscle cells, and a connective tissue matrix composed of thrombi in various stages, as well as calcium deposits.

A person may not know that they have atherosclerosis until a plaque bursts or occludes blood flow, causing ischemic conditions such as stroke or heart attack.

Persons who smoke should be encouraged to cease, as smoking is one of the greatest risk factors for developing atherosclerosis. Nicotine and other chemicals found in cigarette or cigar smoke are toxic to the inner lining of blood vessels. These toxins inflame and scar the vascular endothelium, not only increasing the risk of plaque accumulation, but also causing vasoconstriction. Vasoconstriction in already narrowed blood vessels increases BP and puts the smoker in danger of other life-threatening events, such as clots and TIAs.

Other risk factors for atherosclerosis include hyperlipidemia, diabetes, family history, sedentary lifestyle, obesity, and hypertension.

To confirm a diagnosis of atherosclerosis, the affected blood vessels need to be visualized by imaging techniques such as angiography or ultrasonography.

Modifications in lifestyle such as diet, exercise, and smoking cessation will be encouraged for the patient with atherosclerosis. Drug therapy will include antiplatelets (e.g., aspirin at 100 mg daily) and statins for targeting lipids (e.g., atorvastatin at 40–80 mg daily).

A common venous occlusion is a DVT. Though DVTs may be asymptomatic, the common presentation is redness, pain, and swelling over the site of the clot. Common sites for DVT are the lower extremities, specifically the superficial femoral, popliteal, posterior tibial, or peroneal veins in the calves. Formation of DVTs occurs due to impaired venous return, an injury to the endothelium such as leg fractures, or in states of **hypercoagulability**, in which the body is more apt to form clots. Impaired venous return is common in immobile patients. Therefore, early ambulation is encouraged as well as mobility exercises while the patient is still in bed, to prevent clots.

DVTs in the lower extremities have a high correlation with patients also developing pulmonary embolisms (PEs), or blood clots that travel to the lungs. This is a life-threatening situation. Other complications of DVTs include a chronic insufficiency of the veins and **post-phlebitic syndrome**, in which a patient feels aching, cramping, pain, and other symptoms in the legs that worsen with walking or standing and are relieved by resting.

A **D-dimer** is the test used to help diagnose a DVT. A negative result rules out a DVT, while a positive is not 100 percent conclusive. A positive D-dimer necessitates further testing—usually ultrasonography—to confirm the diagnosis. History and physical examination are also helpful in determining the probability of a DVT.

If left untreated, there is a risk that the patient will develop a life-threatening PE; therefore, prompt detection and treatment are vital. Treatment is usually with anticoagulants, such as subcutaneous heparin for a short period, followed by a longer period of oral warfarin. Pain control with acetaminophen may be included in the treatment plan, along with leg elevation with pillows while the patient is at rest, being careful to avoid venous compression, which could lead to clot dislodgement.

Vascular Interventions

Stents

Peripheral stents are an option to attempt to open occluded arteries in a patient with peripheral arterial disease (PAD). Stent placement occurs at the same time as angioplasty, in which a small thin catheter is threaded into the affected blood vessel, and a tiny balloon is inflated to "pop" open the lumen of the blood vessel. Then, stent placement can occur.

The stent is, in most cases, a tiny metal, mesh-like tube that provides a scaffolding or support structure to keep a blood vessel open. The stent remains in the patient's blood vessel permanently, although it is possible to remove a stent if absolutely necessary.

Antiplatelet and antithrombotic therapies are used in the postoperative period to reduce the risk of stent thrombosis.

Femoropopliteal Bypass

A femoropopliteal (fem-pop) bypass graft is a surgical procedure that reroutes blood in the leg past an occluded section of artery, caused by atherosclerosis. The patient's own vein may be used, or an artificial vein will be used, though this presents a risk for narrowing over time. The vein bypasses the occlusion starting at the femoral artery and ending at the popliteal artery in the knee.

Femoropopliteal Bypass

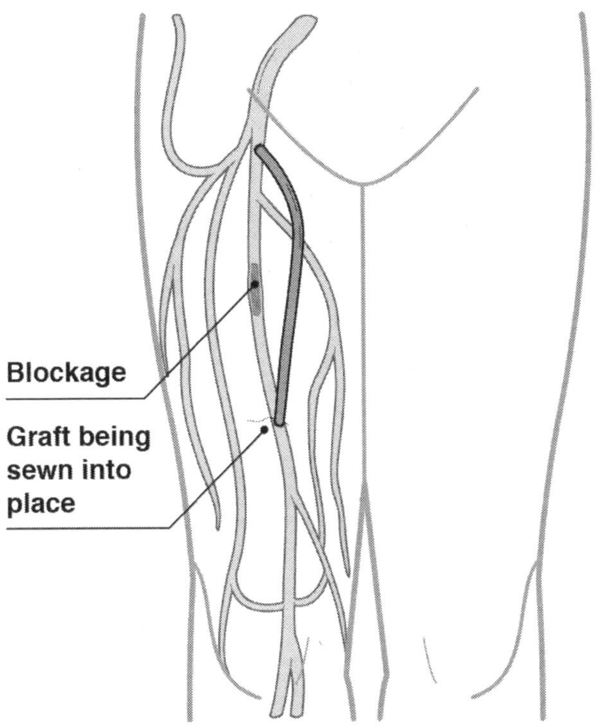

This procedure is used for patients with severe claudication. **Claudication** is a word of Latin origin, originally meaning "limp," but in this case, it means severe pain in the legs caused by restricted blood supply. Claudication may occur in the feet or, most commonly, in the calves. The patient may also be experiencing sores that will not heal or gangrene due to restricted blood flow. The bypass will reinstate healthy blood flow to previously ischemic areas, hopefully alleviating symptoms.

Patients should be encouraged to quit smoking before the procedure to prevent complications and promote overall health. Smoking cessation information and resources should be shared early and often.

Patients will be anesthetized for the procedure. Blood transfusion is a distinct possibility to maintain volume and replace blood loss. The incision made by the surgeon is generally 4 to 8 inches in length, in the groin area where the femoral artery is located. Internal stitches will be made to secure the graft in place. The patient may be in surgery anywhere from 1 to 6 hours depending on the complexity of the surgery.

The nurse in the critical care unit receiving the patient postop will want to monitor the incision site for infection, bleeding, and/or hematoma. Hemodynamic monitoring will be in place to watch for hypotension, which could indicate bleeding, or hypertension, which could put added pressure on the healing graft. Like postoperative therapy for a carotid endarterectomy, the patient will be started on antiplatelet and antithrombotic therapy to prevent clotting and restenosis of the vessels.

Carotid Endarterectomy

The patient with atherosclerosis of the carotid artery may be a candidate for a surgical procedure called an **endarterectomy**. In this surgery, the carotid artery is accessed by a surgeon, incised, and the problematic plaque carefully removed. The artery is then sutured closed, and the patient will likely be sent to an intensive care unit (ICU) to recover.

Endarterectomy

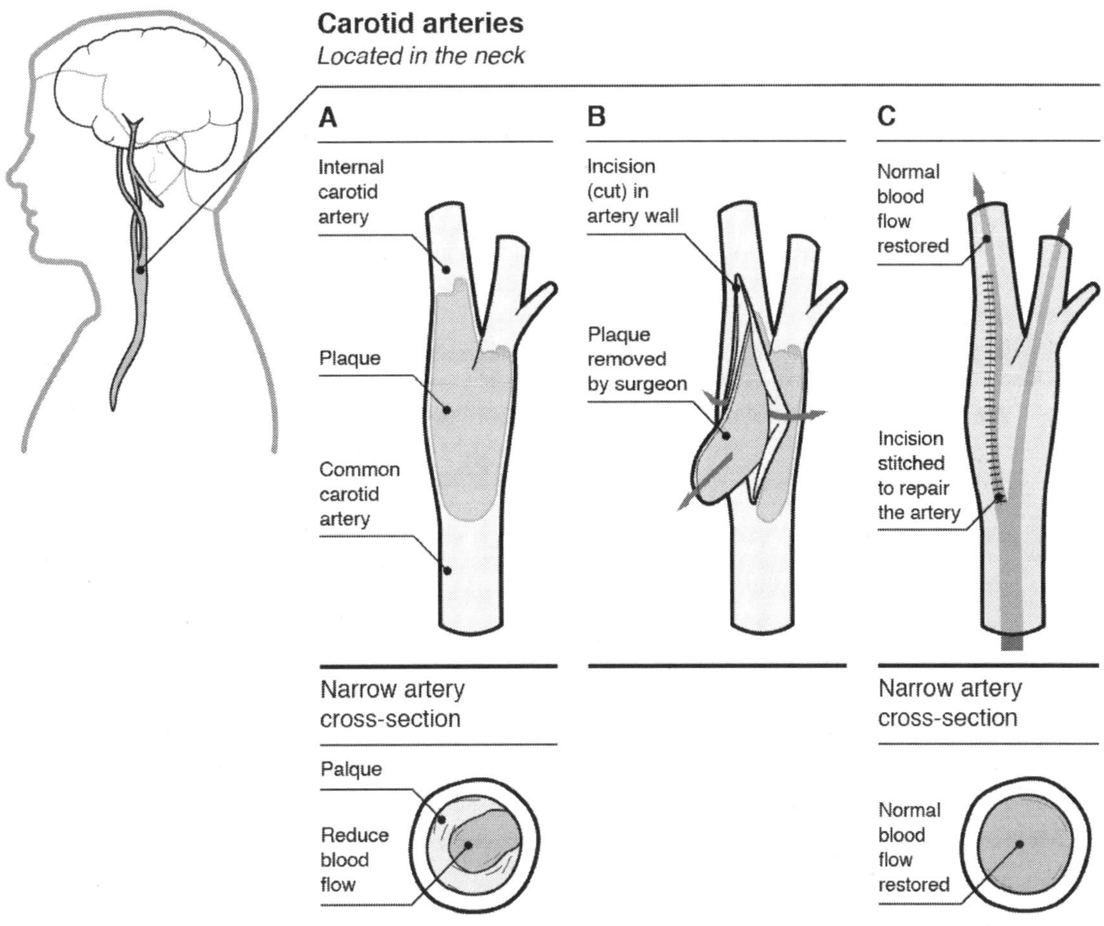

The critical care nurse will be carefully monitoring the patient in the hours and days following the surgery. Since a major artery was accessed, bleeding is the first and most obvious complication to be monitored for. The incision site will be monitored not only for signs of becoming infected, but for hematoma or signs of bleeding. There may be wound drains for which patency needs to be maintained. The patient must be taught to support their head with their hands when moving to minimize strain of the neck muscles. Clots are still a threat to this patient's well-being, so the nurse will monitor for any signs that the carotid artery has become occluded again or that the patient is experiencing a CVA. Signs of a CVA include sudden onset of neurologic deficits such as confusion, dizziness, slurred speech, or paralysis of the arms and/or legs.

Hemodynamic monitoring, already a standard practice in the ICU, will be critical to determine if the patient is developing complications. Hypotension could indicate volume loss or possibly lead to myocardial ischemia. Hypertension puts the patient at risk of developing a CVA, as well as putting added pressure on the recently incised and healing artery.

The critical care nurse will monitor for signs of respiratory distress, such as a change in rate, rhythm, depth, and effort of breath. The nurse will also be mindful of tracheal deviation from the midline and patient restlessness, as well as difficulty swallowing. These could be signs of excessive swelling and could lead to further respiratory distress. It is recommended that a patient who has had an endarterectomy have a tracheostomy kit at their bedside, in case of an emergency.

The patient will likely be put on antiplatelet therapy in the post-op period, including aspirin at 100 mg daily and clopidogrel at 75 mg daily for at least the first thirty days, starting day one post-op. A major complication in the post-operative period is clotting and/or restenosis of the artery, and this therapy aims to prevent that.

Transcatheter Aortic Valve Replacement (TAVR)

Transcatheter aortic valve replacements (**TAVR**) is a procedure used to treat aortic valve stenosis. Aortic valve stenosis is a condition of the heart's aortic valve. The aortic valve regulates blood flow through from the heart into the aorta, the cardiovascular system's primary artery. In patients with aortic valve stenosis, the aortic valve stiffens and narrows, resulting in decreased flow of oxygenated blood throughout the body and increased burden on the heart muscle to pump blood. Patients may experience angina, limb swelling, and difficulty with physical activity; it also significantly increases the patient's risk of heart failure.

The TAVR procedure is considered to be a minimally invasive procedure in which a patient's aortic valve is replaced with a manufactured valve made from animal cardiac tissue. The clinician inserts the new valve with a catheter through a small incision at a less vulnerable blood vessel; most commonly, a TAVR incision is made at the femoral artery in the patient's thigh. However, the catheter can also be inserted near the shoulder, between the ribs, or through the upper chest. The valve is guided to its final location using endoscopic cameras. Post-surgery recovery takes place in intensive care, as the risk for bacterial infection around the new valve is relatively high. However, the TAVR procedure as a whole is much less risky than traditional valve replacement, which is an open-heart surgery that exposes more of the cardiac region to foreign bodies and bacteria.

Most patients are discharged within five days after the procedure, although the wound site will take several weeks to heal. The wound site must be regularly cleaned and monitored for infection. Patients are prescribed blood thinning medication to support blood flow through the new valve. They also undergo cardiac rehabilitation for several months and gradually return to normal cardiovascular activity levels over time.

Practice Quiz

1. Which of the following lifestyle modifications would address the major cause of most aortic aneurysms?

a. Low-fat diet
b. Smoking cessation
c. Exercise program
d. Meditation

2. The perioperative nurse is assessing a 44-year-old male patient with complaints of chest pain and shortness of breath. Examination by the nurse reveals distended neck veins and muffled heart sounds. The patient's blood pressure is 80/55. The nurse should suspect which of the following?

a. Cardiac tamponade
b. Abdominal aortic aneurysm (AAA)
c. Cardiopulmonary arrest
d. Cardiogenic shock

3. A patient presents to the emergency department with the complaint of fever and shortness of breath. During the physical examination, the nurse observes a petechial rash on both hands and a recent nipple piercing on the right chest. The patient reports being on a corticosteroid for a respiratory infection. These findings alert the nurse to the possibility of which of the following?

a. Endocarditis
b. An autoimmune disease
c. Pneumonia
d. Heart failure

4. Which of the following statements made by the patient would cause the nurse to suspect an abdominal aortic aneurysm (AAA)?

a. "I have indigestion when I lie down."
b. "I often have a pulsating sensation in my abdomen."
c. "I get fatigued and short of breath on exertion."
d. "I have extreme pain radiating down my left arm."

5. The patient with decreased level of consciousness is brought to the emergency department by EMS. During the assessment, the nurse observes mottled extremities and distant heart sounds. The nurse demonstrates an understanding of the physician's diagnosis of cardiogenic shock by anticipating which of the following?

a. Arterial blood gas (ABG)
b. Chest x-ray
c. Angiogram
d. Doppler study of the lower extremities

See answers on the next page.

Answer Explanations

1. B: Cigarette smoking is a major cause of atherosclerosis, the most common cause of aortic aneurysms. Following a low-fat diet would help with dyslipidemia, which may be a contributor to atherosclerosis, but it is not as important as stopping smoking, which causes the inflammatory, toxic effects that produce atherosclerosis. Exercise is helpful in coping with stress effectively, as is meditation, but not specific to atherosclerosis that causes aortic aneurysms.

2. A: Beck's triad of muffled heart sounds, distended neck veins, and hypotension are cardinal signs of cardiac tamponade. Chest pain and back pain are the most common presenting symptoms with an AAA. Heart function, breathing, and consciousness are not evident in cardiopulmonary arrest. Cardiogenic shock includes ashen, cyanotic, or mottled extremities; distant heart sounds; and rapid and faint peripheral pulses.

3. A: Fever and petechial rash are signs of endocarditis. Body piercings and corticosteroids are among the risk factors for developing endocarditis. Autoimmune conditions vary, but the most frequent presenting symptoms are fatigue and body aches. Pneumonia presents with fever, chills, and cough. Heart failure (HF) is not associated with a petechial rash or a fever.

4. B: An abdominal aneurysm may present or be found on examination as a pulsating mass in the abdomen. Indigestion when lying down is associated with gastrointestinal reflux disease (GERD) and is not indicative of an AAA. Fatigue and shortness of breath on exertion may be indicative of coronary artery or pulmonary disease. It is not directly associated with an AAA. Pain radiating down the left arm is a classic sign of a myocardial infarction (MI).

5. C: An angiogram to restore coronary blood flow is the priority treatment for cardiogenic shock. ABGs, a chest x-ray, and a Doppler study are not treatments; they are diagnostic tools.

Respiratory

Working in tandem with the cardiac system is the respiratory system, composed of the two lungs, airway, and blood vessels. Airway and breathing are part of the airway, breathing, circulation (ABC) mnemonic representing the patient's most vital functions. The critical care nurse knows that taking good care of the patient's respiratory system using critical thinking and sound clinical judgments is crucial to the patient's overall well-being.

The following is a discussion of the major critical care situations involving the respiratory system, patient presentation, and course of treatment.

Acute Pulmonary Edema

When there is disease and dysfunction in the heart and circulatory system, one of the first systems of the body to be affected is the pulmonary system. The lungs have an intimate relationship with the function of the heart, and when the heart is no longer pumping effectively or the blood vessels are no longer circulating the blood efficiently throughout the body, the lungs bear the brunt of it. **Cardiogenic** is a term that refers to a condition originating in or caused by the heart.

One condition caused by the heart that affects the lungs is cardiogenic **pulmonary edema**. When the heart fails to pump effectively, the pulmonary venous pressure rises. Remember that the pulmonary vein carries oxygenated blood from the lungs back to the left atrium after gas exchange in the pulmonary capillaries. When this pressure rises, fluid begins to build up in the lungs.

There are many different reasons fluid can build up in the lungs in addition to this example, such as an imbalance of Starling forces, alveolar–capillary barrier damage, an obstruction of lymphatic circulation, or even of an idiopathic nature. The critical care nurse will recall that the **Starling forces** entail the Starling equation, in which hydrostatic and oncotic forces work together to move fluid across a capillary membrane, as in the case of oxygen exchange in the alveolar beds of the lungs.

The patient with pulmonary edema will be given supplemental oxygen therapy, diuretics to decrease volume load, and heart medication, depending on their condition. Preload in the heart will be targeted, using diuretics such as furosemide (Lasix®) or nifedipine (Procardia®). If shortness of breath and anxiety are severe, as is the case sometimes, morphine may be prescribed to lessen oxygen demand. The patient may be prescribed agents to reduce afterload, such as nitroprusside, which will cause dilation of the coronary arteries, relieving pressure in the hardworking left ventricle. Blood pressure agents will be used according to the patient's history and clinical presentation, maintaining a normal pressure for optimal blood flow.

The patient experiencing pulmonary edema may have changes in respiratory patterns and decreased oxygenation. The labor of breathing may worsen, increasing fatigue. The patient may require assisted or mechanical ventilation if the condition deteriorates into respiratory distress and failure, until the pulmonary edema has resolved, per the attending physician's discretion.

Acute Pulmonary Embolus

One potential complication for a patient in a critical care unit is a **pulmonary embolus** (**PE**). A PE is a clot that has developed elsewhere in the body, traveled to the pulmonary arteries, and occluded at least one, if not more, of them. PEs often develop in the deep, large, femoral or pelvic veins of the body, become dislodged, and travel up through the right side of the heart, through the pulmonary artery, and into the lungs.

There are three categories of PEs based on severity: small, submassive, and massive. Small PEs may exist without any symptoms. Submassive PEs may slightly impair right ventricular function, but hypotension is absent. A massive PE impairs the function of the right ventricle, causes a hypotensive crisis, and presents a serious risk of death for the patient.

A **saddle PE** is a particularly dangerous type of clot in which the pulmonary embolus has lodged itself in the bifurcation between the main pulmonary artery and the left and right pulmonary arteries. Saddle PEs usually impair right ventricular function with or without hypotension.

Detection of PEs is somewhat difficult. Practitioners may use a D-Dimer test to rule out or indicate the probability of a PE. V/Q scans, in which ventilation and perfusion of the lungs is evaluated, may assist in diagnosis. CT scanning is the best way to image a PE, although patients with renal failure will not be able to tolerate the contrast, and thus, V/Q scanning is used.

Treatment of a PE includes reducing the clot burden in the patient through anticoagulants such as IV heparin, subcutaneous fondaparinux, and/or IV argatroban. Any patient on anticoagulant therapy is at risk for bleeding and should be monitored for such.

Warfarin may be used for long-term anticoagulation therapy in patients at risk for clotting but should be checked for interactions with other medications. Patients on warfarin will also have to have their international normalized ratio (INR) checked periodically to monitor the effectiveness of anticoagulation.

Prevention is key with PEs. Patients who remain immobile and in bed are at risk for developing clots. These clots may start as DVTs and then travel to the lungs to create PEs, a life-threatening event in many patients. Early anticoagulation when PEs or DVTs are possible along with early patient mobilization are key to prevention.

Acute Respiratory Distress Syndrome (ARDS)

When a patient is in respiratory failure that is unresponsive to supplemental oxygen with marked hypoxemia, it is called **acute respiratory distress syndrome** (**ARDS**) or sometimes acute hypoxemic respiratory failure (AHRF). This type of respiratory failure may be caused by acute lung injury (ALI) and can occur in the conditions that predispose a patient to any sort of respiratory distress syndrome (RDS).

When the blood is not adequately oxygenated because of poor oxygen exchange in the alveoli in the lungs, the patient will become dyspneic, and oxygen saturation readings will drop. A pulse oxygenation of below 90 percent is considered below normal in most patients and must be treated. If the patient is not responding to inhaled oxygen therapy through nasal prongs or even high flows of 70 to 100 percent oxygen on a nonrebreather face mask, mechanical ventilation will be the next step in treating ARDS.

Mechanical ventilation can assist in ARDS by relieving the work of the heart and respiratory muscles, distributing cardiac output to other vital tissues in the body while the vent takes over the work of breathing. By maintaining a positive end-expiratory pressure (PEEP), the vent can stave off pulmonary edema, recruiting more alveoli to participate in oxygen exchange.

A patient with ARDS will be diagnosed beginning with pulse oxygenation. When the blood oxygen concentration drops below 90, causes will be investigated, ARDS will be considered, chest x-ray obtained, and arterial blood glasses (ABGs) taken. The chest x-ray may show infiltrates indicating pulmonary edema and/or pneumonia, which are other possible causes of ARDS. The ABGs will indicate oxygenation as well as any acidotic or alkalotic states of the blood. A mild amount of acidosis may be tolerated in the patient when the greater good of ventilation and oxygenation are being maintained. An acidotic pH of less than 7.15, however, may be treated with IV sodium bicarbonate.

ALI can arise from direct and indirect causes. A direct cause would be gastric acid aspiration or pneumonia. Indirect causes of lung injury include sepsis or trauma arising from prolonged hypovolemic shock.

Propofol is a preferred sedative for patients on mechanical ventilation, as breathing with the vent is highly uncomfortable. The patient may become agitated and “fight the vent,” causing uncoordinated breaths and further problems with oxygenation and ventilation. Other analgesics that may be considered are fentanyl and morphine.

Acute Respiratory Failure

Any case in which oxygen exchange in the alveoli of the lungs is impaired, whether due to impaired respiration, weakness of respiratory effort, or obstruction of the airway, is called **respiratory failure**. Though respiratory arrest and cardiac arrest are two different events, one always leads to another if one is left untreated. Lack of oxygen will cause permanent damage to vital organs if respiratory arrest goes on for much longer than five minutes.

Respiratory failure can occur because of an upper or lower **airway obstruction**. Upper airway obstructions include blood, mucus, foreign object, tumor, inflammation, or edema. Lower airway obstructions include aspiration, bronchospasm, pneumonia, pulmonary edema or hemorrhage, or drowning.

Patients with central nervous system deficits may have a decreased respiratory effort, leading to respiratory failure. Examples of this include brain stem injuries, as is the case with strokes and tumors. An adverse medication effect may cause decreased respiratory effort. Alcohol, opioids, and sedatives are all examples of drugs that can depress respiratory effort to the point of failure.

Hypoglycemia and hypotension are examples of metabolic disorders that may weaken respiratory effort.

The critical care nurse will recognize a patient going into respiratory distress by observing lowered respiratory effort, difficulty breathing, unconsciousness, cyanosis, and lowered pulse oxygenation percentages. Patients that may be on the cusp of a respiratory arrest may exhibit signs of decreasing neurologic function such as agitation, confusion, and oxygen hunger. They may be sweating profusely and have a rapid heart rate.

Diagnosis of respiratory failure will be based off clinical observation, and treatment will depend on the cause. If there is an obstruction present, it will need to be removed. If failure was caused by an adverse drug effect, an antidote may be given if appropriate. More than likely, the patient in respiratory failure will be aggressively ventilated using mechanical ventilation if necessary to prevent impending cardiac arrest. Oxygenation and ventilation are the high priority at this point.

Acute Respiratory Infections

Pneumonia

One of the most common and deadly lung infections a patient can succumb to is **pneumonia**. Pneumonia is an inflammation of the lung tissue caused by some sort of infection, whether bacterial, viral, fungal, or parasitic. Most pneumonias are bacterial, usually *Streptococcus pneumoniae*.

Everyone breathes in pathogens daily. The upper airways are colonized with "normal" flora. The difference is when a patient becomes immunocompromised or a particularly virulent pathogen is introduced. The normal responses of mucociliary clearance, cough, and the actions of the white blood cells are no longer effective, and infection results.

There are five categories of pneumonia based on how and where the pneumonia is acquired: community, hospital, healthcare-associated, immunocompromised, and aspiration. Aspiration pneumonia will be discussed in greater detail in a later section.

Community-acquired pneumonia, a leading cause of death globally, occurs in persons with little to no contact with medical settings, such as hospitals or nursing homes, at the time of acquisition. Patients will present with fatigue, dyspnea, cough, fever, chills, and pleuritic chest pain. Diagnosis will be made based upon clinical presentation and chest x-ray films. Antibiotics are the treatment of choice, based on the causative organism. It is important to note that it is often difficult to pin down the exact cause of the pneumonia due to the limited diagnostic methods available at this current time. Antibiotic treatment, as a result, will be based on the clinician's best judgment and empirical evidence.

Hospital-acquired and **healthcare-associated pneumonias** occur in patients in medical settings. These patients are likely to have been infected with gram-negative bacilli, such as *Pseudomonas aeruginosa,* and antibiotic-resistant strains, such as *methicillin-resistant Staphylococcus aureus.* Like the other pneumonias, diagnosis is based on clinical presentation and chest x-ray. Treatment is usually a regimen of broad-spectrum antibiotics.

Patients that are immunocompromised, such as those with HIV infection or those undergoing chemotherapy, may be particularly susceptible to pneumonia. Diagnosis is made after blood cultures have been obtained as well as sputum cultures, chest x-ray, and clinical evaluation. Treatment is the same, with special consideration given to the compromised immune function of the patient.

Aspiration Pneumonia

Aspiration pneumonia occurs when a patient inhales something toxic, usually contents of the stomach or something they are eating. Airway obstruction and pneumonia follow aspiration.

Patients with aspiration pneumonia usually have risk factors that the critical care nurse should be aware of before the event occurs, including impaired cognition, impaired swallowing, or GI devices such as a nasogastric tube in place.

A patient who has aspirated may not always exhibit symptoms of aspiration. This is called "silent aspiration" and can go on for some time without any evidence it is occurring. A patient who is silently aspirating may be constantly clearing their throat or have a cough that sounds wet. Symptoms of aspiration, if evident, include fever, discomfort of the chest, coughing while eating and attempting to swallow, and trouble breathing, especially after eating and drinking.

When gastric contents are aspirated, the acidic nature of the stomach acid burns the lining of the airways and lungs. This chemical burn causes immediate bronchoconstriction, swelling, and hemorrhage of the alveoli. This alveolar bursting is what then leads to the associated aspiration pneumonitis.

A patient is diagnosed with aspiration pneumonia after their clinical presentation is evaluated and a chest x-ray is obtained. If silent aspiration is suspected, a barium swallow study may be performed to confirm. Treatment includes antibiotics and removal of the foreign object if possible.

Preventative interventions for aspiration include elevating the head of the patient's bed to at least 30 degrees (90 degrees if the patient is eating). Diet changes may be necessary, including allowing foods that are easy to chew and swallow, discontinuing straw usage for drinks, and monitoring patient eating times. Patients who are at risk for aspiration should not take in fluids through a straw, since the straw shoots fluid directly onto the back of their throat, not allowing a weakened swallow reflex enough time to "catch" it and direct it down the esophagus. The critical care nurse can encourage the patient to tuck their chin while swallowing to ensure food passes into the esophagus rather than the airway.

Chronic Conditions of the Pulmonary System

Many patients that the critical care nurse will encounter will suffer from long-term diseases of the lungs, falling under the category of chronic obstructive pulmonary disease (COPD), asthma, bronchitis, and emphysema. All four chronic conditions overlap in clinical presentation, diagnosis, exacerbations, and treatment, but it is important to know the distinctions between them as well.

Chronic Obstructive Pulmonary Disease (COPD)

COPD is an umbrella term encompassing various chronic lung conditions—such as emphysema, bronchiectasis, chronic bronchitis, certain cases of asthma, or a combination of these—wherein normal breathing is compromised. Thus, it is possible to be diagnosed with COPD but not emphysema, since there are other diseases—namely, chronic bronchitis—that can be at the root of a patient's COPD. A patient diagnosed with COPD often has emphysema and chronic bronchitis together, but this is not usually the case. In most cases, COPD is progressive and permanent. Symptoms of COPD include shortness of breath and/or wheezing, chest pain, coughing, and excessive mucus in the airways. Smoking cessation should be encouraged to decrease exacerbations and slow the progression of the disease. Smoking is almost always the cause of emphysema, and therefore, also often heavily involved in causing COPD.

Over the course of several years, the disease will worsen, starting with a productive cough and leading to trouble with breathing. Patients with COPD will often complain of a headache that they get every morning. Their chest may become barrel-like in appearance due to hyperinflation of the lungs. Weight loss and muscle wasting are common signs of advanced disease. The patient may breathe with their lips pursed, a sign of "auto-PEEPing." This means they are creating their own PEEP by making the hole their air passes through smaller, like breathing through a straw. As the disease progresses, their exacerbations will increase. A COPD exacerbation occurs when, for a reason that may be unknown, the patient's symptoms worsen, and hospitalization often follows.

Diagnosis of COPD is made based on clinical presentation, pack-a-day history, chest x-ray, and pulmonary function testing. Treatment includes encouragement of smoking cessation, inhaled bronchodilators, corticosteroid use, and supportive care including oxygen therapy and pulmonary rehabilitation.

Asthma

Asthma is an airway disease in which bronchoconstriction occurs in the airways, usually after some triggering stimuli has set in motion the inflammatory responses of the lung tissue. Patients with asthma will have exacerbations that cause them to have trouble breathing, wheezing, a cough, and tightness in the chest. Pulsus paradoxus, or a greater than 10-point fall in systolic BP while breathing in, is a sign of an asthmatic attack, along with tachycardia, tachypnea, and use of accessory muscles to breath.

A diagnosis of asthma will be made based on the patient's clinical presentation, their history of symptoms, and pulmonary function tests. They will be treated with inhaled beta2-agonists and inhaled corticosteroids, as well as monitoring and controlling their exposure to their asthmatic triggers or the substances in their environment that cause exacerbations.

Bronchitis

While chronic bronchitis is a hallmark of COPD, **acute bronchitis** can occur in any patient, most often following an upper respiratory infection (URI). The patient's bronchial tissue has become inflamed because of the URI. The symptoms exhibited are cough, possible fever, and sputum production. A diagnosis of acute bronchitis will be based on clinical presentation, and antibiotics may or may not be used based on the clinician's judgment.

Emphysema

Emphysema usually occurs because of smoking and is defined as a destruction of lung tissue that causes a loss of elasticity, recoil, and alveoli. The airway is more susceptible to collapsing, it hyperinflates, and airflow is limited. Blebs and bullae develop, air trapping occurs, and the airspaces, as a whole, enlarge. All of these physiological effects of emphysema worsen the lungs' functioning capability and can lead to a COPD diagnosis and the exacerbation of such COPD symptoms.

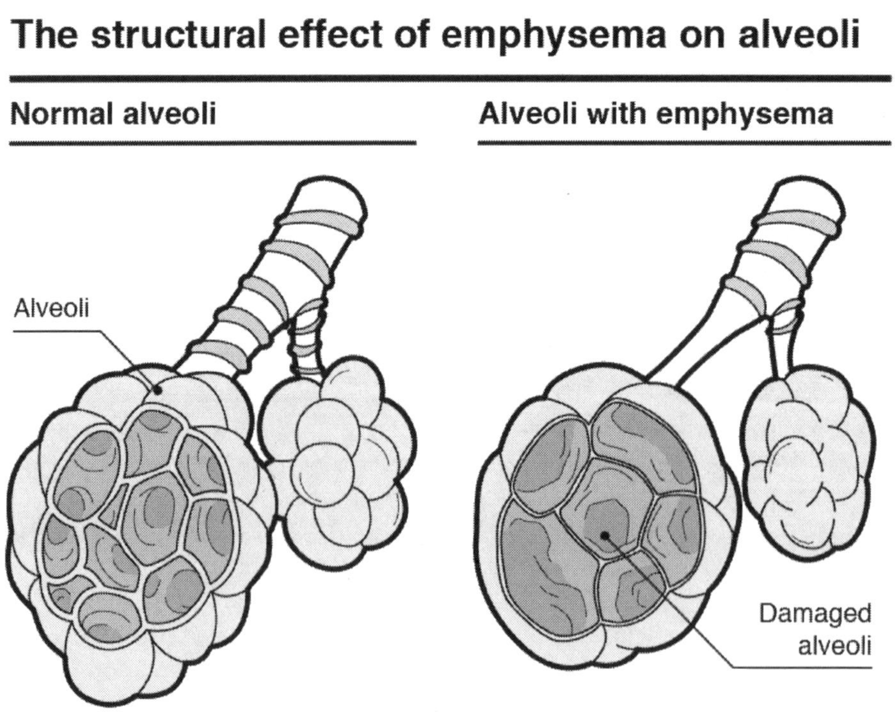

Mechanical Ventilation Complications

Mechanical ventilation is a means to an end, that end being weaning from ventilation and restoring the patient's full ventilatory capacity and functioning. Weaning from the vent can be a difficult task in some patients, especially if their pulmonary system has been weakened by illness. While the critical care nurse will not oversee vent weaning in most facilities, they are there to support the respiratory care team and physicians in achieving this goal.

Vent weaning is achieved through gradual changes in the level of the patient's dependence on the machine. The respiratory therapy team will likely be performing **spontaneous breathing trials** on the patient daily, as these have been shown to assist with weaning. This means they turn off the vent and see how the patient does without it for a few breaths. If the patient is completely apneic and oxygen levels immediately drop off, it is not time, and the vent breathing is resumed.

The critical care nurse is aware that sedative and opioid use on the patient over time, though necessary to keep the patient comfortable while on the vent, may end up prolonging the duration of mechanical ventilation. Caution must then be used when sedating the patient, using enough to keep the patient comfortable, but not so much that the patient is "snowed," meaning overly sedated and unable to wean. Halving the dose may be ordered by the doctor, as well as titrating the dose down regularly and performing sedation vacations. **Sedation vacations** mean the nurse turns off sedation for a period of time, usually once a day for an hour or so. Sedation vacation duration also depends on patient tolerance of the procedure.

Pleural Space Abnormalities

Pneumothorax

Pneumothorax is the abnormal presence of air in the pleural cavity, which is the space between the parietal and visceral pleurae. Pneumothorax can be categorized as:

- **Spontaneous Pneumothorax**: This can be classified as either primary or secondary. Primary spontaneous pneumothorax (PSP) occurs in individuals with no history of lung disease or inciting event. Those at risk for PSP are typically eighteen to forty years old, tall, thin, and smokers. There's also a familial tendency for primary spontaneous pneumothorax. Secondary spontaneous pneumothorax occurs in individuals with an underlying lung disease such as COPD, cystic fibrosis, asthma, tuberculosis (TB), or lung cancer.

- **Traumatic Pneumothorax**: This occurs as a result of blunt or penetrating trauma to the chest wall. The trauma disrupts the parietal and/or visceral pleura(e). Examples of inciting events include: gunshot or stab wounds; air bag deployment in a motor vehicle accident; acute respiratory distress syndrome (ARDS); and medical procedures such as mechanical ventilation, lung biopsy, thoracentesis, needle biopsy, and chest surgery.

- **Tension Pneumothorax**: This is the trapping of air in the pleural space under positive pressure. It causes a mediastinal shift toward the unaffected lung and a depression of the hemidiaphragm on the side of the affected lung. Shortly after, the event is followed by severe cardiopulmonary compromise. Tension pneumothorax can result from any of the conditions or procedures listed for spontaneous and traumatic pneumothorax.

Signs and symptoms of pneumothorax depend on the degree of lung collapse (partial or total) and can include:

- Chest pain
- Dyspnea
- Cyanosis
- Tachypnea
- Tachycardia
- Hypotension
- Hypoxia
- Anxiety
- Adventitious breath sounds
- Unilateral distant or absent breath sounds
- Jugular venous distention (JVD)
- Tracheal deviation away from the affected side (with tension pneumothorax)

Diagnosis of pneumothorax is primarily clinical (based on signs and symptoms), but can involve an upright posteroanterior chest x-ray, chest CT scan (the most reliable imaging for diagnosis), ABG analysis, and ultrasonography of the chest. Treatment of a pneumothorax depends on the severity of the condition and can include:

- Supplemental oxygen
- Thoracostomy (chest tube): standard treatment for all large, symptomatic pneumothoraces
- Observation (a reasonable option for small asymptomatic pneumothorax; multiple series of chest x-rays are needed until resolution)
- Simple needle aspiration (an option for small, primary spontaneous pneumothorax)
- Because they can quickly cause life-threatening cardiopulmonary compromise, the standard of treatment for all tension pneumothoraces is an emergent needle thoracostomy.

Hemothorax

Hemothorax, the presence of blood in the pleural space, is most commonly the result of blunt or penetrating chest trauma. The **pleural space** lies between the parietal pleura of the chest wall and the visceral pleura of the lungs. A large accumulation of blood in the pleural space can restrict normal lung movement and lead to hemodynamic compromise. Common signs and symptoms of hemothorax include chest pain, dyspnea, and tachypnea. When there is substantial systemic blood loss, tachycardia and hypotension can also be present.

Diagnosis of hemothorax primarily involves a chest x-ray, which reveals blunting of the costophrenic angle on the affected side of the lung. A helical CT scan has a complementary role in the management of hemothorax, and it can localize and quantify the retention of blood or clots within the pleural space.

Small hemothoraces usually require no treatment, but need close observation to ensure resolution. Tube thoracostomy drainage is the mainstay of treatment for significant hemothoraces. Needle aspiration has no place in the management of hemothorax. Blood transfusions can be necessary for those with significant blood loss or hemodynamic compromise. Complications from hemothorax can include empyema (secondary bacterial infection of a retained clot) or fibrothorax (fibrosis of the pleural space which can trap lung tissue and lead to decreased pulmonary function).

Empyema

Empyema refers to a condition in which pus, a thick liquid consisting of dead white blood cells, tissue, and other debris as a byproduct of infection, fills the pleural space around the lungs. It results from infection in the lung tissues itself, such as in patients who have bacterial pneumonia, abscesses in the lung, or have foreign bodies in the lungs (e.g., after chest surgery or a traumatic event). Symptoms include a sharp chest pain, difficulty breathing, a dry cough, fever, and night sweats. Treatment includes directly draining pus from around the pleural space through a syringe. Some cases require surgery to drain the pleural space and adjust the pleural membranes which line the lungs. In cases where there is a high volume of pus, pleural membranes can adhere together and prevent the lungs from fully expanding even once the pus is drained. Manual manipulation is required to separate the membranes. In complex cases of empyema, the lung can collapse.

Pleural Effusions

A **pleural effusion** is an abnormal accumulation of fluid in the pleural space. The pleural space is located between the parietal and visceral pleurae of each lung. The **parietal pleura** covers the inner surface of the chest cavity, while the **visceral pleura** surrounds the lungs. Approximately 10 milliliters of pleural fluid are maintained by oncotic and hydrostatic pressures, and lymphatic drainage and is necessary for normal respiratory function. Pleural effusions can be categorized as transudates or exudates. Transudates result from an imbalance between oncotic and hydrostatic pressures, so they are characterized by low protein content. The transudates are often the result of congestive heart failure (CHF), cirrhosis, low albumin blood levels, nephrotic syndrome, and peritoneal dialysis. Exudates result from decreased lymphatic drainage or inflammation of the pleura, so they are characterized by high protein content. The exudates are often the result of malignancy, pancreatitis, pulmonary embolism, uremia, infection, and certain medications.

The main symptoms of a pleural effusion include dyspnea, cough, and chest pain. Diagnosis of a pleural effusion can include chest x-ray, chest CT scan, ultrasonography, and thoracentesis. Thoracentesis can provide pleural fluid for analysis such as LDH, glucose, pH, cell count and differential, culture, and cytology. Pleural fluid should be distinguished as either transudate or exudate. Exudative pleural effusions are characterized by:

- Ratio of pleural fluid to serum protein > 0.5
- Ratio of pleural fluid to serum LDH > 0.6
- Pleural fluid LDH > 2/3 of the upper limit of normal blood value

Treatment of a pleural effusion is usually dictated by the underlying etiology; however, the treatment of a very large pleural effusion can include:

- Thoracentesis
- Chest tube (also known as tube thoracostomy)
- Pleurodesis (instillation of an irritant to cause inflammation and subsequent fibrosis to obliterate the pleural space)
- Indwelling tunneled pleural catheters

Pulmonary Hemorrhage

Pulmonary hemorrhage is characterized by hemoptysis secondary to a variety of conditions, including bronchiectasis, tuberculosis (TB), lung cancer, pneumonia, or lung abscesses. Hemoptysis can be minor, resulting in less than 100mL of blood per day, or massive, resulting in 200 to 1,000mL in 24 hours. Minor pulmonary hemorrhage is typically a symptom of respiratory infection or malignancy. Massive hemorrhage is rare and typically originates from the bronchial vasculature, which is higher pressure than the pulmonary vasculature. Symptoms include the expectoration of blood when coughing, which may be accompanied by other symptoms related to the underlying condition. Assessment should verify that the source of blood loss is respiratory rather than gastric. A complete history and physical examination are vital to diagnosis and should involve an estimate of blood loss, infection symptoms, onset, history of smoking, weight loss, chronic conditions, and TB status. Additional studies such as CBC, blood type, BMP, arterial blood gas, and chest radiography should be obtained to determine the patient's stability and need for transfusion. Chest radiography is the preferred study to determine the exact location of the blood loss, although a CT scan may also be obtained in stable patients. Treatment involves positioning the patient in Trendelenburg or reverse Trendelenburg with the affected lobe down to spare the healthy lung. Intubation may be necessary for patients with uncontrolled bleeding, and an 8mm or greater endotracheal tube should be considered to allow for bronchoscopy if needed. Anticoagulants should be reversed, and tranexamic acid (TXA) may be given to attempt to resolve hemoptysis. Bronchial artery embolization is the first-line treatment for massive pulmonary hemorrhage, with surgical resection being the last resort.

Pulmonary Hypertension

When the pressure in the pulmonary circulation rises, it is termed **pulmonary hypertension**. The blood vessels within the pulmonary beds of circulation become constricted and sometimes even obstructed. This raised BP may cause failure of the right ventricle of the heart.

Causes of pulmonary hypertension may be idiopathic, but left heart failure, diastolic dysfunction, parenchymal lung disease, and a PE have been known to raise the pulmonary pressures.

A patient with pulmonary hypertension may complain of exertional dyspnea and chronic fatigue, experience loss of consciousness, and feel chest discomfort. Diagnosis is made via echocardiography, which estimates the pressures, and confirmed by right heart catheterization.

Pulmonary hypertension can be treated through use of vasodilators and diuretics. Sildenafil is an example of a phosphodiesterase inhibitor used to treat pulmonary hypertension and is helpful in increasing blood flow in the lungs. Amlodipine is an example of a calcium channel blocker, a class of drugs that may be helpful for pulmonary hypertension. Epoprostenol is a drug specifically formulated for use in patients with pulmonary hypertension. Lung transplantation may be an option in advanced disease states.

Status Asthmaticus

Acute severe asthma attacks, also known as **status asthmaticus**, are repeated, back-to-back asthma attacks that are not responding to the usual treatment of bronchodilators. Status asthmaticus is an emergency that requires special medical treatment to resolve.

A patient experiencing a severe asthma attack that is unresponsive to bronchodilators may have chest tightness, severe shortness of breath, a dry cough, and wheezing. Their airway is undergoing bronchospasm, inflammation, and mucus plugging, all of which contribute to difficulty breathing. The patient's lungs may be retaining carbon dioxide, resulting in hypoxemia and respiratory failure.

Often a respiratory illness is the triggering factor in status asthmaticus, occurring a few days before the attack. This weakens the body's immune defenses, leading to exacerbation of asthma. Other triggers may include exposure to allergens or irritants in the environment with an especially potent effect.

In the emergency treatment of a patient with status asthmaticus, subcutaneous epinephrine may be used. Alternatively, terbutaline may be used, as it has fewer cardiac effects such as tachycardia. Albuterol that has been nebulized may be administered alongside nebulized ipratropium. Corticosteroids such as prednisone should be given to decrease the systemic inflammatory response. If a bacterial infection seems to be part of the patient's presentation, antibiotics may be used. Supplemental oxygen will be part of the patient's therapy as well.

If the patient is unresponsive to all the above treatments and respiratory function continues to decline, noninvasive positive pressure ventilation or mechanical ventilation will be considered to stabilize the patient, restore ventilation and oxygenation, and prevent further complications such as cardiac arrest.

Thoracic and Airway Trauma

A **thoracic trauma** can be summarized as an injury to the chest. Frequently, chest trauma results in death within the first few minutes or hours after injury, due to the vitality of the heart and lungs caged within the thoracic cavity. When these organs are damaged, aggressive intervention is necessary to save lives.

A short list of common thoracic traumas includes hemothorax, pneumothorax, disruption of the aorta, flail chest, blunt cardiac injury, lung contusion, and cardiac tamponade. Bone injuries may also occur, such as cracked ribs, clavicle fractures, and fractures of the sternum and scapula.

Hemothorax and pneumothorax may occur at the same time due to their proximity to one another. Hemothorax is a condition in which blood is hemorrhaging and begins filling the pleural space. Pneumothorax occurs when there is an unsealed opening in the thoracic wall, disrupting normal airflow and ventilation. The larger the hole, the worse the respiratory distress and failure. Patients with pneumothorax may have a wound that makes a sucking sound, indicating air moving through an abnormal pathway.

Multiple rib fractures may cause a separating of the chest wall from the thoracic cage, resulting in a disruption to the patient's ability to inspire air. **Flail chest,** the term for this condition, is caused by a blunt force trauma in most cases, which in turn causes significant lung contusion beneath the site of the chest wall separation.

Cardiac tamponade describes the condition in which blood surrounds the pericardial sac, decreasing the heart's ability to fill. Patients experience hypotension, jugular vein distention, and muffled heart tones upon auscultation. A pericardiocentesis is immediately necessary, in which a needle is inserted and the leaked blood aspirated, to relieve pressure surrounding the heart and normalize BP.

Blunt chest injuries may cause a **rib fracture**. Rib fractures often occur simultaneously with other thoracic trauma, such as pneumothorax, flail chest, hemothorax, and tracheobronchial injuries. A rib fracture on its own is painful, but it is not complicated, nor does it need much treatment besides analgesia. Analgesia is achieved using opioids and possibly concurrent NSAID use.

Tracheal perforation refers to a tear in the upper airway of the pulmonary tree. Thoracic trauma may be the cause of a tracheal perforation, but it may also have occurred during a medical procedure such as endotracheal intubation or bronchoscopy. Surgical repair will be necessary to repair the tear after it has been confirmed using CT scanning and chest x-ray.

Thoracic Surgery

In certain conditions of the lung, thoracic surgery may be considered. A thoracic surgeon is one who specializes in operations on the thoracic region of the body, involving the organs of the chest. The heart and lungs are the primary targets of these surgical procedures.

Surgeries may be performed to remove cancerous tumors of the lung. Possible procedures a patient would undergo for this purpose would be a pneumonectomy, lobectomy, wedge resection, or sleeve resection. **Pneumonectomy** removes the entire lung. **Lobectomy** removes the entire lobe containing the cancerous tumor. **Wedge resection** removes part of the affected lobe. **Sleeve resection** refers to "trimming" the affected part of the airway and sewing it back together, like cutting a stain off a sleeve and reattaching the upper and lower portions.

If a thoracic surgeon wishes to visualize the interior of the chest wall and surrounding tissues, they may opt to perform a thoracoscopy. During this procedure, small incisions are made into the chest wall, and a thin tube with a camera at the end, called a **scope,** is inserted. The surgeon then explores the interior cavity and visualizes the area they wish to view. This procedure may be used to biopsy tissue for histological analysis. A more invasive procedure used to visualize the interior chest cavity is called a **thoracotomy,** where the chest is opened directly.

Practice Quiz

1. Which of the following surgeries performed by a cardiothoracic surgeon removes a section of an airway leading to the lung, sewing together the top and bottom of the section removed?
    a. Pneumonectomy
    b. Lobectomy
    c. Sleeve resection
    d. Wedge resection

2. Which of the following is a more invasive procedure performed by a thoracic surgeon involving opening the chest wall to visualize the interior structures?
    a. Thoracotomy
    b. Thoracocentesis
    c. Thoracobronchotomy
    d. Thoracoscopy

3. What emergency surgery is necessary to relieve cardiac tamponade?
    a. Thoracocentesis
    b. Pericardiocentesis
    c. Left heart cardiac catheterization
    d. Open heart surgery

4. Which of the following test results is consistent with pulmonary edema of a non-cardiogenic origin?
    a. Chest x-ray with bilateral pulmonary infiltrates
    b. Elevated blood levels of B-type natriuretic peptide (BNP)
    c. ABG analysis revealing hypoxemia
    d. A pulmonary artery wedge pressure of 12 mmHg

5. A 25-year-old male presents to the Emergency Department complaining of shortness of breath, coughing, and wheezing for two days. His cough is productive, and he reports seeing black material mixed in with his phlegm. Visual examination reveals carbonaceous sputum. At this point in the examination, he develops severe respiratory distress and is subsequently intubated and placed on mechanical ventilation. What is the mostly likely diagnosis for this patient?
    a. Acute bronchitis
    b. Inhalation injury
    c. Community-acquired pneumonia
    d. Hemothorax

See answers on the next page.

Answer Explanations

1. C: Sleeve resection is a thoracic surgery in which an affected part of the airway is removed, with the top and bottom sections being sewn together. This action is similar to cutting a stain off a sleeve and reattaching the top and bottom sections of the sleeve back together—hence, the name "sleeve resection." Pneumonectomy is the removal of an entire lung. Lobectomy is the removal of a lobe. Wedge resection refers to removing a part of an affected lobe.

2. A: A thoracotomy is the opening of the chest by a thoracic surgeon to visualize the interior structures and tissue of the chest. Thoracocentesis is an invasive procedure where small incisions are made in the chest wall with the purpose of removing air or fluid and inserting a chest tube to drain. Thoracocentesis is also called a pleural tap. Thoracobronchotomy is a procedure where an incision is made into the bronchus and thorax, usually to remove a tumor or foreign object. Thoracoscopy is a less invasive procedure involving small incisions and the insertion of a thin tube with a camera affixed to the end, called a scope, to visualize the interior structure and tissues of the chest.

3. B: Pericardiocentesis is indicated in the emergent situation of cardiac tamponade. A needle is inserted, and the hemorrhaging blood is aspirated from the pericardial sac. Thoracocentesis, or pleural tap, can be used for hemothorax or pneumothorax. Left cardiac catheterization is used in acute myocardial infarctions to open obstructed coronary vessels. Open heart surgery can be performed in emergency situations involving thoracic trauma, but not specifically for cardiac tamponade.

4. D: Pulmonary edema can be of cardiogenic or non-cardiogenic origin. There is no single test to differentiate whether the cause of pulmonary edema is cardiac or noncardiac. Bilateral pulmonary infiltrates and hypoxemia are nonspecific symptoms and can occur in both. A pulmonary artery wedge pressure < 18 mmHg is consistent with pulmonary edema of non-cardiogenic origin.

5. B: This scenario depicts an inhalation injury. Although the patient's history is limited, the fact that he produced carbonaceous sputum makes an inhalation injury the most likely diagnosis (specifically smoke inhalation). This scenario emphasizes the point that medical professionals should maintain a high level of suspicion when it comes to inhalation injuries. Treatment of inhalation injuries is largely supportive with an excellent prognosis for complete recovery.

Endocrine/Hematology/Gastrointestinal/Renal/ Integumentary

Major Human Endocrine Glands and Some of Their Hormones

	Gland		Hormone	Chemical Class	Representative Actions	Regulated By
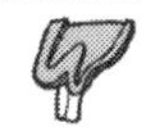	**Hypothalamus**		Hormones released from the posterior pituitary and hormones that regulate the anterior pituitary *see below*			
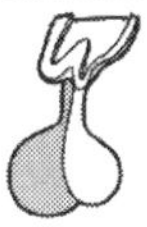	**Posterior pituitary gland** *Releases neurohormones made in hypothalamus*		Oxytocin	Peptide	Stimulates contraction of uterus and mammary gland cells	Nervous system
			Antidiuretic hormone **ADH**	Peptide	Promotes retention of water by kidneys	Water/salt balance
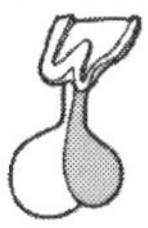	**Anterior pituitary gland**		Growth hormone **GH**	Protein	Stimulates growth (especially bones) and metabolic functions	Hypothalamic hormones
			Prolactin **PRL**	Protein	Stimulates milk production and secretion	Hypothalamic hormones
			Follicle-stimulating hormone **FSH**	Glycoprotein	Stimulates production of ova and sperm	Hypothalamic hormones
			Luteinizing hormone **LH**	Glycoprotein	Stimulates ovaries and testes	Hypothalamic hormones
			Thyroid-stimulating hormone **TSH**	Glycoprotein	Stimulates thyroid gland	Hypothalamic hormones
			Adrenocorticotropic hormone **ACTH**	Peptide	Stimulates adrenal cortex to secrete glucocorticoids	Hypothalamic hormones
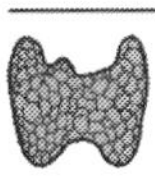	**Thyroid gland**		Triiodothyrocine T_3 Thyrocine T_2	Amine	Stimulate and maintain metabolic processes	TSH
			Calcitonine	Peptide	Lowers blood calcium level	Calcium in blood
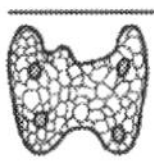	**Parathyroid glands**		Parathyroid hormone **PTH**	Peptide	Raises blood calcium level	Calcium in blood
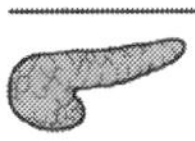	**Pancreas**		Insulin	Protein	Lowers blood glucose level	Glucose in blood
			Glucagon	Protein	Raises blood insulin level	Glucose in blood
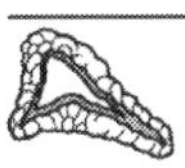	**Adrenal glands**	*Adrenal medulla*	Epinephrine Norepinephrine	Amines	Raises blood glucose level; Increases metabolic activities; Constrict certain blood vessels	Nervous system
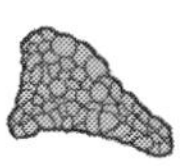		*Adrenal cortex*	Glucocorticoids	Steroid	Raises blood glucose level	ACTH
			Mineralocorticoids	Steroid	Promote reabsorbtion of Na^+ and excretion of K^+ in kidneys	K^+ in blood; angiotensin II
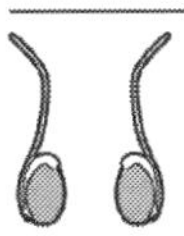	**Gonads**	*Testes*	Androgens	Steroid	Support sperm formation; Promote development and maintenance of male secondary sex characteristics	FSH LH
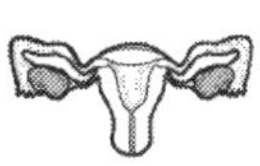		*Ovaries*	Estrogens	Steroid	Stimulate uterine lining growth; Promote development and maintenance of female secondary sex characteristics	FSH LH
			Progestins	Steroid	Promote uterine lining growth;	FSH and LH
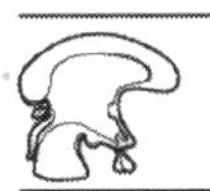	**Pineal gland**		Melatonin	Amine	Involved in biological rhythms	Light/dark cycles

The critical care nurse will encounter several conditions affecting the hormonal regulation of the human body, the blood and its unique chemistry, the digestive tract, the kidneys and their filtration processes and the largest organ of the body, the skin, which protects the interior of the body from the exterior environment. This section comprises a discussion of those body systems, including the endocrine, hematological, neurological, gastrointestinal, and renal systems.

Endocrine

The hormones of the body play a key role in metabolism and the regulation of body processes. Each hormone, produced in various glands throughout the body, has a specific target tissue that it acts upon, producing a specific result. Dysfunction of hormonal regulation can lead to disease states, as will be discussed in the section on the next page.

Adrenal Insufficiency

Adrenal insufficiency may be referred to as **Addison's Disease**. It results when the adrenal glands produce insufficient amounts of glucocorticoids and mineralocorticoids. Mineralocorticoids are another group of steroids influencing electrolyte and fluid balance. This can be the result of an underlying autoimmune disorder or systemic infection. Symptoms include fatigue and skin discoloration. Addison's disease is usually treated with steroid injections but may become a medical crisis if the patient goes into shock, a stupor, or a coma. This can occur if the patient does not realize he or she has the disease, as some of the primary symptoms can be quite generic.

Diabetes Insipidus (DI)

Vasopressin, also known as the antidiuretic hormone, is made in the hypothalamus within the brain and stored in the pituitary gland. It is then secreted by the pituitary gland, targeting the tissue of the kidneys and blood vessels. The role of vasopressin is to help the body concentrate urine and maintain a healthy balance of fluid within the blood.

When the pituitary does not produce enough vasopressin, the kidneys' ability to concentrate urine is significantly decreased, to the point of massive fluid loss through urination.

The term "antidiuretic hormone" should give one a clue as to how this disease works; if the hormone that is supposed to prevent diuresis is inhibited, then severe diuresis will occur.

The condition that results from the inhibition of vasopressin is called **diabetes insipidus**. The onset of the disease may happen slowly over time or quite abruptly. The patient will usually present with symptoms of enormous fluid intake and copious quantities of urine production, termed **polydipsia** and **polyuria**, respectively.

The urine produced by individuals with diabetes insipidus is quite diluted, due to a lack of concentration ability of the kidneys. The patient will require volume replenishment as soon as possible, to prevent further complications of dehydration and hypovolemia.

Since it is difficult clinically to perform tests to detect the amount of vasopressin within the body, the test most often used for diabetes insipidus is the **water-deprivation test**. The patient is carefully monitored while fasting from fluids. Urine output is monitored and analyzed for osmolality and electrolyte concentrations. Toward the end of the testing, vasopressin is administered and the effect it has on the urine measured. If the patient is responsive to the vasopressin and there are signs that without it the urine becomes overly diluted, it is probable that the patient has diabetes insipidus.

Differential diagnoses to be mindful of in a patient with diabetes insipidus are diabetes mellitus and psychogenic polydipsia. A patient with diabetes mellitus, a condition in which insulin regulation of blood glucose is impaired, may present with polyuria like the polyuria present in diabetes insipidus. Patients with psychogenic polydipsia take in enormous quantities of water but not for the same reason as a patient with diabetes insipidus. Their water intake is due to an emotional disturbance or mental illness such as schizophrenia. The critical care nurse will be mindful of this when assessing patients with symptoms of polydipsia and polyuria.

Diabetes Mellitus, Types 1 and 2

Diabetes mellitus is a condition that affects how the body responds to the presence of glucose. Glucose is needed for cellular functions, and all consumable calories eventually are converted to glucose in the body. A hormone produced by the pancreas, called **insulin,** is needed to break down food and drink into glucose molecules. In patients with **type 1 diabetes**, the pancreas fails to produce insulin, leading to high levels of glucose in the bloodstream. This can lead to organ damage, organ failure, or nerve damage. Patients with type 1 diabetes receive daily insulin injections or have a pump that can be programmed to release insulin continuously and/or as needed based on the patient's specific needs and blood glucose levels. These patients need to be careful to not administer excess insulin, as this will cause their blood sugar to become too low. Low blood sugar can lead to fainting and exhaustion and may require hospitalization.

In patients with **type 2 diabetes**, the pancreas produces insulin, but the body is unable to use it effectively. Patients with type 2 diabetes typically need to manage their condition through lifestyle changes, such as losing weight and eating fewer carbohydrate-rich and sugary foods. There are also some medications that help the body use the insulin that is present in the bloodstream. **Gestational diabetes** is a form of diabetes that some women develop during the second to third trimester of pregnancy, when their systems temporarily become resistant to insulin. High blood sugar in a pregnant woman can affect fetal growth and influence the baby's risk of becoming obese. Pregnant women with gestational diabetes are encouraged to exercise daily, avoid excessive weight gain, and carefully monitor their diet. Gestational diabetes is similar to type 2 diabetes in the way symptoms present and in treatment options.

Diabetic Ketoacidosis (DKA)

A patient diagnosed with diabetes mellitus may be prone to a complication of this condition called **diabetic ketoacidosis (DKA)**. The process of developing DKA is a complex metabolic pathway in which the body seeks alternative energy sources to glucose, resulting in an acidotic state.

At the beginning of DKA, the body is in a state of insulin deficiency. This can happen as a result of diabetes mellitus, and the body must compensate to continue operations as usual. The body begins to metabolize triglycerides and amino acids to create energy. In a normal state, the body breaks down glucose as an energy source. However, when insulin is deficient and blood glucose supply is in flux all the time, as is the case with diabetes mellitus, the body searches for alternatives.

The breakdown of triglycerides and amino acids then causes an increase in serum levels of glycerol and free fatty acids as a byproduct of lipolysis, or fat breakdown. Alanine also rises in the serum as a byproduct of muscle breakdown, as another energy source when the body cannot find enough glucose. This rise in alanine and glycerol stimulates the liver to produce its own glucose as an energy source. Glucagon, which is produced in the pancreas and used as an emergency source of energy when outside glucose sources drop, rises to excessive levels and stimulates free fatty acids to be converted to ketones.

This process is called **ketogenesis** and is normally blocked by sufficient levels of insulin. Ketogenesis results in ketoacids, such as acetone, which create the acidic environment of DKA. Acetone is released from the body by way of respiration, which is why a patient with DKA has a "fruity" smell to their breath.

When the blood sugar rises during DKA, this causes substantial amounts of fluids to be excreted through the urine, called **osmotic diuresis**. This leads to fluid and electrolyte imbalances. Potassium levels must be carefully monitored during DKA. They may not initially fall in serum tests because, despite great loss of potassium through the urine, there is also a great release of potassium from the cells into the blood stream. Potassium will be ushered back into the cells when insulin levels return to normal.

Presenting symptoms of DKA include polyuria, polydipsia, nausea, and abdominal pain. Diagnosis will be made based on symptoms and measurements of arterial blood gases. Presence of ketones in the blood stream, an anion gap of >12, and a pH of < 7.30 are considered positive diagnostic signs of DKA.

Treatment of DKA will include insulin administration, correction of fluid and electrolyte imbalances, and possibly bicarbonate to correct severe cases of acidosis.

Hyperglycemia

Hyperglycemia, or a random blood sugar reading not affected by a recent meal that is greater than 200 mg/dL, is often a symptom of insulin resistance or insulin deficiency. Insulin resistance and deficiency are the key factors producing diabetes types I and II, hence hyperglycemia is a trademark of these two diseases.

When insulin does not properly regulate the level of blood glucose circulating, blood sugar rises to unhealthy levels. This produces a sequela of complications, as well as some unpleasant symptoms in the patient experiencing hyperglycemia.

The most commonly-associated symptoms of hyperglycemia are polydipsia and polyuria, in which a person is drinking and then urinating copious amounts of fluids. A patient might also experience nausea, warmth, and blurred vision. The high level of circulating blood sugar puts the patient at risk for bacterial and fungal infections, as these organisms feed on and thrive in environments where there are high levels of glucose.

Prolonged polyuria will result in dehydration, as evidenced by tachycardia, hypotension, fatigue, and weakness in the patient. These are serious complications that will be treated with fluid resuscitation and electrolyte correction if imbalances exist. High blood glucose will be treated with insulin therapy, including oral antihyperglycemics, and injectable glucagon.

Hyperglycemic Hyperosmolar Nonketotic Syndrome (HHNK)

A patient with Type II diabetes still produces insulin, though insulin response and efficacy are limited as the cells have developed a resistance to insulin. When blood sugar rises to unhealthy levels, it stimulates the kidneys to drop large amounts of urine, a condition called polyuria. The blood volume is thus depleted, causing a state of dehydration and abnormal concentration of the blood. Concentration of the blood creates a hyperosmolar state in the blood stream. When the blood is concentrated yet not acidotic as a result of fat cells breaking down, this is called **hyperglycemic hyperosmolar nonketotic syndrome**.

HHNK can result from a patient not taking their prescribed diabetic medications appropriately, causing a hyperglycemic state. At other times, an infection or illness unrelated to diabetes mellitus may cause a hyperglycemic state. Corticosteroids are known to cause a rise in blood sugar; thus, their use must be administered with caution. If the patient also suffers from high blood sugar and has been prescribed diuretics, this may also cause a hyperosmolar state.

The concentrated blood of HHNK will primarily cause neurological deficits such as confusion, disorientation, drowsiness, and even coma. Certain patients will experience seizures or stroke-like syndromes. Death may occur if HHNK is left untreated.

HHNK will be diagnosed based on symptoms of confusion and blood tests to look for hyperosmolarity of the blood, as well as decreased blood volume signaling dehydration. Treatment will occur via intravenous (IV) therapy to correct fluid and electrolyte imbalances.

Syndrome of Inappropriate Secretion of Antidiuretic Hormone (SIADH)

Antidiuretic hormone, or vasopressin, is released by the pituitary gland to signal the kidneys to retain fluid in the body. When too much vasopressin is released, as is the case in **SIADH**, fluid is retained and sodium levels become diluted, resulting in hyponatremia.

SIADH may occur in some cases of cancer where vasopressin is being produced outside of its normal pituitary gland location. Hospitalized and elderly populations are also susceptible to SIADH.

A patient with SIADH will present with confusion and fatigue, common hyponatremic symptoms. Diagnosis will be made based on clinical presentation and after analysis of blood tests, which will uncover the hyponatremia.

Fluid intake will be restricted to prevent further volume dilution. Hypertonic saline, which has a high concentration of sodium, will be used to correct the hyponatremia. Drugs that reduce the effects of vasopressin may be used, such as demeclocycline or lithium.

Thyroid Disorders

Hyperthyroidism

When patients are diagnosed with **hyperthyroidism**, they may also be referred to as having an overactive thyroid, which results in the overproduction of T4 and/or T3 hormones. Symptoms include feelings of anxiety, trouble focusing, feeling overheated, gastrointestinal problems such as diarrhea, insomnia, elevated heart rate, and unexplained weight loss. Hyperthyroidism is commonly caused by **Grave's disease**, an autoimmune disorder. The extent to which symptoms of Grave's disease manifest can be broad, depending on the severity of the disease. Family history, stress, smoking, and pregnancy can increase the risk of developing Grave's disease. Women under the age of forty are most likely to be diagnosed.

Medical treatment options can include methimazole and propylthiouracil, two common antithyroid medications. Prescription corticosteroids may also be used. In nonpregnant patients, radioactive iodine may be used. This is a long-term, repeat-dose solution that can sometimes result in hypothyroidism, which can be easier to treat. In serious cases, some or all of the thyroid may be removed, although this also usually results in hypothyroidism. It is also recommended that most patients with Grave's disease modify their lifestyle to limit stress, eat a healthy diet, and exercise regularly.

Hypothyroidism

When patients are diagnosed with **hypothyroidism**, they may also be referred to as having an underactive thyroid, which results in the underproduction of T4 and/or T3 hormones. Symptoms include depression, excessive fatigue, chills, dry skin, lowered heart rate, gastrointestinal problems such as constipation, and unexplained weight gain. Hypothyroidism is commonly caused by **Hashimoto's disease**, another autoimmune disease that affects thyroid function. This disease is usually treated with synthetic thyroid hormone replacement therapy, which involves taking a daily dose of the T4 hormone. T3 supplementation is rare, as it is derived from T4. Hypothyroidism can also be caused by the presence of too much iodine. The thyroid uses iodine to make T4 and T3 hormones. If there is too much iodine in the blood, the pituitary gland releases less TSH. The low levels of TSH can later result in the thyroid not producing enough T4 and/or T3 hormones. In some cases of hypothyroidism, surgery is required.

Hematology/Immunology

Anemia

There are certain components in the blood that have the capacity to carry oxygen to the tissues of the body. These components are called the red blood cells (RBCs), hematocrit, and hemoglobin. When any of these three components drops in number, oxygen-carrying capacity also drops. A hemoglobin of less than 14 g/dL, a hematocrit of less than 42%, or a red blood cell count of less than 3.4 million/mL are all general ranges of what is considered anemic.

Often **anemia** is not a disease in and of itself but rather a symptom of an underlying disorder. The practitioner will investigate for underlying causes of anemia to make sure nothing is missed.

There are three broad categories of anemias, not including blood loss: microcytic anemias, normocytic anemias, and macrocytic anemias. In **microcytic anemias**, including iron-transport deficiency, lead poisoning, and thalassemia, the heme and globin synthesis is defective or deficient. Testing for microcytic anemias will include an analysis of the patient's iron stores. In **normocytic anemias**, the RBC is normal in size but deficient in number. Examples of normocytic anemias include anemia of chronic disease and aplastic anemia acquired from primary bone marrow disorders. **Macrocytic anemias**, caused by abnormal DNA synthesis, lead to large RBCs that do not have sufficient oxygen-carrying ability.

The commonly-seen symptoms in a patient with anemia include fatigue, weakness, difficulty breathing during exercise, and a pale skin tone. Pallor, or paleness, can be assessed in a dark-skinned patient by looking at the bottoms of their feet, palms, lips, buccal mucosa, and conjunctiva of the eye. Dark-skinned patients will usually have a warm tone, but when anemic or cyanotic, they will have a more gray or ashen hue.

As mentioned, there are a variety of different types of anemias. **Thalassemia**, common in those of Mediterranean descent, is one type in which the amount of oxygen-carrying hemoglobin is decreased causing pallor, weakness, fatigue, and poor growth. **Folate deficiency anemia**, associated with alcoholism, is a result of poor absorption of nutrients and decreases the amount of folate available to RBCs, thus decreasing oxygen delivery to tissues. Infections, cancers, and many other illnesses may destroy RBCs, hemoglobin, and/or hematocrit, causing an anemia.

The treatment of anemia will depend on the underlying cause and the severity of the patient's condition. If the patient is anemic because of massive blood loss, blood transfusions will be required. If the anemia is caused by deficient **erythropoiesis**, the process by which blood is formed, drugs like erythropoietin will be used to stimulate blood production.

Autoimmune Disorders

Guillain-Barre Syndrome

Guillain-Barré syndrome is an autoimmune disorder in which the immune system progressively attacks the peripheral nervous system. The exact cause of Guillain-Barré syndrome is currently unknown, but it has been correlated with recent viral infection, *Campylobacter* infection, trauma, surgery, and recent vaccinations. Symptoms of Guillain-Barré syndrome tend to start with neuropathy in the lower extremities, progress into weakness in the legs, and can eventually progress into paralysis, including the diaphragm.

Initially, diagnosis of Guillain-Barré syndrome involves a thorough clinical assessment and past medical history. The patient will likely have a CBC and CMP drawn to rule out other causes of neurological symptoms, but these tests will likely be normal and not definitive in diagnosing Guillain-Barré syndrome. **Lumbar puncture** may be performed during the acute phase, which may show elevated protein in the cerebral spinal fluid. The patient may also have **electromyography** to test motor nerve function, which will likely indicate demyelination of the nerves.

While there is no cure for Guillain-Barré syndrome, there are several treatments that can slow its progression; as a result, most patients are able to recover much of their motor nerve function within a year of diagnosis. One treatment is **plasmapheresis**, a procedure in which the plasma is filtered through a machine to remove particles, such as antibodies, that are causing negative symptoms in the patient. Prior to the procedure, the patient should drink plenty of fluids to maintain their fluid and electrolyte balance, and they should be encouraged to eat. The patient is at risk of electrolyte imbalances following plasmapheresis, including hypocalcemia and hypomagnesemia. Therefore, serum electrolytes should be monitored and potentially replaced, and the patient should be on continuous cardiac monitoring in case of arrythmia. The patient may also become hypotensive due to fluid loss, which may be treated with fluid resuscitation or blood products. Finally, the nurse should monitor for hypothermia, providing warming measures to reduce potential worsening outcomes.

Immunoglobulin therapy, in which healthy antibodies are infused into the blood, may also be helpful. Patients will also benefit from routine physical therapy to reduce muscle atrophy and regain function. In more severe cases (when the disease progresses to the diaphragm), treatment may become supportive, including respiratory support through mechanical ventilation.

The first priority of nursing management of the patient with Guillain-Barré syndrome is to monitor for progression of the disease. The nurse should monitor for difficulty breathing, aspiration risks, and urinary incontinence or retention. Analgesics may be administered as needed to improve the patient's comfort, especially in anticipation of physical therapy. Additionally, because of their immobility, these patients are at an increased risk of blood clots. Therefore, the nurse should administer prophylactic anticoagulation therapy as ordered, encourage mobility where possible, and provide sequential compression devices as needed.

Myasthenia Gravis

Myasthenia gravis is also an autoimmune disease of the CNS that is manifested by severe muscle weakness resulting from altered transmission of acetylcholine at the neuromuscular junction due to antibody formation. Relapses and remissions are common; examples of relapse triggers include infection, stress, pregnancy, and increases in body temperature due to immersion in hot water. Subjective manifestations include weakness, diplopia, dysphagia, fatigue on exertion, and bowel and bladder dysfunction. Objective manifestations include unilateral or bilateral ptosis of the eye, impaired respiratory function, impaired swallowing, and decreased muscle strength. Tensilon testing and electromyography, which measures muscle activity over time, are used to diagnose this disorder, while anticholinesterase agents and immunosuppressant agents are the mainstays of treatment. Additional treatments include plasmapheresis to decrease circulating antibodies and removal of the thymus gland to slow T-cell production.

Patients in myasthenic crisis due to a lack of cholinesterase may present in the emergency department with hypertension and severe muscle weakness that requires mechanical ventilation. Tensilon therapy may temporarily reduce the symptoms. Patients in cholinergic crisis due to an excess of cholinesterase exhibit hypotension, hypersecretion, and severe muscle twitching, which eventually results in respiratory muscle fatigue requiring ventilatory support. Atropine is used to control manifestations of this complication.

Systemic Lupus Erythematosus (SLE)

Systemic lupus erythematosus (SLE) is an autoimmune disease in which the immune system attacks tissues throughout the body, causing damage and widespread inflammation. This can affect any of the organs in the body, including the skin, heart, lungs, liver, kidneys, nervous system, and digestive system. Because of this, symptoms can be varied and systemic. For example, should the disease attack the nervous system, the patient may present with fatigue, headaches, seizures, and memory problems. Should it attack the heart, the patient may present with palpitations, murmurs, and arrythmias.

Diagnosis of SLE can be a lengthy process, as the patient may present with many seemingly unrelated symptoms. Depending on presentation, the patient may have basic laboratory work, imaging of various organs, ECG, EEG, or biopsies completed. SLE is more definitively diagnosed with a positive antinuclear antibody test along with clinical findings.

Treatment for SLE is much like that of other autoimmune disorders, in that it involves suppression of the overactive immune system along with treatment of the damage it has caused to the body. Patients with SLE may be given NSAIDs for pain management and to decrease inflammation. They may also be placed on steroids for inflammation and immunosuppressants to decrease immune response. Those at risk of blood clots may also be placed on anticoagulants. Treatment beyond this varies significantly depending on the organs affected. For example, if the disease is affecting the heart, the patient may require antihypertensives, antiarrhythmics, or even procedures like valve replacements. Those who have had kidney damage due to lupus may end up requiring hemodialysis or kidney transplantation.

Nursing management of the SLE patient is also multifaceted. The patient may be admitted to the progressive care unit for disruption of any number of their organ systems. This will require thorough head-to-toe assessment and continuous monitoring. Additionally, nurses should be aware that those on immunosuppressants are at greater risk of infection, and thus, nurses should be especially careful about infection prevention with SLE patients. Finally, nurses should provide thorough education to the SLE patient, informing them about infection prevention, the need to wear protective garments, when to seek emergency care, and how to decrease adverse outcomes by maintaining a healthy diet, exercising (when possible), and avoiding drugs, alcohol, and smoking.

Coagulopathies

Coagulation is the process by which the blood clots to prevent excessive bleeding when an injury occurs. The process of coagulation is orchestrated by several different components of the blood. Injury first occurs, followed by action from the platelets, activation of proteins and a cascade of other coagulation components, conversion of prothrombin to thrombin, then fibrinogen to fibrin, and finally **hemostasis**, or stopping of bleeding, is achieved.

When a step in this complicated process is interrupted and hemostasis is not adequately achieved, it is called a **coagulopathy**. Idiopathic thrombocytopenia purpura (ITP), disseminated intravascular coagulation (DIC), and heparin-induced thrombocytopenia (HIT) are three such examples and will be discussed here.

Idiopathic Thrombocytopenia Purpura (ITP)

Thrombocytes are cells in the blood that help with the clotting process that achieves hemostasis. A lack of thrombocytes is called a **thrombocytopenia**. ITP, then, is a type of thrombocytopenia that occurs in the absence of systemic disease, is marked by bleeding, and often has no known cause, hence the idiopathy.

ITP is a chronic condition in adults but usually resolves spontaneously in children. Typically, the patient will present with petechiae, purpura, and mucosal bleeding. **Petechiae** are small red or purple spots that appear on the skin and mark small points of bleeding in the capillary beds. **Purpura** is a slightly larger point of collected blood under the skin that indicates uncontrolled bleeding in the capillary beds. **Ecchymosis**, or bruising, is the largest of the bleeding lesions and may also be present in ITP.

Diagnosis of ITP is made via blood tests, with other causes of thrombocytopenia excluded to confirm diagnosis. Corticosteroids will be used to try and stop bleeding. In very severe cases of ITP, a splenectomy, in which the spleen is removed, is considered to resolve ITP. In the case of severe, uncontrolled bleeding, the patient may be given a platelet transfusion.

Disseminated Intravascular Coagulation (DIC)

DIC is a medical emergency in which the coagulation cascade has been activated by exposure to a tissue factor. The fibrinolytic pathway is also activated. Usually onset of DIC is rapid, with bleeding and occlusion of the small blood vessels present. The result of a sudden onset of DIC is thrombocytopenia, a prolonged PT and PTT time, high d-Dimer, and lowered plasma fibrinogen.

Causes of DIC can include obstetric complications such as abruptio placentae, retained dead fetus, or amniotic fluid embolism. Infections with gram-negative organisms can result in the release of an endotoxin and tissue factor that may cause DIC. Cancers usually produce a slow-onset DIC in which more clotting activities are part of the clinical presentation.

Treatment of DIC will include replacement therapy of platelets, cryoprecipitate, and fresh frozen plasma. In patients with a slower onset of DIC, heparin may be used to treat the condition.

Heparin-Induced Thrombocytopenia (HIT)

HIT is a condition in patients receiving heparin therapy in which platelet aggregation occurs in excessive amounts leading to blockage of blood vessels. These vessel obstructions may lead to other life-threatening events such as stroke, acute MI, and occlusion of arm or leg arteries. If HIT is suspected, heparin therapy should be stopped immediately. Alternative anticoagulants such as argatroban, bivalirudin, and fondaparinux will be used until platelet count has returned to normal.

Myelosuppression

Thrombocytopenia

In the blood, there are cells called thrombocytes that play a key role in clotting, as previously mentioned. Literally meaning "blood clot cell," a thrombocyte can also be called a platelet. Thrombocytes arise from the bone marrow and are shed off of a cell called a megakaryocyte. Thrombocytes are irregularly shaped, making them excellent at clumping together and assisting with the formation of clots.

When the number of thrombocytes is lowered in the blood, a condition called thrombocytopenia occurs. This condition puts patients at increased risk for bleeding as they do not have an essential component of clotting present in adequate numbers.

There are a number of different ways thrombocytopenia can occur, arising from numerous different causes. Two main categories of thrombocytopenia are those that occur as a result of immunologic causes and those that occur as a result of nonimmunologic causes. An immunologic cause of thrombocytopenia could include a viral infection, side effects of drugs, blood transfusions, or connective tissue disorders. Nonimmunologic causes include sepsis or acute respiratory distress syndrome.

A normal count of thrombocytes or platelets is 140,000 to 440,000, though that number can vary in the case of pregnant women or persons with inflammatory conditions. A significant drop below that number is considered thrombocytopenia.

A patient with thrombocytopenia will likely exhibit signs of bleeding, the classic signs being petechiae, purpura, and ecchymoses scattered across the body. Bleeding from the mucosal regions of the body, such as the mouth, is common.

Based on clinical observations of the above signs and symptoms, as well as the patient's history and laboratory findings, diagnosis will be made. The treatment will be based on the underlying cause.

Neutropenia

When the white blood cells drop to a count of less than four thousand cells per microliter of blood, it is termed **leukopenia**. A person experiencing leukopenia will be more susceptible to invasive organisms and, as a result, infections, because their normal defenses are compromised. The term leukopenia may sometimes be used interchangeably with the term neutropenia. **Neutropenia** refers to a drop in the number of circulating neutrophils within the blood. Neutrophils are the most numerous components of the white blood cells; thus, leukopenia and neutropenia are very similar in concept.

There are numerous causes of leukopenia within the body. A severe infection may lower the count of white blood cells, as can the side effects or abuse of certain drugs. Patients with cancers involving malignant tumors that destroy the immune system will show a lowered white blood cell count and thus be leukopenic. An enlarged spleen, termed splenomegaly or hypersplenism, may cause leukopenia.

Diagnosis of leukopenia or neutropenia will be made based upon clinical presentation of the patient and blood test measuring the count of the white blood cells. Treatment will be aimed at the underlying cause, be it infection, malignancy, or otherwise. Antimicrobial therapy may be used to target a systemic infection causing the leukopenia.

Oncologic Complications

Tumor Lysis Syndrome

Tumor lysis syndrome can occur in some cancer patients undergoing treatment. If a large number of cancerous cells are broken down by treatments such as radiation or chemotherapy, they burst and release their toxic contents into the patient's bloodstream. This can cause a significant imbalance in the patient's blood electrolyte levels. Notably, the patient may show high levels of potassium, phosphate, uric acid, and urea in the blood, and low calcium. This results in metabolic dysfunction and symptoms including seizures, heart arrhythmias, nausea and vomiting, and kidney failure. It can also result in patient death. Patients receiving treatment for leukemias and lymphomas are at highest risk of experiencing tumor lysis syndrome, as these cancers tend to present larger tumors with more cells.

Transfusion Reactions

Transfusion reactions occur when a patient has an adverse response to receiving a blood transfusion. Blood transfusions are routinely administered to patients who have experienced significant blood loss. Generally, donated blood is matched to a patient based on blood type. If a patient does not receive blood that matches their own blood type, they will experience an adverse reaction due to the mismatch in protein markers that denote each blood type. Patients will experience a strong immune response that will cause their immune cells to attack the transfused blood. Additionally, they may have an allergic response to an entity in the donated blood. Transfusion reactions typically occur within twenty-four hours. Patients may experience symptoms such as physical pain, dark urine, fever, dizziness, shortness of breath, widespread itching, organ failure, lung injury, or death. Based on the intensity of the reaction, treatment can range from administering an antihistamine to performing emergency surgery.

Transfusion-Related Acute Lung Injury (TRALI)

Transfusion-related acute lung injury (**TRALI**) is a syndrome in which a patient experiences acute respiratory distress syndrome (ARDS) after a blood transfusion. While TRALI is a rare syndrome that is not yet well understood, it is the leading cause of death associated with blood transfusion in the United States. TRALI is believed to result when a patient has a strong immune response to anti-leukocyte antibodies in a donor's blood. Some theories also indicate that donor blood storage methods may also play a role. The syndrome generally presents within six hours after a transfusion. Symptoms include erratic breathing, shortness of breath, fever, blue-tinged skin, and abnormally low blood pressure. Lung imaging may show fluid in the lungs and pulmonary edema, while blood oxygen levels may rapidly drop. Patients generally require immediate airway management and assisted ventilation. In otherwise healthy patients who experience TRALI, there is a twenty percent mortality rate; in more ill patients, the mortality rate is around sixty percent. Measures to prevent TRALI include testing blood donor samples for the antibodies that are associated with the response and not administering samples that have these antibodies present to patients requiring blood transfusion.

Transfusion-Associated Circulatory Overload (TACO)

Transfusion-Associated Circulatory Overload (**TACO**) typically occurs within six hours of a blood transfusion and is characterized by acute pulmonary edema. TACO, along with transfusion-related acute lung injury (TRALI), accounts for the highest number of transfusion-related events that end in morbidity. Pulmonary edema from TACO results due to circulatory overload and is typically accompanied by elevated BNP, high central venous pressure, positive fluid balance, and left heart failure. Symptoms of TACO include tachypnea, hypoxia, and tachycardia within the first six hours post-transfusion. TACO commonly occurs perioperatively in patients with a history of chronic kidney disease (CKD) and congestive heart failure. Diagnosis involves obtaining an echocardiogram to determine any abnormalities congruent with circulatory and pulmonary overload. Elevated BNP levels are also an important diagnostic marker, as they can indicate circulatory overload. It is also vital to determine the total number of units of blood that the patient received during the transfusion, as well as amount of maintenance fluids. Patients with a history of malignancy or those undergoing chemotherapy are also at a higher risk of developing TACO due to the high volume of fluids and transfusions required for treatment. Active surveillance is vital to the prevention of TACO, including assessment of renal and cardiac function prior to transfusion in high-risk patients. By assessing this risk prior to transfusion, providers can choose to administer a diuretic or consider an alternative route to transfusion.

Gastrointestinal

The abdomen holds within its walls almost all the vital organs of the body, save the heart, lungs, and brain. These organs are prone to injury and disease, with one organ's ailment occasionally affecting nearby organs. The following will be a discussion of injuries and diseases affecting the abdominal region of the body, as well as the processes of the gastrointestinal tract.

Abdominal Compartment Syndrome

Abdominal compartment syndrome occurs when excess fluid in various tissues of the torso results in increased intra-abdominal pressure. The syndrome most commonly results from trauma to the region, sepsis, or an illness. As intra-abdominal pressure increases, it disrupts blood flow to the visceral organs in this region. Multiple organs are vulnerable to hypoxia and failure; this can significantly disrupt the patient's internal homeostasis to the point of death. This syndrome has a high mortality rate of approximately seventy percent, generally caused by heart and lung failure. Initial symptoms of abdominal compartment syndrome include a distended, swollen abdomen, pain upon palpitation of the abdomen, limited urine output, and abnormally low blood pressure. Early treatment interventions include treating the primary cause of the increased intra-abdominal pressure (e.g., if a patient is septic, administering systemic antibodies; if a patient is hemorrhaging, managing the bleed). Other responses include balancing the patient's fluids and electrolytes and decompressing the bowels and bladder.

Acute Abdominal Trauma

When an injury occurs that affects the abdomen, it is called an **abdominal trauma**. Since there are a vast number of ways in which the abdomen can be traumatized, it is helpful for the practitioner to categorize the injury. One method of categorizing abdominal trauma is by the area of the abdomen affected: the abdominal wall, one of the major solid organs, one of the hollow organs, or the vasculature of the abdomen. Examples of solid organs include the liver, spleen, pancreas, and kidneys. The hollow organs are the stomach, small intestine, colon, ureters, and bladder. The abdominal aorta would be the most serious component of the vasculature to be injured, as it carries the majority of the blood pumped out of the heart to supply the lower half of the body.

A trauma to the abdomen can be blunt or penetrating. A blow such as a kick, a fall down a set of stairs, or hitting the steering wheel in a car accident are all examples of blunt force trauma. A penetrating wound, such as a gunshot or stab wound, is one in which the abdominal wall is penetrated.

An abdominal trauma may also affect the structures surrounding it, such as the spinal cord, the vertebrae, or the pelvis.

The common manifestations of abdominal trauma are lacerations, hemorrhage, hematoma, and perforation of the contents of the abdomen, depending on where the injury occurs and the severity of the force. When a hollow viscus such as the stomach or the colon are perforated, their contents seep out into the peritoneal cavity, causing acute peritonitis.

A patient who has suffered an abdominal trauma may develop delayed complications such as rupture of a hematoma, development of an intra-abdominal abscess, an obstruction or ileus within the bowel, a leakage of bile, or compartment syndrome of the bowel.

The chief complaint of those who have abdominal injuries is abdominal pain. Blood in the urine, radiating pain to the left shoulder indicating splenic injury, and signs of hypovolemia are all indicative of abdominal injury. Tachycardia, low blood pressure, diaphoresis, pallor or duskiness, as well as altered level of consciousness are all signs that an abdominal trauma has occurred.

Depending on the injuries incurred and the severity of the patient's condition, emergency laparotomy to repair damage and stop bleeding may be necessary. In other cases, however, the patient may simply be put under observation and visual imaging tests run to determine damage and treatment plan.

Acute GI Hemorrhage

Bleeding along the gastrointestinal (GI) tract can be insidious or acute in onset, occurring anywhere along the tract from the mouth to the anus. Acute GI bleeding is more serious in nature and needs to be addressed sooner in order to prevent hypovolemic shock.

A patient experiencing an **acute GI hemorrhage** will present differently based on the origin of the bleed. If it is an upper GI bleed, hematemesis or bloody vomit will appear with either a coffee ground (older blood) or bright red (new blood) appearance. Bleeding originating in the lower GI tract will appear in fecal matter as black or tarry stool (old blood), dark blood, or bright red blood. It is important to note that bright red blood in the stool is sometimes a result of hemorrhoids, not a GI hemorrhage.

The hemorrhage itself is not a disease but rather a sign of underlying disease, which will determine the target of treatment. Peptic ulcers, tears in the esophagus, diverticulitis, or cancers of the GI tract are all possible culprits of an acute GI bleed.

In order to target the source of the bleed, a tool called an endoscope will often be used. Depending on the suspected region of the GI tract, an upper or lower endoscopy may be used. **Colonoscopy** refers to a scope of the colon, part of the lower GI tract, while **esophagogastroduodenoscopy** (EGD) looks at the esophagus, stomach, and duodenum, or the upper GI tract.

In endoscopy, a thin tube with a camera affixed to the end of it is threaded into the body and images are produced. During endoscopy, areas that are bleeding may be cauterized to stop bleeding. **Cauterization** is the application of heat to the lesion to bring about hemostasis.

Bowel Infarction/Obstruction/Perforation

Almost one-quarter of the blood that is pumped out of the heart with each beat is required to supply the mucosa of the intestine with oxygen and other nutrients required for the metabolic activity that takes place there. An interruption to this blood flow, therefore, could lead to profound consequences. Ischemia, as discussed in the cardiac section, describes such an interruption of blood flow to tissue, which, over time, will lead to tissue death.

Mesenteric Ischemia

Acute mesenteric ischemia describes an ischemic condition of the bowel in which blood flow has been interrupted. This is a medical emergency that leads to inflammation and, eventually, infarction. **Infarction** describes total tissue death. The interruption in acute mesenteric ischemia is often caused by a blood clot. It may also be caused by a state of low blood flow, such as hypotension caused by shock.

The patient with acute mesenteric ischemia will often complain of abdominal pain. An exploratory laparotomy or angiography will be necessary to diagnose this condition. Once diagnosed, the patient may be treated by an embolectomy, in which the clot is removed. Other treatment options include resection of the bowel, in which the affected region is removed and the remaining segments reattached. Vasodilators and revascularization therapies will also be used when appropriate. This condition has a high mortality rate.

Bowel Obstruction/Adhesions

Within the bowels, obstructions may occur, causing cramping, vomiting, constipation, and decreased flatulence leading to bloating. An obstruction may be complete or partial. Diagnosis of intestinal obstruction is made by X-ray images of the abdomen as well as clinical presentation. A patient with an abdominal obstruction will be treated using fluid resuscitation, suction via nasogastric tube or, in severe cases, surgery to remove the obstruction.

The most common causes of mechanical obstruction in the bowel are adhesions, hernias, or cancerous tumors. Gallstones, diverticulitis, twisting of the bowel or volvulus, intussusception, and fecal impaction are also potential causes of obstruction.

Adhesions are bands of sticky, fibrous tissue within the bowel that cause surrounding tissues and organs to stick together, resulting in obstruction and ischemic conditions of the bowel. An adhesion must be removed surgically.

Illustration of an Adhesion

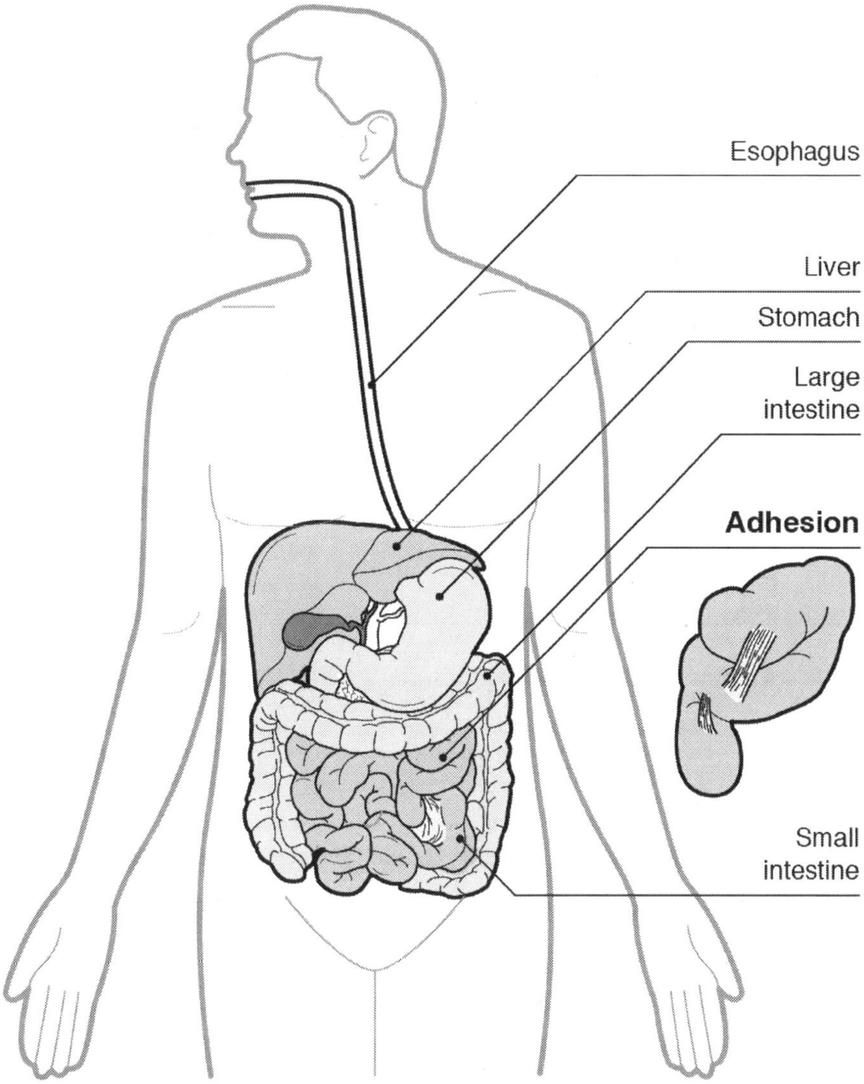

Bowel Perforation

A **gastrointestinal perforation** refers to a hole or tear that has formed through the entire wall of an intestine, whether small or large. Symptoms of this condition include abdominal pain, vomiting, and fever. The hole must be surgically repaired and is an emergency situation. Contents of the bowel may leak out when perforation has occurred resulting in an inflammatory condition called peritonitis.

GI Surgeries

Cholecystectomy

A **cholecystectomy** is a procedure in which the entire gallbladder is removed. The **gallbladder** is a pear-shaped organ that is positioned below the liver and adjacent to the stomach. The decision to take out the gallbladder is based on patient condition and, specifically, if gallstone formation is causing pain.

Cholecystectomy begins with the physician inflating the abdomen for a clear view with which to work. After this, the physician makes small incisions and insets a thin tube with a camera at the end into the abdomen. The physician visualizes the gallbladder and then removes it. This type of surgical procedure, in which there is minimal invasion, a camera or scope is used, and smaller incisions are made, is called a laparoscopic procedure.

Illustration showing cholecystectomy using the minimally-invasive laparoscopic procedure

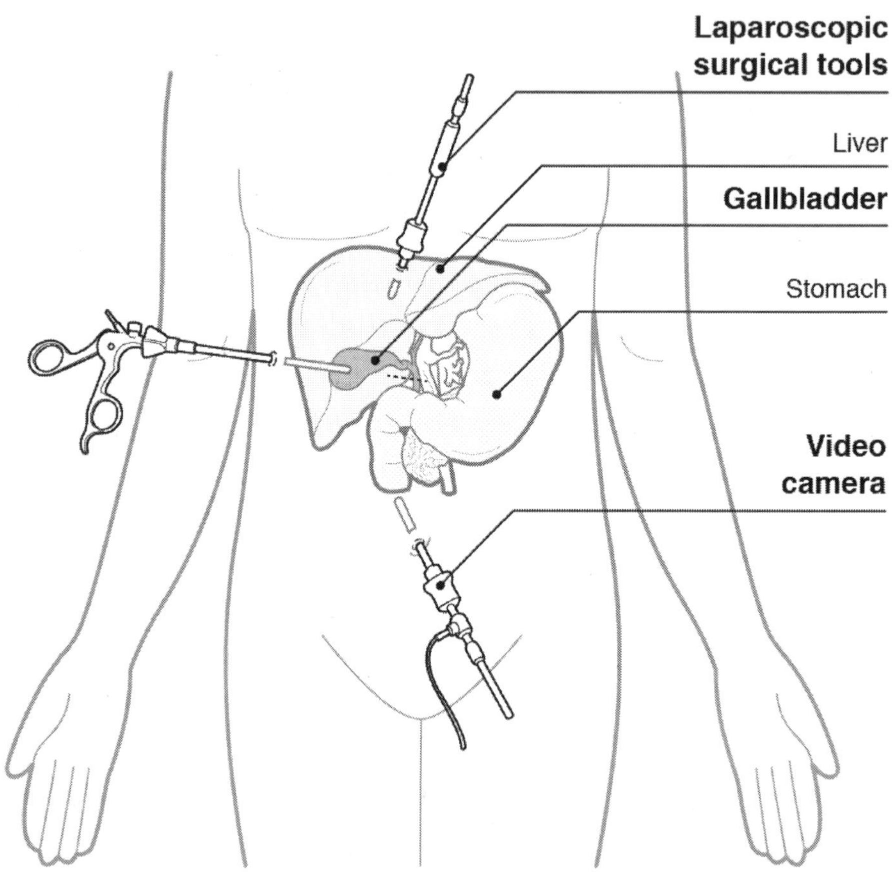

A **JP drain** is placed after a cholecystectomy to remove excess bile and blood that may drain and collect in the abdomen. Removing these fluids is thought to allow for better healing and prevent infection, although results of its efficacy are mixed.

Nurses should assess the drain site for patency and any signs or symptoms of infection, including redness, pain, or purulent discharge from the site. This involves double checking that the bulb is properly compressed to allow suction to pull fluid from the abdominal space. Additionally, the drain should be emptied when it becomes full to encourage proper drainage, and the output should be recorded at least once each shift. This measurement provides a trend of how much fluid is being pulled out of the space and is often used to determine how long a drain will remain in place.

Esophagectomy

An **esophagectomy** is a surgical removal of the esophagus. It is typically performed to treat esophageal cancer or Barrett's esophagus if precancerous cells are present. In an esophagectomy, an incision is made in the neck, chest, or abdomen to remove the affected parts of the esophagus and reconstruct it with a portion of stomach or intestine. Enteral nutrition is used after surgery until the patient can tolerate a regular diet without losing weight or requiring supplementation. Since the esophagus is often rebuilt with a portion of the stomach, the remaining smaller stomach size results in the need for frequent, smaller meals afterwards.

Post-surgically, patients may be given an epidural or a patient-controlled analgesic (PCA) pump to manage pain. Early mobility is encouraged to minimize complications associated with sedentary behavior, such as pneumonia and pressure ulcers. Patients and caregivers will need education on proper nutrition strategies, including care of the feeding tube. Consults from physical and occupational therapy are helpful to assist with strategies for ADLs upon discharge. Patients should be reminded it may be months until their functional status returns to near baseline.

Gastrectomy

A **gastrectomy** is a surgery performed to remove all or a portion of the stomach. It is typically performed to treat stomach cancer; however, it is also used to treat ulcers, obesity, and polyps. It can be a total gastrectomy, partial gastrectomy, or sleeve gastrectomy. In the event of a partial gastrectomy, only a portion is removed, typically the lower part of the stomach, and the intestine will be reconnected to the portion of the stomach that remains. In a total gastrectomy, the entirety of the stomach is removed, and the esophagus will be connected to the intestine instead. In a sleeve gastrectomy, the left side of the stomach is removed.

The surgery can be performed as either an open surgery, where a large incision is made into the abdomen or chest, or laparoscopically, where several smaller incisions are made for surgical tools and insertion of a camera.

With the removal of all or a portion of the stomach, patients need counseling on nutritional changes and considerations. Patients will receive parenteral nutrition for several days until some healing has occurred, followed by a slow progression from a liquid diet to a soft diet, and then to light meals. Consulting with a nutrition specialist is vital in order to maximize nutrition and avoid complications, such as **dumping syndrome**.

Colectomy

A **colectomy** is the surgical removal of the large bowel. It can include the removal of a portion of the colon, or the totality of it, and may or may not include the rectum. A colectomy is performed to treat colon cancer, a blockage, or diseased areas of the colon from conditions such as ulcerative colitis. The surgery can be open or laparoscopic in nature.

An **anastomosis** (to connect the ends of the portions of healthy large intestine) will be created if there is enough left after surgery. If there is not enough healthy bowel, a colostomy will be created by making a **stoma**, or opening, in the abdominal wall, and attaching the colon to the stoma. This allows for the body to continue to excrete waste through the large intestine. The colostomy may only be temporary if there is enough viable bowel left that needs time to heal, and the reconnection will happen later.

After surgery, nurses should encourage early mobilization as tolerated. The patient should be assessed for return of bowel function, and their diet should be progressed as bowel function returns. Patients will require education and encouragement to participate with ostomy care if a colostomy was created, as it is often an emotionally distressing event. Collaboration with a nurse specialized in wound and ostomy care (WORN nurse) can be helpful in troubleshooting, providing correct supplies, and ensuring proper fit of the ostomy bag. The nurse should frequently assess and document the surgical sites and stoma appearance. The stoma should appear moist, pink or red, and above the skin level. If the stoma takes on a dusky appearance or retracts, the surgical team should promptly be made aware.

Ileostomy and Colostomy

Ileostomy and colostomy are surgical procedures in which a portion of the bowel is rerouted up through a hole in the abdomen. **Ileostom**y involves the small intestine or ileum, while **colostomy** involves the large intestine or colon. These two procedures are performed in the cases of severe bowel disease, such as bowel cancer, diverticulitis, and inflammatory bowel disease.

The patient with a stoma as a result of an ileostomy or colostomy will need to be educated on how to care for it. A bag is attached to the stoma for the purpose of collecting fecal matter. This bag can be taken off and replaced as needed. The stoma needs to be assessed regularly to make sure it has not become infected. The stoma should be pink, and the area surrounding it should be kept clean and dry.

Healthy stoma site postcolostomy

Stoma is pink; area surrounding is clean and dry

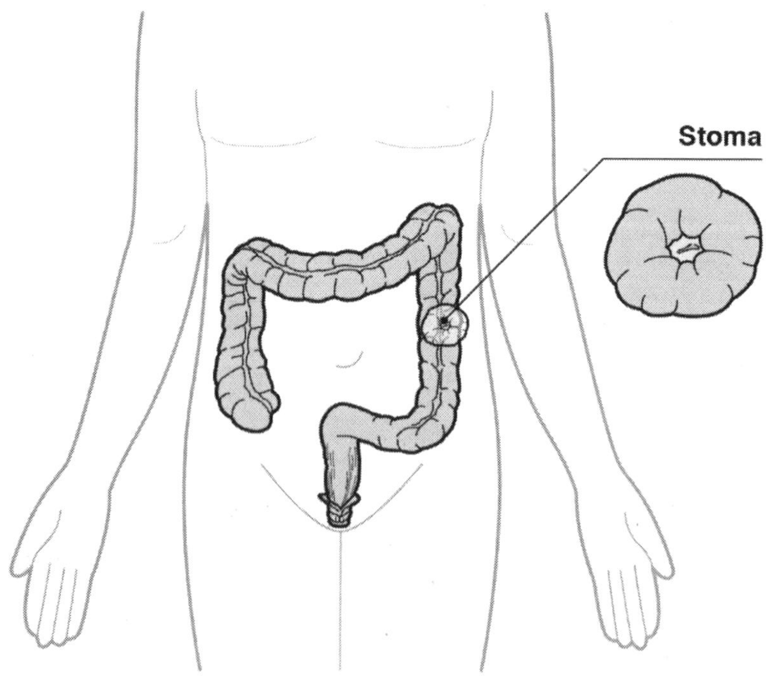

Whipple Procedure

Pancreaticoduodenectomy, also known as the **Whipple procedure**, is characterized by the surgical resection of the duodenum, gallbladder, pancreatic head, bile duct, and occasionally a portion of the stomach. This procedure is commonly performed on patients suffering from tumors in this area to effectively cure malignancy and may be accompanied by radiation and chemotherapy. This procedure holds significant risk with a high mortality rate, making proper patient selection, surgical technique, and postoperative care imperative to positive patient outcomes. Several non-malignant conditions may also require a Whipple procedure to be performed, such as severe trauma to the area or chronic pancreatitis. If malignancy is present, it is imperative that the tumors are shown to have clearly defined borders and no distant metastasis. If distant metastasis or aortic involvement are apparent, this case would be classified as unresectable and not a viable candidate for this procedure. Outcomes have improved since the development of minimally invasive methods such as laparoscopy and robotic surgery techniques, but morbidity rates remain high. Significant risks exist postoperatively, including delayed gastric emptying, exocrine and endocrine insufficiency, pancreatic fistulas, and bile leakages. In the postoperative period, closed suction drains will be monitored for output and tested for elevated amylase levels, which may indicate a leak in the pancreas. A nasogastric tube may be used to decompress and relieve pressure in the stomach. When drainage is minimal, the patient will regain the ability to eat a regular diet, and once a pancreatic fistula has been ruled out, the suction tubes can be removed.

Liver Disease

Hepatitis is an inflammatory condition of the liver, which is further categorized as infectious or noninfectious. Causative infectious agents for hepatitis may be viral, fungal, or bacterial, while noninfectious causes include autoimmune disease, prescription and recreational drugs, alcohol abuse, and metabolic disorders. More than 50 percent of the cases of acute hepatitis in the United States are caused by a virus. Transmission routes include fecal-oral, parenteral, sexual contact, and perinatal transmission. There are four phases of the course of viral hepatitis. During phase one, which is asymptomatic, the host is infected, and the virus replicates. The onset of mild symptoms occurs in phase two, while progressive symptoms of liver dysfunction appear in phase three. Finally, recovery from the infection occurs in phase four. These phases are specific to the causative agent and the individual.

The most common viral agents are hepatitis A (HAV), hepatitis B (HBV), and hepatitis C (HCV). Less commonly, hepatitis D (HDV), hepatitis E (HEV), CMV, Epstein-Barr virus, and adenovirus may cause hepatitis. HAV and HBV often present with nausea, jaundice, anorexia, right upper quadrant pain, fatigue, and malaise. HCV may be asymptomatic or, alternatively, may present with similar symptoms. Approximately 20 percent of acute infections with HBV and HCV result in chronic hepatitis, which is a risk factor for the development of cirrhosis and liver failure. The care of the patient with acute hepatitis due to HAV and HCV is focused on symptom relief, while the antiviral treatment for HBV is effective in decreasing the incidence of adenocarcinoma.

Chronic hepatitis is a complication of acute hepatitis and frequently progresses to hepatic failure, which is associated with deteriorating coagulation status and the onset of hepatic encephalopathy due to alterations in the blood-brain barrier that result in brain cell edema. Care of the patient with hepatic failure is focused on fluid volume and coagulation homeostasis and reduction of encephalopathy.

Hepatic Failure/Coma

Acute hepatic failure is a condition in which the liver is no longer performing at its normal level of metabolic function, often caused by drug toxicity or viral infection. For instance, acetaminophen is known to cause liver damage and failure in toxic overdoses. The common viral culprit of liver failure is hepatitis B, with hepatitis C being less common.

A patient experiencing liver failure will exhibit signs of encephalopathy—including confusion—as well as jaundice and ascites. **Jaundice** is a yellowing of the skin, and **ascites** is a bloating of the abdomen resulting from an accumulation of free fluid. In severe cases, this fluid will be drained off the abdomen to relieve pressure.

Portal Hypertension

Portal hypertension is a condition most often caused by cirrhosis or scarring of the liver in which the pressure of the portal vein is elevated. The portal vein drains blood from the organs of the upper GI tract, such as the spleen, intestines, and pancreas, into the liver. When the liver cannot receive the normal amount of blood due to scarring or disease, the resistance to the incoming blood rises, resulting in the higher pressure. Complications of portal hypertension include ascites, splenomegaly, and acute variceal bleeding. Variceal bleeding has a high mortality rate as it is difficult to control.

Treatment of portal hypertension includes monitoring, banding via endoscopy, and pharmacologic therapy, such as beta-blockers.

Cirrhosis

Cirrhosis is a scarring of the liver tissue over time and is an associated condition of acute liver failure. Chronic alcoholism is a leading cause of cirrhosis. The scarring of the liver can be slowed with treatment and alcohol abuse cessation, but ultimately is irreversible.

Esophageal Varices

Esophageal varices are dilated veins located in the esophagus and are a result of portal hypertension. These varices are highly vulnerable to massive bleeding, but are otherwise asymptomatic. Esophageal varices may be treated with banding procedures as well as intravenous administration of octreotide.

Fulminant Hepatitis

Fulminant hepatitis is a type of acute liver failure that occurs without the presence of pre-existing, chronic disease states. This type of liver failure is usually preceded by hepatic viruses, exposure to toxins, or drug injury. Fulminant hepatitis causes a large amount of necrosis or tissue death in the liver. As a result, liver transplantation may be needed in order for the patient to fully recover.

Biliary Atresia

Biliary atresia is a condition of the bile duct in which it is blocked or possibly even absent. This condition occurs in newborns because of abnormal fetal development. Newborns with biliary atresia are jaundiced because of the bile-duct atresia. A procedure called the **Kasai procedure** is often used to repair biliary atresia. In this procedure, the small intestine is attached to the liver to create a new pathway for bile to drain. The intestine is then reattached to a lower portion of the small intestine to reconnect it with the GI tract. Many infants with biliary atresia will develop liver failure later in life and will likely need liver transplants.

Illustration of the Kasai procedure performed for biliary atresia

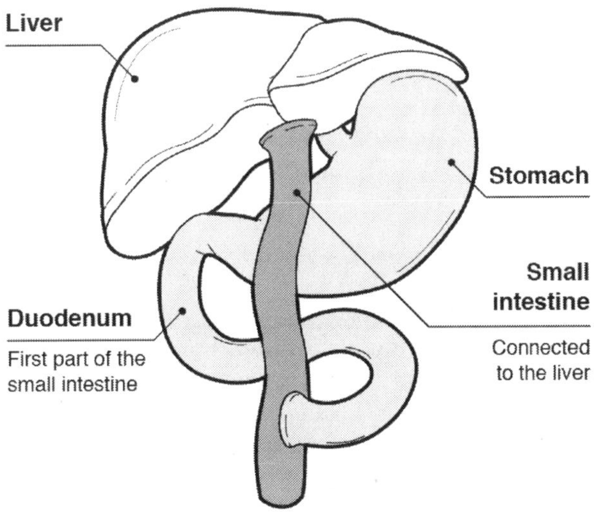

Malnutrition and Malabsorption

Malnutrition is a disorder that includes overnutrition and undernutrition. **Overnutrition** is a form of malnutrition that is associated with obesity and metabolic syndrome, in which a person is consuming far more calories from food than needed for healthy body function. **Undernutrition** is a result of deficient consumption of necessary nutrients for the body's function. Nutrients can be lost as a result of diarrhea or vomiting, leading to an undernourished state. **Anorexia**, a psychological condition in which a person refrains from eating in order to lose weight to achieve an unrealistic body image, is another form of undernutrition.

Progression of malnutrition may be slow or rapid, depending on the case. Anorexia is a slow decline in nourishment, while the body wasting, or cachexia, associated with cancers may result in rapid undernourishment.

Undernutrition often manifests as weakness, muscle wasting, weight loss, and irritability. The patient may become pale and fatigued.

Treatment of undernutrition includes diet control, correction of fluid and electrolyte irregularities, and correction of complications that may have developed.

Malabsorption is a disorder of the small intestine in which nutrients are not properly absorbed into the blood stream, resulting in a malnourished state of the body. Chronic diarrhea is the most common manifestation of malabsorption. **Steatorrhea**, or fatty stools, is a common sign of malabsorption, reflecting the fat loss of the body. Treatment of malabsorption will be aimed at correcting the cause. Common causes of malabsorption include bacterial overgrown syndrome, celiac disease, Whipple disease, and short-bowel syndrome.

Pancreatitis

Pancreatitis is an inflammation of the pancreas. The pancreas functions as both an exocrine and an endocrine gland. Inflammation results in a decrease in the pancreas's ability to function in these capacities. The condition can be either chronic or acute, with chronic pancreatitis leading to irreversible damage, fibrosis, and strictures of the ductal systems of the pancreas.

Major risk factors for developing chronic pancreatitis include alcohol abuse and smoking cigarettes. A patient will likely present with severe abdominal pain, centered around the epigastric region of the abdomen, that may be relieved or partially relieved by leaning forward or sitting up.

Treatment of pancreatitis will target control of the pain associated with flare-ups. Enzymes of the pancreas may be supplemented and complications such as diabetes will be managed.

Peritonitis

Peritonitis is an inflammatory process affecting the peritoneum, which is the serosal membrane that lines the abdominal cavity. The normally sterile environment of the peritoneum can become infected by a pathogen, irritated by bile from a perforated gallbladder or lacerated liver, or from secretions from the perforation of the stomach. The onset, severity, and course of the condition vary according to the precipitating event. Presenting manifestations may include abdominal pain, nausea and vomiting, diarrhea, fever and chills, altered peristalsis, abdominal distention, and possible encephalopathy. Diagnosis is based on the patient's history, in addition to the results of routine lab studies and blood cultures; ultrasound, computerized tomography (CT), and x-ray studies of the abdomen; and paracentesis. Emergency care of peritonitis is focused on eliminating the source of infection or irritation, controlling the infection and inflammatory process with aggressive antibiotic therapy as appropriate to prevent progression to generalized sepsis, and maintaining organ function of the abdominal organs.

Renal/Genitourinary

The kidneys are responsible for maintaining a healthy fluid and electrolyte balance in the body through filtration, reabsorption, and excretory processes. Urine is formed in the kidney, drained through the ureters to the bladder, and then excreted via urination. When these vital processes are interrupted by diseases, disorders, and injuries, imbalances occur. The following will be a discussion of diseases of the renal and genitourinary tract.

Acute Kidney Injuries (AKIs) and Acute Renal Failure (ARF)

An **acute kidney injury** and **acute renal failure** are essentially interchangeable terms referring to a rapid decline in kidney function. The course of dysfunction may last for days to weeks, with a build-up of nitrogenous waste products in the blood stream as a result. The cause of acute injury or failure may be a severe blow, such as blunt force trauma. Illnesses and surgical procedures may also cause the kidneys to fail.

Patients experiencing AKI or ARF may present with symptoms of nausea, anorexia, and vomiting, which are all reactions to the excessive waste products polluting the body. In severe cases, the patient may experience seizures or coma. When the kidney is no longer performing at capacity, fluid, electrolyte, and acid-base imbalances will develop. AKI is treated based on cause, with fluid and electrolyte rebalance being the target. In some cases, dialysis may be necessary.

Acute Tubular Necrosis (ATN)

One of the most common causes of ARF is **acute tubular necrosis**. The tubular cells of the kidney are key to its function. They absorb and filtrate vital fluid and electrolytes, as well as help form urine. When the kidney is hypoperfused or injured, such as is with hypotensive crises or use of nephrotoxic drugs, the tubular cells begin to die and kidney failure results.

Symptomology is like that of ARF and AKI, since ATN is a causative factor. **Oliguria**, or little to no urine production, is a sign of ATN that has developed into ARF. Correcting the cause of ATN, as well as neutralizing nephrotoxins and correcting fluid and electrolyte imbalances, will help bring the patient's kidney function back to normal.

Chronic Kidney Disease (CKD)

While acute injury and failure of the kidney can often be corrected, **chronic kidney disease** is a slow, progressive, and irreversible decline in function of the kidney. The most common causes of CKD are diabetes, hypertension, and diseases of the glomerulus. **Metabolic syndrome**, in which the patient has both diabetes and hypertension, is a major factor in CKD development.

Over time, these causative factors slowly destroy vital cells in the renal tissue. Renal function first becomes insufficient and then fails altogether, which is called **end-stage renal disease** (**ESRD**).

As the kidney fails, waste products build up in the body. Creatinine and urea are markers for kidney decline, though they are not the only waste products that cause the symptoms of **uremia**, or "urine in the blood." Sodium, water, potassium, and other fluid and electrolyte imbalances will occur as a result of CKD.

The kidney is responsible for releasing **erythropoietin**, a hormone that stimulates the production of red blood cells. When kidneys fail, as is the case in CKD, erythropoietin release is decreased as well, resulting in decreased erythropoiesis, or RBC production. Thus, anemia results. Patients with CKD often must be treated for anemia along with many other conditions.

A patient with CKD will present with weight loss, anorexia, nausea, vomiting, and stomatitis. They may have a yellow-brown tint to their skin, as well as itchiness and crystallization of their sweat called **uremic frost.**

Treating a patient with CKD is a complicated matter, as so many other systems are involved as a result of the kidneys failing. Management of diabetes and hypertension is crucial, as these are often the underlying causes. Heart failure and anemia must be addressed. Dialysis will likely be an option in the future of the CKD patient to replace the function of the kidney.

Infections

Urinary Tract Infection (UTI)

Urinary tract infections or **UTI**s can be divided into two categories: lower and upper. Upper UTIs affect the kidneys and can be called pyelonephritis. Lower UTIs affect the bladder, urethra, or prostate and can be called cystitis, urethritis, or prostatitis. Differentiating between the specific types of UTIs in clinical practice can be difficult to do and thus the broad term of UTI usually refers to an infection of the kidneys or bladder.

There are many causative organisms involved in UTIs, but the most commonly seen UTIs are caused by a bacterial infection. Fungal infections, usually arising from the candida species, are also a possibility, as well as parasites and viruses.

An infection that affects the urethra specifically, called **urethritis**, is likely a result of a sexually transmitted disease (STD).

A urinary tract infection that was caught as a result of a urinary catheter insertion is called a **catheter-associated urinary tract infection (CAUTI)**. These are of special interest to the critical care nurse as so many patients have catheters inserted while in critical care. The critical care nurse must take special care to use proper aseptic technique when inserting a catheter, remove catheters as soon as they are no longer needed, and follow facility procedure when deciding if a patient actually needs a catheter in the first place. Many patients have catheters that may not need them, setting them up for a hospital-acquired infection.

Patients who have contracted a UTI may be asymptomatic for some time before the UTI is detected. When they are symptomatic, they may present with a fever, altered mental status, hypotension, dysuria, and lower abdominal pain.

Urine will be cultured and, in the case of patients with indwelling catheters, the catheter tip will be cultured as well to obtain diagnosis of UTI. Antibiotic therapy is common in the treatment of UTI, depending on the cause.

Urosepsis

Urosepsis is characterized by an infection in the urinary tract such as pyelonephritis, cystitis, post-renal obstruction, bladder infection, or kidney infection, which can lead to sepsis or systemic inflammatory response syndrome (SIRS). Sepsis can result in organ failure and even death when not diagnosed and managed properly. *Escherichia coli* is the most common bacterium that leads to sepsis from urinary tract infections. Bacteria, typically from fecal matter, ascends from the urethra to the bladder and potentially to the kidneys, causing pyelonephritis. Symptoms depend on the specific cause of the urinary tract infection but typically involve fever, chills, hematuria, and dysuria, as well as suprapubic or flank pain. Pyelonephritis also presents with possible nausea, vomiting, and costovertebral angle tenderness (CVAT). Diagnosis of urosepsis typically follows SIRS criteria, including tachycardia, elevated body temperature, changes in white blood cell counts, and respiratory rate, along with the suspicion of urinary tract infection. Organ dysfunction, such as low urine output from kidney dysfunction, is also an indication of sepsis. Laboratory studies including CBC, CMP, blood cultures, urinalysis, urine culture, and lactate levels should be obtained. Ultrasound or CT imaging is also frequently used to confirm diagnosis of prostate abscess or other causes of urinary tract infection. Treatment involves the initiation of antibiotics within one hour of diagnosis following the collection of blood and urine cultures. Crystalloid fluid resuscitation is also typically used, along with a vasopressor such as norepinephrine to maintain a MAP of 65 mmHg or greater.

Integumentary

The largest organ of the body is the skin, protecting the internal environment of the body from the external environment. To prevent infections and promote healing, the critical care nurse needs to be knowledgeable about the conditions that compromise the skin's integrity.

Cellulitis

Cellulitis is a bacterial skin infection that can become life-threatening without early treatment intervention. It is most commonly seen on the lower body. Group A streptococcus bacteria is one of the most common causes of cellulitis, but any bacteria that is able to enter the body and reach the deeper layers of skin tissue can cause cellulitis. The bacteria enter the body through any opening in the skin, such as a cut, wound, surgical incision, or insect bite. Symptoms include skin that appears red and inflamed, is hot to the touch, and painful.

Some people may experience blisters, skin dimpling, chill, and fever. Cellulitis is typically not spread between people, but it can spread quickly through a single individual's body. When the bacteria reach the patient's lymph nodes or blood stream, critical care is needed. Treatment includes intravenous antibiotics. Risk factors for cellulitis include poor hygiene, a surgical procedure, a history of edema, chronic injuries, chronic skin conditions, and a weakened immune system.

IV Infiltration

Most patients in the critical care unit will require an IV infusion of some kind. A complication of peripheral IV therapy that the nurse must be watchful for is IV infiltration. An **infiltration** of an IV means that the IV catheter has become dislodged or misplaced within the tissue and IV fluid or medications are leaking into the surrounding tissue as a result. This also can be caused by a sudden movement or jerking motion by the patient.

Patients with an altered mental status are prone to IV infiltration due to their, at times, compulsive, uncontrolled movements. This behavior can lead to dislodgment of the IV catheter and result in IV infiltration.

When an IV has infiltrated, the tissue surrounding the site may become puffy, tight, cool, and swollen. The patient, if alert, may complain of discomfort and burning. The IV pump infusing the fluids or medications may begin to beep due to line occlusion; when normal interventions in these cases are ineffective, infiltration should always be suspected.

Some fluids and medications can be toxic to the tissues and must be carefully monitored for infiltrations. An example of this is toxic chemotherapy drugs, which are often infused through a centralized port for just this reason.

Prevention of IV infiltration includes proper IV placement technique, educating the patient on signs of infiltration, and frequent monitoring and assessment of the IV sites. Most IVs and dressings must be changed frequently to prevent infiltration, and the critical care nurse must follow related facility policies.

Necrotizing Fasciitis

Necrotizing fasciitis is a rare bacterial skin infection in which serious complications are likely to occur. Also known as "flesh-eating bacteria," it occurs when bacteria enter connective tissues of the skin and rapidly spread, destroying muscle, skin cells, and fat tissue in the process. Bacteria enter the skin tissue through a cut or other open wound, and most symptoms begin within twenty-four hours. Symptoms include flu-like feelings, inflammation, fever, nausea, dehydration, and severe pain around a cut. Symptoms rapidly progress to large, fluid-filled rashes and gangrene. Within days, a patient may experience toxic shock. Even early in its clinical presentation, necrotizing fasciitis is considered a medical emergency. Necrotizing fasciitis is most commonly caused by Group A streptococcus bacteria but can also be caused by staphylococcus (of which several strains are antibiotic resistant) and other less common bacteria. Treatment includes intravenous antibiotics, blood pressure support, blood transfusions, and amputation of the affected area.

Pressure Injury

Most critical care nurses that have had to deal with immobile, bedridden patients who are very ill are familiar with pressure injuries. Because of immobility, pressure against vulnerable parts of the body results in tissue necrosis and ulceration. Bony prominences are especially susceptible to ulceration.

Risk factors for developing **pressure ulcers** include increased age, immobility, undernutrition, and urinary and/or fecal incontinence. Factors that contribute to pressure ulcers include shear, friction, pressure, and moisture. Increased exposure in compromised patients results in ulceration.

Ulcers can be staged into several categories, including stages I, II, III, and IV, unstageable, and suspected deep tissue injury (DTI). Each category looks at depth of wound and tissues affected. Wounds do not necessarily progress from one stage to the next; they can sometimes develop very quickly, skipping stages.

Prevention is obviously the best intervention when addressing pressure ulcers. The critical care nurse can help prevent pressure ulcers by turning the patient every two hours, reducing pressure where possible with pillows and supports, encouraging early mobilization and proper nutrition, and meticulously caring for wounds that do develop to prevent infection and loss of tissue.

Skin Failure (Perfusion Injuries)

Acute skin failure related to perfusion injury is characterized by the acute necrosis of tissue due to reduced blood flow to the skin and hemodynamic instability. Severe illness involving multi-organ failure often leads to acute skin failure due to the hemodynamic alterations and increased intolerance in the tissue. Cardiogenic shock is a leading cause of acute skin failure due to the rerouting of blood supply from the skin to the organs to maintain function. Signs and symptoms of acute skin failure include decreased oxygen saturation readings from fingertip monitors, skin mottling, and large ulcers (typically purple in color), which can occur all over the body. These ulcers are known to have a horseshoe or pear shape and occur due to hypoperfusion. This differentiates them from pressure injuries, which occur from skin shearing or prolonged pressure on a specific area rather than lack of blood flow. Assessment and prompt intervention are vital to ensuring positive outcomes for this condition. Medical staff must be able to differentiate acute skin failure from pressure injuries to ensure that the condition does not progress. Acute skin failure has a high mortality rate of 42 percent, often related to the severity of the illness that causes the condition. Treatment involves increasing tissue perfusion and treating the underlying cause of hemodynamic instability and hypoperfusion.

Wounds

Knowing how to care for each wound type is crucial to restoring the patient back to their normal functioning ability. There are three distinct types of wounds that a critical care nurse may encounter in their practice: infectious, surgical, and traumatic:

Infectious

A wound that has become infected is called an **infectious wound**. This means that bacteria and other microorganisms have invaded and colonized. This infection can delay healing and spread to other tissues of the body or even to the body's internal system. Any wound that a patient develops, whether a pressure ulcer, trauma wound, or surgical wound, may become infected; thus, the critical care nurse must be aware of signs and symptoms.

An infectious wound may become reddened or painful, swell as a result of inflammation, discharge a pus-like fluid that is green or yellow, be malodorous, and not heal as a result of the infection.

Staphylococcus aureus is a common bacterial invader of wounds, as it is often found on normal skin. The wound is its entryway to becoming a full-blown infection.

Those at risk for developing infectious wounds are the elderly, diabetics, and those who are immunocompromised, such as patients with the HIV infection.

Surgical

A **surgical wound** is a natural byproduct of any surgery. Whether a small or large incision, the surgeon has to open the body cavity in some way, shape, or form to access the internal tissue or organ he/she needs to operate on. Surgical wounds will usually be dressed by the operating room (OR) team, but the critical care nurse will be in charge of monitoring the wound and changing the dressing while the patient is in the critical care unit. A surgical wound will often have **sutures**, or tiny stitches that are sewn onto the patient's skin, in place. Sometimes these sutures will dissolve and be absorbed by the patient, and sometimes they will need to be removed after a certain amount of time, depending on the procedure, the surgeon, and the facility policy on the subject.

Signs of an infected surgical wound include redness, swelling, discharge of pus, odor, pain, and lack of healing.

Trauma

A **trauma wound** differs from a surgical wound in that its openings will usually be irregular and large. Bleeding is a major factor in traumatic wounds due to their depth and size. Bleeding must be stopped, and the wound must be closed before any dressing may be placed and healing can begin. Typically, this will be handled in the emergency department or the surgical suite, but the critical care nurse receiving the patient in the critical care unit will be responsible for further monitoring of the wound, dressing changes, and assessing for healing.

Most dressing changes are recommended daily, usually to be administered with an antibiotic cream. Dressing changes may be more or less frequent depending on the wound and the surgeon's orders.

Practice Quiz

1. The nurse is preparing a discharge plan for a patient with risk factors for acute pancreatitis. Which of the following information should be included in this plan?
    a. Endoscopic retrograde cholangiopancreatography (ERCP) imaging is required to confirm the diagnosis.
    b. Ultrasonography is the most useful imaging study when significant abdominal distention is present.
    c. Current research confirms the efficacy of rectal administration of indomethacin to reduce the incidence of pancreatitis due to the ERCP procedure.
    d. There is no scientific rationale to explain why some individuals with chronic ETOH abuse develop acute pancreatitis, while others do not develop pancreatitis.

2. Which treatment intervention should be implemented in the plan of care for a patient with acute renal failure?
    a. Sulfonylureas
    b. Intravenous contrast studies
    c. Bed rest
    d. High-protein diet

3. The nurse is developing a teaching plan for a patient with newly diagnosed type 2 diabetes. Which of the following symptoms of hyperglycemia would the nurse include?
    a. Tremors, fatigue, dizziness
    b. Excessive urination, excessive thirst, confusion
    c. Anxiety, blurred vision, headache
    d. Slurred speech, sweating, fainting

4. An 18-year-old female comes in with a gunshot wound to the abdomen. Which of the following takes highest priority when caring for this patient?
    a. Fluid resuscitation
    b. Stopping the bleeding
    c. Monitoring for infection
    d. Assessing internal damage

5. Which of the following anemia categories, in which heme and globin do not synthesize appropriately, does thalassemia fall into?
    a. Thrombocytic
    b. Macrocytic
    c. Normocytic
    d. Microcytic

See answers on the next page.

Answer Explanations

1. D: Chronic alcohol abuse and biliary tract dysfunction are the most frequent causes of acute pancreatitis; however, there are no identified criteria that explain why some individuals will experience pancreatitis while others do not. Acute pancreatitis is most often diagnosed by the presenting history and physical examination. ECRP is only indicated in patients with acute pancreatitis and concomitant biliary disease; therefore, Choice *A* is incorrect. Ultrasonography is generally less useful than CT imaging for pancreatitis, and its efficacy is significantly decreased in the presence of abdominal distention, which distorts the images; therefore, Choice *B* is incorrect. Although rectal indomethacin is used commonly to treat acute pancreatitis resulting from ERCP imaging, controversy remains regarding the efficacy of the therapy; therefore, Choice *C* is incorrect.

2. C: Choice *C* is a key intervention for patients with acute renal failure due to the importance of monitoring the progression of the condition. Choices *A*, *B*, and *D* all should be avoided in this patient's treatment plan.

3. B: Hyperglycemia occurs when the patient's blood sugar level is greater than 200 milligrams per deciliter. Common symptoms of hyperglycemia include polyuria (excessive urination), polydipsia (excessive thirst), nausea, abdominal pain, fruity-scented breath, and confusion. Choices *A*, *C*, and *D* describe symptoms of hypoglycemia.

4. B: The highest priority in this patient is stopping the flow of blood out of her body. Nothing else can be addressed until this is performed. Fluid resuscitation is highly important, but useless if the bleeding continues. Monitoring for infection will happen later. Assessing for organ damage is ongoing but ultimately secondary to stopping active bleeding.

5. D: Thalassemia is considered a microcytic anemia, in which heme and globin do not synthesize appropriately and oxygen-carrying capacity is compromised. Normocytic anemias are those that include normally-sized red blood cells that are deficient in number. Aplastic anemia is an example of a normocytic anemia. Macrocytic anemias are defined as red blood cells that are quite large in shape, leading to abnormalities in oxygen-carrying ability and oxygen delivery. Thrombocytic refers to a platelet, a different component of the blood, and is thus irrelevant in this scenario.

Musculoskeletal/Neurological/Psychosocial

Musculoskeletal

Compartment Syndrome

Compartment syndrome affects muscles and connective tissues. In this context, compartment refers to a grouping of individual muscle cells muscle cells, muscle fibers, and groups of muscle fibers, encased in a sheath-like structure of connective tissue known as fascia. Compartment syndrome occurs when a section of muscle is exposed to excessive fluid buildup, leading to increased pressure within the compartment. This causes the fibers to expand to a level beyond what the fascia can accommodate, resulting in the inability for adequate blood circulation to take place.

As fluid and waste byproducts accumulate, the patient will experience excruciating pain and swelling. Compartment syndrome can take place in any part of the body. When it is not treated in the hand, forearm, and arm, it can progress to a condition referred to as **Volkmann Contracture** in which the muscle remains permanently contracted and causes permanent joint damage. This will often lead to a visible deformity of the arm. Volkmann Contracture can render the hand, arm, or forearm permanently useless in both moderate and severe cases.

Compartment syndrome can come on suddenly, such as in a traumatic event resulting in the shattering of bone. This is referred to as acute compartment syndrome. It is considered an emergency situation requiring immediate surgery to relieve the compartment and allow circulation to resume. Without this procedure, permanent nerve damage will occur within hours. Acute compartment syndrome is common after fractures, crushing injuries, the placement of a tight cast, and from abusing certain drugs that cause tissue swelling.

Chronic compartment syndrome normally results from heavy exertion that places a demand on muscle tissues that are unable to be healthfully managed. Individuals who participate in sports that require constant repetitive motions, such as swimming and running, are at a higher risk of developing chronic compartment syndrome. Failing to adequately rest between heavy workouts can also contribute to developing this condition. Chronic compartment syndrome is characterized by painful cramping, immobility and numbness in the affected compartment, and visible swelling or concentrated bulging in the area. Stopping activity immediately normally causes symptoms to subside within 30 minutes. However, if symptoms consistently present with particular activities, the individual may require surgery in that area to help the body deal with this load. Untreated, the individual is likely to ultimately experience a sports-related injury to the compartment. Chronic compartment syndrome is not well understood; it can affect people with excellent health and fitness, and most commonly affects younger people under the age of forty.

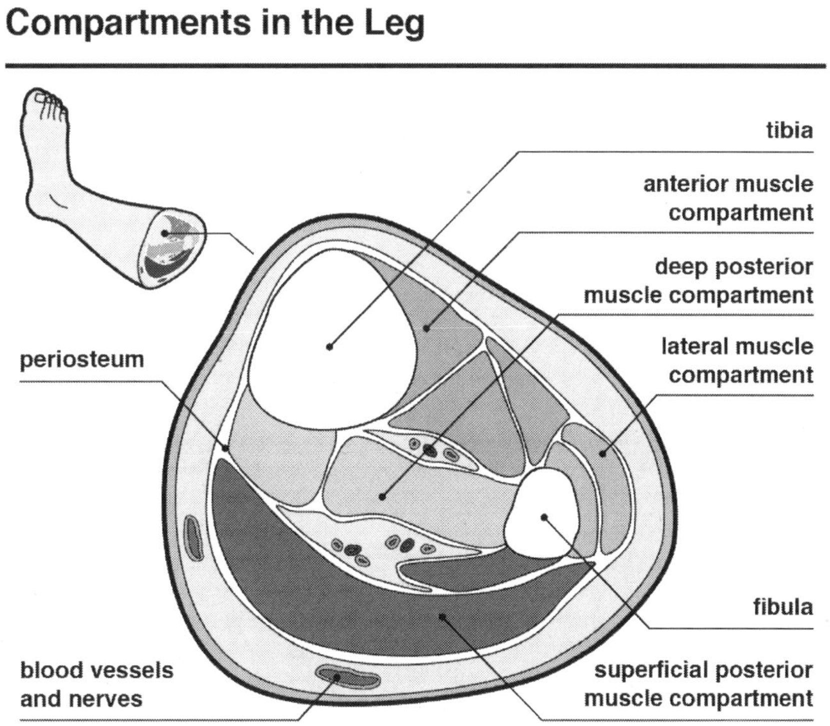

Fractures

Fractures refer to a break in any of the bones in the human body. Symptoms of a bone fracture include pain, swelling, partial or total loss of mobility at the site, and visible deformity in the region. There are a number of different kinds of fractures that can occur. Closed fractures occur without any breakage in the skin. Open fractures occur when the broken portion of the bone pierces through the skin. Pathologic fractures occur when normally-tolerable levels of force are able to break a bone; this normally occurs in the case of bone diseases that cause the structure to weaken, such as osteoporosis or bone cancer cases.

Stress fractures occur from occurrences of force placed over the same area of bone repetitively, and are commonly seen in athletes. In general, fractures take place when a single forceful blow occurs. This blow can be direct, occurring directly at the place of fracture, or indirect, where the force occurs elsewhere but travels to another bone. Finally, the shape of the fracture can be categorized in different ways. Simple fractures refer to a single break line in the bone. Avulsion refers to a chunk of bone breaking away from the main structure. Comminuted refers to a bone with multiple simple breaks in it.

Dislocations refer to separations of bone at a joint and always occur as a result of spontaneous force applied to the joint. The sudden and forceful nature in which dislocations occur usually means that the entire area will require medical attention. For example, a dislocated shoulder would not only affect bones of the shoulder joint, but also may affect adjacent bones, connective tissues, and nerves. A dislocated joint is likely to remain fragile even after it has been treated and reset.

Spinal fractures and dislocations are especially serious due to the housing of the nervous system. While pediatric patients often experience bone fractures and joint dislocation, it usually takes a serious blow to cause these conditions. In elderly patients, a fall or bump can cause serious musculoskeletal injury from which recovery can take months. The incidence of hip fractures doubles every five years after the age of 60 in both sexes.

Types of Fractures

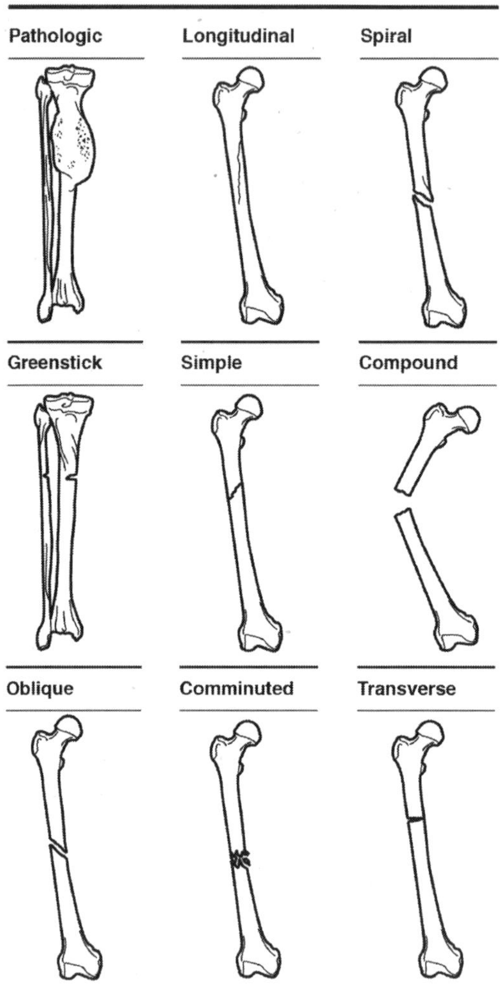

Muscular Deconditioning

Patients who experience prolonged sedentary or immobile periods are at risk of developing **muscular deconditioning**. The potential impacts of deconditioning span a range of body systems, including weakening of the patient's cardiovascular, musculoskeletal, and respiratory function. Clinical studies have shown that the bedbound patient suffers a 20% decrease in muscle strength per week and a 50% decrease in muscle strength after a month in bed. There is also a 3% loss of muscle mass within the thigh muscles within 7 days. While bedbound, the muscle fibers and connective tissues are maintained in a shortened position, and contractures begin within 3 weeks.

Musculoskeletal Trauma

Amputation

Amputation refers to the removal of a body part due to infection, trauma, or illness. It is often needed in cases where the region in question is no longer living and cannot be rescued, is ravaged by cancerous cells, or is susceptible to a life-threatening infection. The most common cause of amputation in the United States is due to poor circulation, which results in cell death and gangrene. If these areas are not removed, wide-spread infection in the blood (sepsis) can occur. However, removing cancerous bones, extra limbs or fingers, or deformed limbs and fingers also comprises a large number of amputations.

Amputation can also be spontaneous (such as the result of a traumatic accident where a limb is severed, construction injuries where fingers are cut or falling injuries where a limb is crushed). Spontaneous amputations are at high risk for infection and hemorrhage. These incidents are most likely to be emergency situations, and emergency surgeons use the Mangled Extremity Severity scale to determine whether amputation is needed. This scale produces a score based on factors such as the patient's age, tissue necrosis, shock, and what caused the injury.

Surgical amputations are performed by sectioning off blood vessels that will be affected, and sawing through muscle and bone. The remaining edge of bone is smoothed, and the surrounding muscle and bone are neatly sutured around it. After this, the patient may choose to wear a prosthetic limb or utilize a tool such as a cane or crutch to support their movements. Regardless, most patients suffer severe emotional and psychological distress as they adjust post-surgery. Adjusting to changed or limited mobility and a new appearance can reduce quality of life for many patients. A large majority experience sensory discomfort, such as itching, burning, or an unpleasant sensation of the limb still existing (phantom limb syndrome). This may reduce over time if the brain is able to adjust its neural signaling for the missing limb, or if the patient becomes comfortable with a prosthesis.

Most common amputations involve the legs, feet, arms, and hands; however, reproductive organs may also be amputated in late-stage cancer cases. In some countries outside of the United States, amputations can be performed as acts of war, punishment, or cultural mutilation. These types of amputations can extend to the face and reproductive organs.

Dislocations

Dislocations refer to separations of bone at a joint and always occur as a result of spontaneous force applied to the joint. The sudden and forceful nature in which dislocations occur usually means that the entire area will require medical attention. For example, a dislocated shoulder would not only affect bones of the shoulder joint, but also may affect adjacent bones, connective tissues, and nerves. A dislocated joint is likely to remain fragile even after it has been treated and reset.

Ligament Tendon Injuries

Ligaments are soft tissues that stabilize a joint by connecting bone to bone, while tendons are soft tissues that connect muscle to bone. Ligaments can be sprained, meaning that they are stretched past their natural point of extension (e.g., from blunt force or some other trauma). They can tear if they are overstretched. Strains are similar injuries that take place in tendons or muscles. Sprains and strains most commonly occur as a result of falls or sports injuries, especially in close contact and high impact sports such as wrestling or football. Most ligament or tendon injuries are characterized by pain, swelling, inflammation, and bruising.

Ligament injuries are classified as Grade I (a mild overstretch with minimal instability at the site), Grade II (a moderate overstretch or incomplete tear that results in some joint instability), or Grade III (a complete tear resulting in significant instability). Ligament injuries are graded based on damage to connective tissue around a joint. Tendon injuries are also categorized as Grade I, II, or III, but the tendon injury scale refers to the level of muscle fiber damage. Initial tendon injuries may not cause major symptoms at first, resulting instead in mild inflammation and microtears that do not limit range of motion. Over time and without proper rest, mild cases tend to worsen and result in more significant symptoms such as extreme pain, stiffness, and immobility.

Ligament and tendon injuries that occur without an open wound are called closed injuries. Open tendon or ligament injuries refer to instances where an open wound (e.g., laceration) results in extensive soft tissue damage. This most commonly occurs along the back of the hand and tops of the fingers. These injuries may not look extensive at first sight, but open wounds along the back of hand almost always require significant tendon repair due to their superficial location, along with extensive follow-up with specialized hand therapy. Fat embolisms occur in a large percent of musculoskeletal trauma cases. Trauma to long bones can cause fat globules to pass into the vascular system and can result in respiratory distress and other systemic inflammatory complications.

Neurological

Acute Spinal Cord Injury

Injuries to the spinal cord are associated with severe and often irreversible neurological deficits and disabilities. **Spinal cord injuries** (SCIs) may be due to one or a combination of the following types of injury: direct traumatic injuries of the spinal cord, compression of the spinal cord by bone fragments or hematoma formation, or ischemia resulting from damage to the spinal arteries. The anatomical location of the SCI predicts the degree of sensory and motor function that will be lost. In addition, the injury will be labeled as **paraplegia** if the lesion is at the T1 to the T5 level, affecting only the lower extremities, or **tetraplegia** if the lesion is at the C1 to the C7 level, affecting both the upper and lower extremities in addition to respiratory function.

SCIs may be categorized as complete or incomplete depending on the degree of impairment. While complete SCIs are associated with complete loss of sensory-motor function, incomplete lesions are determined by the actual portion of the spinal cord that is affected. Central spinal cord syndrome is an incomplete SCI that involves upper extremity weakness or paralysis with little or no deficit noted in the lower extremities. Anterior spinal cord syndrome is also an incomplete SCI that is associated with loss of motor function, pain, and sensation below the injury; however, the sensations of light touch, proprioception, and vibration remain intact. In addition, Brown-Sequard syndrome is an incomplete lesion of one-half of the spinal cord, which results in paralysis on the side of the injury and loss of pain and temperature sensation on the opposite side of the injury.

Emergency providers understand that the injury to the spinal cord is an evolving process, which means that the level of the injury can rise one to two spinal levels within 48 to 72 hours after the initial insult. An incomplete injury may progress to a complete injury during this time due to the effects of altered blood flow and resulting edema and the presence of abnormal free radicals. Essential interventions aimed at minimizing or preventing this progression include establishing and maintaining normal oxygenation, arterial blood gas (ABG) values, and perfusion of the spinal cord.

Neurogenic Shock

SCIs are also associated with three shock syndromes, including hemorrhagic shock, spinal shock, and neurogenic shock. Hemorrhagic shock from an acute or occult source must be suspected in all SCIs below the T6 level that present with hypotension. Spinal shock refers to the loss of sensory-motor function that may be temporary or permanent depending on the specific injury. At the same time, the patient must be monitored for signs of **neurogenic shock**, which presents with a triad of symptoms that include hypotension, bradycardia, and peripheral vasodilation. This complication is due to alterations in autonomic nervous system function, which causes loss of vagal tone. Most often, it occurs with an injury above the T6 level, resulting in decreased vascular resistance and vasodilation. Neurogenic shock may also be associated with hypothermia due to vasodilation; rapid, shallow respirations; difficulty breathing; cold, clammy, pale skin; nausea; vomiting; and dizziness.

Emergency treatment of neurogenic shock includes IV fluids and inotropic medications to support the BP and IV atropine and/or pacemaker insertion, as needed, to treat the bradycardia. If a patient presents with neurological deficits 8 or more hours after sustaining an SCI, high-dose prednisone may be administered to reverse the manifestations of neurogenic shock.

Emergency management of SCIs is focused on preventing extension of the injury and long-term deficits with immobilization and interventions based on the Airway, Breathing, and Circulation protocol. Cervical SCIs result in an 80 to 95 percent decrease in vital capacity, and mechanical ventilation is often required for lesions at this level. Support of the circulation is addressed in the treatment of neurogenic shock. Other supportive treatment interventions are aimed at minimizing the effects of immobility. Emergency providers are aware that patients with complete SCIs have less than a 5 percent chance of recovery; however, more than 90 percent of all patients with SCIs eventually return home and regain some measure of independence.

Brain Death

When the functioning capacity of the brain is lost but the heart and the lungs continue artificially, this is called **brain death**. The cerebrum and brain stem no longer signal spontaneous respiration, and there are no brain stem reflexes. The concept of brain death developed because ventilators and drugs can continue cardiopulmonary and other body functions despite complete cessation of all cerebral activity. The concept that the brain determines a person's death has been accepted legally and culturally in most of the world. The following, which is the American Academy of Neurology's Guidelines for Brain Death Determination, is the pathway most hospitals use for their policy:

1. Establish proximate cause and irreversibility of coma and monitor the patient for an appropriate waiting period in order to exclude the possibility of recovery.

2. Initiate the hospital policy for notifying the patient's Surrogate Decision-maker.

3. Conduct and document the clinical assessment of brain stem reflexes.

4. Perform and document the apnea test. An **apnea test** of a minimum of 8 min shows no respiratory movements with a documented increase in $PaCO_2$ of > 20 mm Hg from pretest baseline. Apnea testing is done by disconnecting the ventilator from the endotracheal tube. Oxygen (6 L/min) can be supplied by diffusion from a cannula placed through the endotracheal tube. Despite the ventilatory stimulus of the passively rising $PaCO_2$, no spontaneous respirations are seen over an 8 to 12-min period.

5. Perform ancillary testing, if indicated. Sometimes EEG, brain vascular imaging, or both.

6. If the individual's religious or moral objection to the brain death standard is known, implement hospital policies for reasonable accommodation.

7. Certify brain death.

8. Discontinue cardio-respiratory support in accordance with hospital policies, including those for organ donation. Brain death is loss of function of the entire cerebrum and brain stem, resulting in coma, no spontaneous respiration, and loss of all brain stem reflexes. Spinal reflexes, including deep tendon, plantar flexion, and withdrawal reflexes, may remain. Recovery does not occur.

After brain death is confirmed, all supporting cardiac and respiratory treatments are ended. Terminal arrhythmias result, and spinal motor reflexes may occur during terminal apnea; they include arching of the back, neck turning, stiffening of the legs, and upper extremity flexion. Family members who wish to be present when the ventilator is shut off need to be warned of such reflex movements. A patient diagnosed as brain dead is removed from all cardiopulmonary support and palliation is given until the patient expires.

Encephalopathy

Encephalopathy is a general term that means brain disease, damage, or malfunction, with the major symptom being an altered mental state. Encephalopathy is often considered a complication of a primary problem. In most cases, the word encephalopathy is preceded by a term that describes the reason, cause, or special conditions of the patient that leads to brain malfunction. For example, anoxic encephalopathy means brain damage due to lack of oxygen, and hepatic encephalopathy means brain malfunction due to liver disease.

A broad spectrum of symptoms occur that can range from mild (some memory loss or subtle personality changes) to severe (dementia, seizures, coma, or death). In general, encephalopathy shows itself as an altered mental state sometimes accompanied by physical manifestations.

Chronic traumatic encephalopathy (CTE) describes a gradual degeneration in brain function due to repeated head injuries that causes both symptomatic and asymptomatic concussions. Once the initial symptoms of concussion have faded, months and years later, new symptoms occur. CTE symptoms start slowly and creep up on the patient. Initially, there may be concentration and memory problems with episodes of disorientation and confusion, dizziness, and headache. It is as if the concussion symptoms were starting to return even without a new head injury. This type of encephalopathy is usually irreversible. CTE is common in athletes such as boxers and football players who have received several blows to the head during their career. Symptom management and improving quality of life for the patient and the caregivers is the priority.

Although numerous causes of encephalopathy are known, the majority of cases arise from several major categories: infection (HIV, Neisseria meningitides, herpes, and hepatitis B and hepatitis C), liver damage (alcohol and toxins), brain anoxia, or brain cell destruction (including trauma), and kidney failure (uremic).

Metabolic Encephalopathy

Metabolic encephalopathy (ME) occurs when there is an alteration to the brain function as a result of conditions that alter electrolyte or vitamin balance in the body. Examples of these conditions include diabetes, liver disease, and renal failure. ME occurs acutely or sub-acutely and is usually reversable if the underlying condition is treated. However, if left untreated, ME can lead to secondary structural damage, resulting in permanent changes to neurologic function.

With ME, patients present with confusion, drowsiness, irritability, difficulty concentrating, fatigue, depression, anxiety, or loss of consciousness. Diagnostic tests include basic blood tests (e.g., CMP), arterial blood gas testing, urine testing, and spinal fluid testing to determine the root cause of symptoms. Radiological tests, such as CT or MRI, may rule out structural conditions, while an EEG is used to rule out subclinical seizures.

Interventions focus on treatment of the underlying cause. Electrolyte imbalances caused by renal impairment (e.g., hyponatremia, hypernatremia, hypercalcemia, hypocalcemia, hypomagnesemia, and hypophosphatemia) can be readily treated through the correction of electrolyte levels. Uncontrolled diabetes is a leading cause for hyperglycemia and can be addressed with appropriate use of insulin. Liver disease, as well as alcoholism, can lead to hypoglycemia-related encephalopathy, which can be treated through administration of glucose.

Haloperidol can be given to treat severe agitation. Medications that can worsen delirium caused by encephalopathy and should be avoided include diphenhydramine, lorazepam, zolpidem, metoclopramide, promethazine, prochlorperazine, famotidine, and fentanyl.

Nursing care involves keeping the environment as quiet as possible, such as by bundling care to allow for more periods of uninterrupted rest at night. Patients should also be encouraged to mobilize and spend time out of bed as appropriate. Nurses should perform neurological exams regularly to detect changes from baseline. Fall prevention is important, as confusion can result in unsafe ambulation. Education provided to caregivers should encourage safe practices and prevention of subsequent events once the patient is discharged. Many patients, especially alcoholics and newly diagnosed diabetics, can benefit from education on management of the condition at home and potential nutritional impacts. To provide support, nurses can arrange a nutrition consult and provide ongoing assistance during hospitalization.

Infectious Encephalopathy

Infectious encephalopathy is an inflammatory condition of the brain caused by a viral, bacterial, or protozoal infection. The damage may either be caused by the organism directly invading the central nervous system (neurotropism) or peripherally through a secondary inflammatory response of the brain (neuroinflammation). While the incidence is low (with approximately 20,000 new cases each year in the United States), immunocompromised patients are at higher risk of acquiring such infections. Often those with infectious encephalopathy have also had exposure to a mosquito or tick bite. Symptoms often begin similarly to the flu, presenting with fever, chills, headaches, body aches, and neck stiffness. As time progresses, however, patients will develop neurological symptoms, such as changes in balance, coordination, mood, cognition, sensitivity to light, and seizures. Although treatment of the underlying cause can prevent further damage, some of these symptoms may continue after treatment.

As with other types of encephalopathy, correct diagnosis is vital in resolving the condition. Blood and spinal fluid tests are used to determine the type of organism causing the infection. While the primary focus is on treating the underlying cause with antibiotics or antivirals, there is a significant role for nursing and supportive care services in rehabilitation.

Many patients will continue to have symptoms of fatigue, depression, memory loss, coordination, and balance issues after the infection has resolved. Therefore, a multidisciplinary approach is essential for managing the various effects. Physical and occupational therapy are utilized to assist patients in regaining strength and participation in activities of daily living. Speech therapy may be useful if the patient is experiencing difficulties with speaking, swallowing, and/or cognition (e.g., organizing thoughts, attention span, remembering, and planning). Caregiver education is essential to ensure they understand that the patient may need long-term assistance due to chronic impact of the disease.

Hepatic Encephalopathy

Hepatic encephalopathy (HE) occurs as a result of liver dysfunction, when neurotoxins are no longer being removed from the blood and thereby impact the function of the brain. Two forms are recognized: acute and chronic. Acute hepatic encephalopathy is seen in patients with acute onset hepatic failure, which is often caused by viral hepatitis, sepsis, or exposure to toxic substances, and is associated with pronounced cerebral edema. Chronic hepatic encephalopathy occurs in patients with chronic liver disease and those with a portosystemic shunt. While serious, HE may be reversable.

Patients often present with confusion, lethargy, personality changes, disorientation, altered levels of consciousness, and symptoms suggestive of liver failure (e.g., jaundice and pruritis). Disruptions in the sleep-wake cycle, where patients are awake during the night and asleep during the day, often occur in early stages. In advanced stages, coma can occur.

With impairment of liver function, ammonia accumulates in the bloodstream and disrupts normal neuronal function. Tests to confirm diagnosis should include blood tests (to identify abnormal liver function and ammonia levels); radiologic imaging (to rule out stroke, seizure, lesions, or masses); and ultrasound (to determine the presence of a portosystemic shunt).

Treatment of HE requires addressing the underlying cause and therapies to lower the ammonia levels in the blood. Other critical aspects include supporting nutrition, adequate hydration, management of electrolyte abnormalities, and ensuring a safe environment. Patients should meet caloric goals and avoid protein restriction. Additionally, they should consume small, frequent meals to prevent fasting, which can cause an increase in ammonia production. Sedative medications, such as benzodiazepines, can worsen encephalopathy and should be avoided. Lactulose is an ammonia-lowering therapy that is highly effective in 70 to 80 percent of patients with HE. It works by facilitating the conversion of NH_3 ammonia to NH_4^+ ammonia in the gut, therefore reducing the amount of NH_3 being diffused into the blood stream. Lactulose also has an osmotic effect in the colon and promotes the excretion of NH_3 in the stool; ideally, the goal is to have two to three soft stools daily.

Patients who have chronic liver disease have a risk of HE recurrence. Patients and caregivers should be educated on the early signs of HE and when to seek medical attention. They should be made aware of potential triggers and hepatotoxins to avoid as well as counseled on the importance of adherence to prescription medications.

Stroke

A **stroke** is defined as the death of brain tissue due to ischemic or hemorrhagic injury. Ischemic strokes are more common than hemorrhagic strokes; however, the differential diagnosis of these conditions requires careful attention to the patient's history and physical examination. In general, an acute onset of neurological symptoms and seizures is more common with hemorrhagic stroke, while ischemic stroke is more frequently associated with a history of some form of trauma. The National Institutes of Health (NIH) Stroke Scale represents an international effort to standardize the assessment and treatment protocols for stroke. The scale includes detailed criteria and the protocol for assessment of the neurological system. The stroke scale items are to be administered in the official order listed, and there are directions that denote how to score each item.

Ischemic Stroke

Ischemic strokes result from occlusion of the cerebral vasculature as a result of a thrombotic or embolic event. At the cellular level, the ischemia leads to hypoxia that rapidly depletes the ATP stores. As a result, the cellular membrane pressure gradient is lost, and there is an influx of sodium, calcium, and water into the cell, which leads to cytotoxic edema. This process creates scattered regions of ischemia in the affected area, containing cells that are dead within minutes of the precipitating event. This core of ischemic tissue is surrounded by an area with minimally-adequate perfusion that may remain viable for several hours after the event.

These necrotic areas are eventually liquefied and acted upon by macrophages, resulting in the loss of brain parenchyma. These affected sites, if sufficiently large, may be prone to hemorrhage, due to the formation of collateral vascular supply with or without the use of medications such as recombinant tissue plasminogen activator (rtPA). The ischemic process also compromises the blood-brain barrier, which leads to the movement of water and protein into the extracellular space within 4 to 6 hours after the onset of the stroke, resulting in vasogenic edema.

Nonmodifiable risk factors for ischemic stroke include age, gender, ethnicity, history of migraine headaches with aura, and a family history of stroke or transient ischemic attacks (TIAs). Modifiable risk factors include hypertension, diabetes, hypercholesterolemia, cardiac disease (e.g., atrial fibrillation, valvular disease, and heart failure), elevated homocysteine levels, obesity, illicit drug use, alcohol abuse, smoking, and sedentary lifestyle. The research related to the occurrence of stroke in women indicates the need to treat hypertension aggressively prior to and during pregnancy, as well as prior to the use of contraceptives, to prevent irreversible damage to the microvasculature. In addition, it is recommended that to reduce their risk of stroke, women with a history of migraine headaches preceded by an aura should ameliorate all modifiable risk factors, and all women over seventy-five years old should be routinely assessed for the onset of atrial fibrillation.

Heredity is associated with identified gene mutations and the process of atherosclerosis and cholesterol metabolism. Hypercholesterolemia and the progression of atherosclerosis in genetically-susceptible individuals are now regarded as active inflammatory processes that contribute to endothelial damage of the cerebral vasculature, thereby increasing the risk for strokes. There are also early indications that infection also contributes to the development and advancement of atherosclerosis.

The presenting manifestations of ischemic stroke must be differentiated from other common diseases, including brain tumor formation, hyponatremia, hypoglycemia, seizure disorders, and systemic infection. The sudden onset of hemisensory losses, visual alterations, hemiparesis, ataxia, nystagmus, and aphasia are commonly, although not exclusively, associated with ischemic strokes. The availability of reperfusion therapies dictates the emergent use of diagnostic imaging studies, including CT and MRI scans, carotid duplex scans, and digital subtraction angiography to confirm the data obtained from the patient's history and physical examination. Laboratory studies include CBC, coagulation studies, chemistry panels, cardiac biomarkers, toxicology assays, and pregnancy testing as appropriate.

The emergency care of the patient who presents with an ischemic stroke is focused on the stabilization of the patient's ABCs, completion of the physical examination and appropriate diagnostic studies, and initiation of reperfusion therapy as appropriate, within 60 minutes of arrival in the emergency department. Reperfusion therapies include the use of alteplase (the only fibrinolytic agent that is approved for the treatment of ischemic stroke), antiplatelet agents, and mechanical thrombectomy.

Emergency providers must also be alert for hyperthermia, hypoxia, hypertension or hypotension, and signs of cardiac ischemia or cardiac arrhythmias.

Hemorrhagic Stroke

Hemorrhagic strokes are less common than ischemic strokes; however, a hemorrhagic stroke is more likely to be fatal than an ischemic stroke. A hemorrhagic stroke is the result of bleeding into the parenchymal tissue of the brain due to leakage of blood from damaged intracerebral arteries. These hemorrhagic events occur more often in specific areas of the brain, including the thalamus, cerebellum, and brain stem. The tissue surrounding the hemorrhagic area is also subject to injury due to the mass effect of the accumulated blood volume. In the event of subarachnoid hemorrhage, ICP becomes elevated with resulting dysfunction of the autoregulation response, which leads to abnormal vasoconstriction, platelet aggregation, and decreased perfusion and blood flow, resulting in cerebral ischemia.

Risk factors for hemorrhagic stroke include older age; a history of hypertension, which is present in 60 percent of patients; personal history of stroke; alcohol abuse; and illicit drug use. Common conditions associated with hemorrhagic stroke include hypertension, cerebral amyloidosis, coagulopathies, vascular alterations including arteriovenous malformation, vasculitis, intracranial neoplasm, and a history of anticoagulant or antithrombotic therapy.

Although the presenting manifestations for hemorrhagic stroke differ in some respect from the those associated with ischemic stroke, none of these such manifestations is an absolute predictor of one or the other. In general, patients with hemorrhagic stroke present with a headache that may be severe, significant alterations in the level of consciousness and neurological function, hypertension, seizures, and nausea and vomiting. The specific neurological defects depend on the anatomical site of the hemorrhage and may include hemisensory loss, hemiparesis, aphasia, and visual alterations.

Diagnostic studies include CBC, chemistry panel, coagulation studies, and blood glucose. Non-contrast CT scan or MRI are the preferred imaging studies. CT or magnetic resonance angiography may also be used to obtain images of the cerebral vasculature. Close observation of the patient's vital signs, neurological vital signs, and ICP is necessary.

The emergency management of the patient with hemorrhagic stroke is focused on the ABC protocol, in addition to the control of bleeding, seizure activity, and increased ICP. There is no single medication used to treat hemorrhagic stroke; however, recent data suggests that aggressive emergency management of hypertension initiated early and aimed at reducing the systolic BP to less than 140 millimeters of mercury may be effective in reducing the growth of the hematoma at the site, which decreases the mass effect. Beta-blockers and ACE inhibitors are recommended to facilitate this reduction. Endotracheal intubation for ventilatory support may be necessary; however, hyperventilation is not recommended due to the resulting suppression of cerebral blood flow. While seizure activity will be treated with AEDs, there is controversy related to the prophylactic use of these medicines. Increased ICP requires osmotic diuretic therapy, elevation of the head of the bed to 30 degrees, sedation and analgesics as appropriate, and antacids. Steroid therapy is not effective and is not recommended.

Patients who present with manifestations of hemorrhagic stroke with a history of anticoagulation therapy present a special therapeutic challenge due to the extension of the hematoma formation. More than 50 percent of patients taking warfarin who suffer a hemorrhagic stroke will die within thirty days. This statistic is consistent in patients with international normalized ratio (INR) levels within the therapeutic range, with increased mortality noted in patients with INRs that exceed the therapeutic level. Emergency treatment includes fresh frozen plasma, IV vitamin K, prothrombin complex concentrates, and recombinant factor VIIa (rFVIIa). There are administration concerns with each of these therapies that must be addressed to prevent any delays in the reversal of the effects of the warfarin.

Transient Ischemic Attack

A **transient ischemic attack** (**TIA**) is defined as a short-term episode of altered neurological function that lasts for less than one hour; in some cases, it may be imperceptible to the patient. The deficit may be related to speech, movement, behavior, or memory and may be caused by an ischemic event in the brain, spinal cord, or retina. The patient's history and neurological assessment according to the NIH Stroke Scale establish the diagnosis. Additional diagnostic studies include CBC, glucose, sedimentation rate, electrolytes, lipid profile, toxicology screen, 12-lead ECG, and CSF analysis. Imaging studies include non-contrast MRI or CT, carotid Doppler exam, and angiography.

Emergency care of the patient with a TIA is focused on the assessment of any neurological deficits and the identification of comorbid conditions that may be related to the attack. Hospital admission is required in the event that an attack lasts greater than one hour, the patient has experienced more than a single attack in a one-week period, or the attack is related to a cardiac source (e.g., atrial fibrillation or myocardial infarction). The **ABCD2 stroke risk score** calculates the patient's risk for experiencing a true stroke within two days after the TIA based on five factors (see the table below). Interventions aimed at stroke prevention in relation to the risk stratification as calculated by the ABCD^2 score are specific to underlying comorbidities; however, treatment with ASA and clopidogrel is commonly prescribed.

ABCD^2 Stroke Risk Score		
	1 Point	2 Points
***A*ge**	≥ 60 years	
***B*lood Pressure**	SBP ≥ 140 mmHg DBP ≥ 90 mmHg	
***C*linical Features**	Speech impairment but no focal weakness	Focal weakness
***D*uration of Symptoms**	≤ 59 minutes	≥ 60 minutes
***D*iabetes**	Diagnosed	
Total Score (denotes risk for stroke (CVA) within 2 days after TIA)	0-3 points = 1% risk 4-5 points = 4.1% risk 6-7 points = 8.1% risk	

Increased Intracranial Pressure

Under normal circumstances, there is a dynamic equilibrium among the bony structure of the cranium, brain tissue, and extracellular fluid that comprise approximately 85 percent of the intracranial volume; the blood volume that comprises 10 percent of the volume; and the CSF that occupies the remaining 5 percent of the volume of the cranium. If any one of these volumes increases, there must be a compensatory decrease in one or more of the remaining volumes to maintain normal intracranial pressure (ICP) and optimal cerebral perfusion pressure (CPP). The CPP represents the pressure gradient for cerebral perfusion and is equal to the difference between the mean arterial pressure (MAP) and the ICP ($MAP - ICP = CPP$).

The process of autoregulation maintains optimal CPP by dilation and constriction of the cerebral arterioles; however, if the MAP falls below 65 millimeters of mercury or rises above 150 millimeters of mercury, autoregulation is ineffective, and cerebral blood flow is dependent on blood pressure (BP). Once this mechanism fails, any increase in volume potentially will cause an increase in the ICP. For instance, normal ICP may be maintained in the presence of a slow-growing tumor; however, a sudden small accumulation of blood will cause a sharp increase in the ICP. Eventually, all autoregulatory mechanisms will be exhausted in either circumstance, and the ICP will be increased. In an adult in the supine position, the normal ICP is 7 to 15 millimeters of mercury, while an ICP greater than 15 millimeters of mercury is considered abnormal, and pressures greater than 20 millimeters of mercury require intervention.

Conditions associated with **increased ICP** include space-occupying lesions such as tumors and hematomas; obstruction of CSF or hydrocephalus; increased production of CSF due to tumor formation; cerebral edema resulting from head injuries, strokes, infection, or surgery; hyponatremia; hepatic encephalopathy; and idiopathic intracranial hypertension. Early manifestations of increased ICP include blurred vision with gradual dilation of the pupil and slowed pupillary response, restlessness, and confusion with progressive disorientation as to time, then to place, and finally to person. Later signs include initially ipsilateral pupillary dilation and fixation, which progresses to bilateral dilation and fixation; decorticate or decerebrate posturing; and Cushing's triad of manifestations that include bradycardia, widening pulse pressure, and Cheyne-Stokes respirations.

ICP monitoring will be used to assess all patients requiring emergency care for any condition that is potentially associated with increased ICP. Depending on the underlying pathology, common interventions for increased ICP include sedation and paralysis, intubation and hyperventilation to decrease the $PaCO_2$, infusion of mannitol, an osmotic diuretic, and hypertonic saline IV solutions. Emergency providers understand that sustained elevations of ICP are associated with a poor prognosis, and therefore, the underlying cause and manifestations must be treated aggressively.

Hydrocephalus

Hydrocephalus is the abnormal buildup of cerebrospinal fluid in the ventricles of the brain, which leads to increased intracranial pressure and neurological impairments from damage to the brain tissue. The condition is characterized as either communicating, which means it's caused by impaired absorption of cerebrospinal fluid (e.g., impaired arachnoid villi or a blockage in the subarachnoid space), or noncommunicating, which means it's caused by physical obstruction or occlusion (e.g., tumor or congenital malformation). Hydrocephalus can be congenital or acquired through infections like meningitis or tumors. A third type, normal pressure hydrocephalus, is most often seen in elderly patients who present with gait problems, incontinence, and cognitive deficits.

Symptoms present differently at different ages. Infant patients will present with enlarged head circumference, irritability, and bulging fontanel. In children into elderly adulthood, symptoms include headaches, nausea and vomiting, blurred vision, gait problems, urinary incontinence, and cognitive deficits. Diagnosis is made via CT scan or MRI, while a lumbar puncture can rule out infections and determine the cerebrospinal fluid pressure. Medical management includes the placement of a ventriculoperitoneal shunt to divert cerebrospinal fluid from the ventricles into the peritoneal cavity. Diuretics may also be used to temporarily aid in reducing cerebrospinal fluid and intracranial pressure.

Neurologic Infectious Diseases

Encephalitis

Encephalitis, an inflammation of the parenchyma of the brain, should be suspected in patients with unexplained alterations in mental status. Acute disseminated encephalomyelitis is brain and spinal cord inflammation caused by a hypersensitivity reaction to a foreign protein. Both disorders are usually triggered by viruses and are classified as follows: Epidemic (arbovirus, echovirus, coxsackievirus); sporadic (cytomegalovirus, herpes simplex, varicella-zoster, rabies, or mumps virus); or mosquito-borne (West Nile, St. Louis, Eastern and Western equine, Zika).

Clinical presentation may be preceded by a gastrointestinal or respiratory illness and typically involves fever, headache, and changes in mental status, with the possibility of accompanying seizures and focal neurologic deficits. Meningeal signs are typically mild and less prominent than other manifestations. In severe cases, status epilepticus or coma may be present. In severe cases, status epilepticus or coma may be present.

Diagnosis requires CSF analysis and neuroimaging. Treatment is supportive and may include antiviral drugs. Additional diagnostic testing often includes MRI, analysis of CSF, and serologies with the goal of identifying the specific infectious cause. Some cases of encephalitis may be idiopathic with the cause unknown.

Meningitis

Meningitis is inflammation of the meninges and subarachnoid space that may result from infections, other medical disorders, or reactions to drugs. Meningitis may be classified as acute, subacute, chronic, or recurrent and by its cause; bacteria, viruses, fungi, and protozoa. The most clinically useful categories of meningitis will be used here: acute bacterial, viral, noninfectious, recurrent, subacute, and chronic.

Acute bacterial meningitis is serious and rapidly progressive. Aseptic meningitis is an older term used synonymously with viral meningitis; however, it usually refers to acute meningitis caused by anything other than meningococcus or streptococcus. Viral and noninfectious infections are usually self-limited. Subacute and chronic meningitis usually follows a slower course and makes diagnosis difficult. Symptoms vary in severity and acuity; however, all types of meningitis present with headache, fever, nuchal rigidity, and lethargy. **Nuchal rigidity** can be distinguished from neck stiffness because the neck can usually be rotated but cannot be flexed. Additional treatment priorities include seizure management (e.g., antiseizure medications), reduction of brain inflammation (e.g., corticosteroids), as well as intravenous fluid and/or nutritional support as needed. Various types of therapy may also be necessary to address any resulting mental, physical, or speech deficits.

Neurological Storming

Paroxysmal sympathetic hyperactivity (PSH), also known as **neurological storming**, is characterized by the dysfunction of the sympathetic nervous system commonly following traumatic brain injury (TBI), brain tumor, and stroke. Symptoms of PSH include tachycardia, tachypnea, diaphoresis, hypertension, hyperthermia, dystonia, and posturing. Males and young adults who have suffered from brain trauma carry a higher risk for PSH. Diagnosis of PSH can be difficult, as the signs and symptoms often mimic other conditions such as septicemia, epilepsy, or even pulmonary embolism. PSH episodes typically last between a few minutes to two hours long and may continue to occur for weeks or months after the initial TBI or stroke. There are no laboratory studies that can confirm the diagnosis of PSH; instead, conditions such as seizures, rhabdomyolysis, infection, and dehydration should be ruled out. The presence of focal lesions on CT scan within 48 hours of the traumatic event is an indication for increased risk of developing PSH. Treatment involves supporting symptoms such as dehydration with adequate fluid intake and taking measures to reduce the sympathetic nervous system activity. While there is no definitive treatment for PSH, there are pharmacologic treatments to manage symptoms. In some cases, sedation and muscle relaxation may be required; however, prolonged sedation and ICU stays are often linked to negative neurological outcomes.

Neuromuscular Disorders

Amyotrophic Lateral Sclerosis (ALS)

Amyotrophic lateral sclerosis (ALS) is a degenerative disease of the central nervous system, mainly affecting the body's motor nerve function. The most common initial symptoms involve the large muscle groups, resulting in difficulty walking, foot drop, and decreased muscle tone. In some cases, patients may also have difficulty talking and swallowing food. Other patients may develop symptoms similar to dementia, with changes in cognitive function and personality. As the disease progresses, the patient will increasingly lose muscle function, have clear atrophy to the limbs, more advanced changes to speech or loss of speech, and drooling. Eventually, the patient will likely require mechanical ventilation. ALS is incurable and fatal; only in rare cases do patients live beyond five years after diagnosis.

Diagnosis of ALS can be difficult, requiring months of data collection to confirm the cause of the patient's symptoms. MRI and CT may be done to rule out structural neurological changes, but these results will appear normal in the ALS patient. Various laboratory tests may also be done but will likely only rule out other conditions. Electromyography can be assistive in testing neuromuscular function.

Since ALS has no cure and is a terminal illness, treatment is mostly supportive and dependent upon the patient's symptoms and needs for quality-of-life improvement. The medication riluzole may be given to extend the patient's life and delay the need for mechanical ventilation. Muscle relaxers may be given to decrease contractions and pain from muscle spasms, while anticholinergics can decrease drooling. Physical therapy and range of motion exercises can help with muscle atrophy. As the disease progresses, the patient will likely require mobility aids, tube feeding, and mechanical ventilation.

Nursing management of the ALS patient prioritizes maintenance of their airway and ventilation. Even in the earlier stages of the disease process, the nurse should be mindful of aspiration risks, ensuring the patient is eating upright as well as chewing and swallowing effectively. The nurse may need to modify the patient's diet for aspiration risks by providing softened foods or thickened liquids. Eventually, the nurse may also need to maintain the patient's gastric tube. Additional care responsibilities include monitoring for signs of difficulty breathing in the earlier stages, followed by eventual management of a chronic mechanical ventilator. Upon discharge, patients and their families should be provided education on what to expect with disease progression and ways to improve the patient's quality of life throughout the disease process.

Neurosurgery

Neurosurgery, the practice of surgery on the neurological system and its structures, may be performed for numerous different diagnoses. Procedures can be performed via stereotactic techniques, conventional open surgery, and microsurgery. Microscopic surgeries can include laminectomy, microdiscectomy, and artificial disc replacement. There are hundreds of different types of neurosurgery procedures ranging from the minor to complicated. The critical care nurse might see patients recovering from the following surgeries.

- Anterior Cervical Discectomy and Fusion: Because it is not generally safe to access herniated discs in the neck from the back, treatment of these usually requires this anterior approach.
- Craniotomy: Surgical treatment of some brain diseases or tumor removal
- Epilepsy Surgery: When a patient does not respond adequately to medications, there are different types of procedures that are used to diagnose and treat epilepsy.
- Laminectomy: A procedure to access and decompress the spine
- Lumbar Puncture: The gold standard test for diagnosing meningitis, a lumbar puncture may be used in the diagnosis of a number of different diseases of the nervous system.
- Microdiscectomy: One of the most common procedures used to treat a disease of the nervous system, this procedure is the way that most herniated discs in the lumbar spine are treated.
- Pituitary Tumor Surgery: Most pituitary adenomas, benign tumors of the pituitary gland, are treated by surgery through a route called the transsphenoidal approach.
- Spinal Fusion: Fusion of the spine may be necessary in a number of spinal disease conditions, from degenerative disease to trauma.
- Ventriculoperitoneal Shunt: One of the classic treatments for hydrocephalus, a **shunt** is an internal implant that helps divert fluid from the brain.
- Ventriculostomy: A tube placed into the fluid spaces within the brain, is a common procedure that may be used in a number of different clinical situations

Neurological surgery management

The nurse plays an important role for patients undergoing neurological surgery. Pre-operatively, they ensure the patient is well-equipped to have a successful surgery. Post-operatively, the nurse monitors the patient's healing and recovery, along with encouraging collaboration of the interdisciplinary team to ensure resources are available to be successful upon discharge.

Pre-operatively, the nurse should perform a thorough history and assessment, including allergies, current medications, vital signs, and laboratory results. They will assist in educating the patient and caregivers on the surgery, expected outcomes, and recovery process. While not responsible for obtaining informed consent, the nurse should provide education to ensure patient and caregiver understanding of the process, risks, and post-operative care. The nurse should also ensure administration of pre-operative antibiotics and anxiety medications as indicated.

Post-operatively, the nurse is responsible for monitoring the patient for complications, encouraging healing and activities for recovery, and preparing them for discharge. Regular assessments to monitor vital signs, changes in neurological status, and surgical sites should be completed for early detection of any complications, which leads to lessened risk of morbidity and mortality. Such complications include increased intracranial pressure and infection, but other risks may be present depending on the type of surgery.

Nurses should follow physician orders for timely medication administration and necessary laboratory tests. Once appropriate, mobilization should be encouraged to reduce risk of pneumonia, maintain skin integrity, and rebuild strength and stamina. Nurses should collaborate with supportive services, such as physical therapy, occupational therapy, and speech therapy, to assist in the transition to discharge. Referrals to social work or patient navigation may be necessary for nursing care facilities, depending on the patient's function and outcomes.

Pharmacologic methods to reduce cerebral edema include osmotherapy, diuretics, and corticosteroids. An external ventricular drain is a temporary measure to aid in the reduction of intracranial pressure by redirecting the CSF fluid from the ventricles of the brain. Surgical interventions aim to remove the lesion and necrotic tissue in order to reduce the pressure on surrounding tissues and prevent further damage to healthy brain tissue.

Nursing interventions should be implemented based on the type of lesion and therapy used to treat it. For medical management, nurses should administer medications as ordered and assess the patient for changes in neurological status at frequent intervals. Frequent monitoring of vital signs should include watching for **Cushing's triad**, a signal of high intracranial pressure that is characterized by three clinical symptoms: bradycardia, irregular respirations, and widened pulse pressure (large gap between systolic and diastolic blood pressures). It is considered a medical emergency if identified.

The clinical environment should remain calm and quiet to reduce agitation and, thereby, intracranial pressure. The head of the bed should be maintained between 30 and 45 degrees. If an external ventricular drain is placed, the color, clarity, and volume should be documented along with an assessment of the insertion site to ensure it is working properly and not infected. For patients receiving surgical intervention, the nurse should be sure to assess the surgical sites for signs of infection. Pain should be adequately controlled with adherence to a pain regimen in order to promote patient comfort and lower intracranial pressure.

Neurovascular Abnormalities

Arteriovenous Malformation

Arteriovenous malformations (**AVM**s) are blood vessel misconnections in which arteries flow directly into veins, with the most common site of misconnection involving the cerebral arteries. An AVM can bleed or directly compress brain tissue, resulting in seizures or ischemia. Neuroimaging may detect them incidentally; contrast or non-contrast CT can usually detect AVMs over one centimeter, but the diagnosis is confirmed with MRI. Occasionally, a cranial bruit suggests an AVM. Conventional angiography is required for definitive diagnosis and determination of whether the lesion is operable. Superficial AVMs over three centimeters in diameter are usually removed with microsurgery, radiosurgery, and endovascular surgery. AVMs that are deep or less than three centimeters in diameter are treated with stereotactic radiosurgery, endovascular therapy or coagulation with focused proton beams.

Cerebral Aneurysm

Bulging or ballooning in a blood vessel within the brain is the second most common site for an aneurysm in the body. Another common site for aneurysms is where the internal carotid artery (ICA) enters the cranium; it branches into a system of arteries that provide blood flow to the brain, known as the **circle of Willis**. Most small brain aneurysms do not rupture and are found during various tests. An aneurysm may press on brain tissue and present with ocular pain or symptoms. However, a rupture is a medical emergency that can lead to stroke or hemorrhage. The most common symptom described by patients is "the *worst* headache of my life." A sudden, severe headache, stiff neck, blurred or double vision, photophobia, seizure, loss of consciousness, and confusion may also be reported.

Seizure Disorders

A **seizure** is an abnormal, unregulated electrical discharge that occurs within the brain's cortical gray matter and interrupts normal brain function. A seizure typically causes altered awareness, abnormal sensations, and convulsions. Diagnosis may be clinical and involves results of neuroimaging, laboratory testing, and EEG for new-onset seizures or anticonvulsant levels for previously diagnosed seizure disorders. Treatment includes elimination of the cause, if possible, anticonvulsants, and surgery.

Epilepsy (also called epileptic seizure disorder) is a chronic brain disorder characterized by recurrent ($\geq$ 2) seizures that are unprovoked and that occur > 24 h apart. A single seizure is not considered an epileptic seizure. Epilepsy is often idiopathic, but various brain disorders, such as malformations, strokes, and tumors, can cause symptomatic epilepsy. Symptomatic epilepsy is epilepsy due to a known cause (brain tumor, stroke). The seizures it causes are called symptomatic epileptic seizures and are most common among neonates and the elderly.

Nonepileptic seizures are provoked by a temporary disorder or stressor, such as metabolic disorders, CNS infections, cardiovascular disorders, drug toxicity or withdrawal, or psychogenic disorders. By age of onset, the common causes of seizures are: before age 2, fever, birth or developmental defects, birth injuries, and metabolic disorders; ages 2 to 14, idiopathic seizure disorders; adults, cerebral trauma, alcohol withdrawal, tumors, strokes, and an unknown cause in 50%; the elderly, tumors and strokes.

Seizures are classified as generalized or partial. **Generalized seizures** result from electrical discharges across both hemispheres of the brain and typically lead to loss of consciousness. Generalized seizures result most often from metabolic disorders and sometimes from genetic disorders. **Partial seizures** result from electrical discharges in one hemisphere of the brain and are typically attributed to deviations from normal brain structure. Partial (focal) seizures may evolve into a generalized seizure (called secondary generalization), which causes loss of consciousness. Secondary generalization occurs when a partial seizure spreads and activates the entire cerebrum bilaterally. Activation may occur so rapidly that the initial partial seizure is not clinically apparent or is very brief.

Auras are simple partial seizures that begin focally. Auras may consist of motor activity or sensory, autonomic, or psychic sensations. Most seizures end spontaneously in one to two minutes. A **postictal state** often follows generalized seizures; it is characterized by deep sleep, headache, confusion, and muscle soreness; this state lasts from minutes to hours. Sometimes the postictal state includes **Todd paralysis**, a transient neurologic deficit, usually weakness, of the limb contralateral to the seizure focus. Most patients appear neurologically normal between seizures, although high doses of the drugs used to treat seizure disorders, particularly anticonvulsants, can reduce alertness. Any progressive mental deterioration is usually related to the neurologic disorder that caused the seizures rather than to the seizures themselves.

Testing is done routinely, but normal results do not necessarily exclude a seizure disorder. Thus, the diagnosis may ultimately be clinical. Testing depends on results of the history and neurologic examination. If patients have a known seizure disorder and examination results are normal or unchanged, little testing is required except blood anticonvulsant levels. Additional testing is indicated if patients have symptoms or signs of a treatable disorder such as trauma, infection, or a metabolic disorder. If seizures are new-onset or if examination results are abnormal for the first time, neuroimaging is required. Patients with new-onset seizures or atypical manifestations also require laboratory testing, including blood tests (serum electrolytes, BUN, creatinine, glucose, Ca, Mg, and K levels), and liver function tests. Other tests may be done based on disorders that are suspected clinically.

Unreported use of recreational drugs can cause or contribute to seizures. Drug screens may be done, although this practice is controversial because positive results do not indicate causality, and test results can be inaccurate.

Follow-up MRI is recommended when CT is negative. It provides better resolution of brain tumors and abscesses and can detect cortical dysplasias, cerebral venous thrombosis, and herpes encephalitis. MRI can detect some common causes of seizures, such as malformations of cortical development in young children and mesial temporal sclerosis, traumatic gliosis, and small tumors in adults.

EEG is critical in the diagnosis of epileptic seizures, particularly of complex partial or absence status epilepticus, when EEG may be the most definitive indication of a seizure. EEG may detect epileptiform abnormalities (spikes, sharp waves, spike and slow-wave complexes, polyspike and slow-wave complexes). Epileptiform abnormalities may be bilateral, symmetric, and synchronous in patients with primarily generalized seizures and may be localized in patients with partial seizures.

With treatment, seizures are eliminated in one-third of patients with epileptic seizures, and frequency of seizures is reduced by > 50% in another third. About 60% of patients whose seizures are well-controlled by drugs can eventually stop the drugs and remain seizure-free. Epileptic seizures are considered resolved when patients have been seizure-free for 10 years and have not taken anticonvulsants for the last five years of that time period.

If the cause cannot be corrected or identified, anticonvulsants are often required, particularly after a second seizure; usefulness of anticonvulsants after a single seizure is controversial, and risks and benefits should be discussed with the patient. Because the risk of a subsequent seizure is low, drugs may be withheld until a second seizure occurs, particularly in children. In children, certain anticonvulsants cause important behavior and learning problems.

Most seizures remit spontaneously in several minutes or less and do not require emergency drug treatment. However, **status epilepticus** and most seizures lasting > 5 min require drugs to terminate the seizures, with monitoring of respiratory status. Endotracheal intubation is necessary if there is any indication of airway compromise. The sooner anticonvulsant therapy is started, the better and the more easily seizures are controlled. IV access should be quickly obtained, and patients are given lorazepam 0.05 to 0.1 mg/kg IV (typically a 4-mg IV dose for adults) at a rate of 2 mg/min. Larger doses are sometimes required. After lorazepam is given, a second, longer-acting anticonvulsant is indicated.

There is no consensus or evidence-based guideline indicating which longer-acting anticonvulsant is preferred. Many experts choose fosphenytoin 15 to 20 PE (phenytoin equivalents)/kg IV, given at a rate of 100 to 150 PE/min.

Anticonvulsants may be required indefinitely, but many types of seizures (most febrile seizures, seizures due to alcohol withdrawal, and seizures that do not recur) do not require treatment with anticonvulsants. No single drug controls all types of seizures, and some patients require multiple drugs. The drugs preferred vary according to type of seizure.

About 10 to 20% of patients have intractable seizures refractory to medical treatment and are potential surgical candidates. If seizures originate from a focal, resectable area in the brain, resection of the epileptic focus usually improves seizure control markedly. If the focus is in the anteromesial temporal lobe, resection eliminates seizures in about 60% of patients. After surgical resection, some patients remain seizure-free without taking anticonvulsants; however, many still require the drugs in reduced doses and possibly as monotherapy. Because surgery requires extensive testing and monitoring, these patients are best treated in specialized epilepsy centers.

Space-Occupying Lesions

Space occupying lesions (SOLs) of the central nervous system can pursue a serious clinical course even when they are inflammatory or benign. SOL are growths within the skull, which present with common symptoms and signs. The most common causes are metastatic brain tumors. The primary brain tumors are astrocytoma, glioblastoma, oligodendroglioma, and ependymoma, which all have less than a five-year survival rate. Meningioma is a benign tumor which is twice as common in women. Brain aneurisms, abscesses, and subdural hematomas are all benign.

The presenting symptoms of SOL are those of increased intracranial pressure: focal neurological signs, seizures, headache, nausea and vomiting, behavioral changes, paralysis, and visual disturbances. Loss of vision and combinations of symptoms can also occur, depending upon the brain region involved in the process. Localizing syndromes differentiate lesions in the occipital, temporal, frontal, and parietal regions. Other symptoms that may be present depending on the location of the lesion include:

- **Frontal lobe lesion**: may result in agitation; mood swings; changes in attention span, learning, or motor function; and loss of smell
- **Temporal lobe lesion**: may lead to trouble understanding words, hallucinations, and difficulty processing sounds
- **Parietal lobe lesion**: may present with the inability to write, do math, recognize own hands and fingers, and confusion of left and right
- **Occipital lobe lesion**: may result in loss of vision, color blindness, or difficulties recognizing visual objects
- **Cerebellum lesion**: may result in loss of coordination, dizziness, shaking/tremors, paralysis, and difficulty controlling eye movement
- **Brainstem lesion**: may cause changes in heart rhythm, blood pressure, and breathing

Radiology is the primary assessment method prior to a surgical diagnosis. Radiological techniques allow precise localization for a stereotactic biopsy. When there is a radiologic impression of an SOL, histological confirmation is required.

The treatment of the brain tumor is based on severity of the tumor. Mannitol is helpful in treating brain herniation and Dexamethasone may be prescribed to decrease the intracranial pressure. Depending on the location of the tumor and intensity of the disease, excision may be necessary. Radiation therapy and/or chemotherapy and stereotactic radiosurgery are also treatment options.

Abscess

An **abscess** is a localized collection of pus in the brain that results from an infection elsewhere in the body. Paranasal sinus infections and dental infections are the most common causes of brain abscess, while pulmonary infections and endocarditis are the most common causes from distant sites. Brain abscesses are uncommon, making up 8 percent of SOL cases. Patients who are immunocompromised, such as those with AIDS, are at higher risk of developing a brain abscess.

Approximately 66 percent of patients will present with symptoms occurring for two weeks or less. Because of the nonspecific nature of symptoms, diagnosis is often delayed. Frequent symptoms include intense localized headache not relieved by over-the-counter medications, changes in mental status, fever, seizures, nausea/vomiting, focalized neurologic deficits, and neck stiffness. A sudden worsening headache followed by meningismus (stiff neck, sensitivity to light, and nausea/vomiting) is typically associated with rupture of the abscess, which is a fatal complication.

Diagnostic workup involves laboratory work, including CBC, ESR, CRP, and blood cultures. Preferred imaging modality is an MRI; however, a CT scan is often used in an emergency due to availability. Once an abscess is identified, a biopsy through aspiration or surgical drainage is often performed to identify the organism causing the infection.

Because a brain abscess can lead to increased intracranial pressure and therefore an increased risk of damage and death, large abscesses (typically larger than 2 cm) are treated with aspiration or excision. Multiple abscesses are treated with a 4–8 week course of high-dose antibiotics, sometimes in addition to aspiration. The antibiotic regimen is determined based on results of the biopsy.

In addition to typical nursing management of patients with SOL, nurses should provide education to patients and their caregivers emphasizing the importance of adherence to the antibiotic administration schedule. They should also be given strict return precautions if there is new onset of fever, worsening of symptoms, or development of symptoms indicating rising intracranial pressure.

Spinal Surgeries

There are several spinal disorders that, in severe cases, may require surgical intervention. The following conditions are associated with a variety of treatment options, ranging from pharmacological to surgical based upon disease progression.

Herniated Disc Disease

Herniated disc disease, also called a slipped or ruptured disc, occurs when the nucleus pulposus (gel in the center of the disc) leaks through a weak area or tear in the annulus fibrosus (outer layer of the disc). This leads to the compression of neighboring nerves, causing numbness, weakness, and pain. Herniated discs are most commonly seen in the lumbar and cervical spine. Causative factors include degeneration of the discs through age, trauma, forceful injury, repetitive stress, or overuse. The patient's chief complaint is most often shooting pain that follows the distribution of the affected nerve (e.g., a patient with a lumbar herniated disc would experience sciatica). Other symptoms include numbness, weakness, a positive straight leg raise, and symptoms that worsen with sitting or bending and improve with laying down or walking.

Physical examination for diagnosis should include a thorough neurological exam, assessing for any motor weakness, sensory deficits, or abnormal reflexes (e.g., L5 radiculopathy with a weak foot dorsiflexion or decreased sensation to foot). The preferred imaging option for diagnosis is an MRI, as it is able to highlight the size, location, and severity of the herniation. Electromyography and nerve conduction studies may be helpful to assess the severity of nerve damage or for patients with persistent symptoms despite treatment.

For most patients, medical management will be conservative with rest and activity modification or reduction. NSAIDs can help to reduce pain and inflammation. Physical therapy may also be beneficial to strengthen the surrounding supportive muscles. Corticosteroids can be injected into the epidural space to reduce severe inflammation and/or pain. Muscle relaxers are beneficial to help reduce muscle spasms associated with herniated discs. Approximately ninety percent of patients see improvement within six to twelve weeks with conservative treatment measures. However, when these interventions are unsuccessful and symptoms persist, surgical intervention via a discectomy, laminectomy, or spinal fusion may be necessary.

Kyphosis

Kyphosis is an abnormal curvature of the thoracic spine, which in turn causes a significant forward curve of the spine usually greater than forty to forty-five degrees. It is most common in older adults due to degenerative changes like osteoporosis; however, the condition can occur at any age, especially if caused by trauma or certain conditions like spinal tumors. It can also be caused by Scheuermann's disease, congenital anomalies, spinal trauma, infections (e.g., tuberculosis or Pott's disease), and tumors. The characteristic symptom of kyphosis is a hunched or rounded back; other symptoms include pain, numbness, tingling, and weakness. Physical assessment should look for tenderness, deformities, decreased spinal mobility, and the possibility of nerve compression. X-rays are the imaging option of choice for diagnosis, as it can confirm the angle of kyphosis and possible vertebral fractures. An MRI can be used to assess for possible infections or tumors, while a CT scan can visualize fractures or tumors.

Medical management is usually conservative and may include physical therapy, pain management with NSAIDs and muscle relaxants, weight management, and smoking cessation. If these interventions are unsuccessful or in severe cases (e.g., severe pain, progressing deformities, and neurological symptoms), surgical intervention via a spinal fusion, vertebroplasty, kyphoplasty, or osteotomy may be necessary. Routine follow-up visits are recommended to monitor symptoms and progression of the disease.

Scoliosis

Scoliosis involves an abnormal spinal curvature of more than ten degrees. It is most often diagnosed in children or teens; however, the condition can present in adulthood, especially in cases where neuromuscular or degenerative disorders are present. Multiple causes of scoliosis exist, including idiopathic (which is the most common). Neuromuscular scoliosis is caused by weakened muscles due to neurological disorders like cerebral palsy and polio. Degenerative (adult-onset) scoliosis is caused by the degenerative spinal changes associated with age, leading to decreased structural integrity of the spine. Congenital scoliosis occurs during fetal development, during which vertebral anomalies like hemivertebrae occur. Other causes of scoliosis include infections (e.g., Pott's disease), tumors, and trauma (e.g., fractures).

Patients with scoliosis will present with an abnormal posture, including uneven shoulders, unilateral rib hump, and uneven hips; these deformities are most noticeable when the patient bends over (referred to as the Adam's test). Patients may also complain of back pain, numbness, tingling, and weakness in more severe cases. X-rays are the imaging option of choice to diagnose scoliosis, where the Cobb angle is used to determine the degree of the curvature (greater than ten degrees is abnormal, indicating scoliosis). An MRI may be used to assess for the presence of neurological damage and to rule out any spinal tumors or infections.

Medical management is conservative for mild cases and may only require observation. For teenagers with moderate scoliosis (Cobb angle of twenty-five to forty-five degrees), a brace, such as a Boston brace or thoracolumbosacral orthosis, may be used to prevent the spinal curvature from progressing. Physical therapy, including Schroth therapy, is also used to improve posture and muscle strength. NSAIDs are recommended for mild to moderate pain, while muscle relaxers are recommended for severe pain. For severe cases of scoliosis (Cobb angle of forty-five to fifty degrees), surgical intervention in the form of spinal fusion, vertebral osteotomy, or growing rods may be necessary. Routine follow up visits to monitor disease progression are recommended.

Spinal Stenosis

Spinal stenosis refers to the narrowing of the spinal canal, which most commonly occurs in the lumbar and cervical spine as a result of structural changes and places pressure on the spinal cord and/or nerves. There are three categories of change that contribute to spinal stenosis: degenerative, congenital, and acquired. Examples of degenerative changes include intervertebral disc degeneration, face joint arthritis, and/or ligamentum flavum hypertrophy. Congenital factors may not present with symptoms until later in life, when degenerative changes associated with age exacerbate the already restricted spinal area. Acquired factors include trauma (e.g., spinal fractures), spinal tumors, infection, and inflammation. The most common symptoms include pain in the affected region of spine, neurogenic claudication, and cervical myelopathy.

Physical assessment to confirm diagnosis should look for postural abnormalities, spinal tenderness, muscle atrophy, nerve root compression, positive straight leg raise test, and gait or balance troubles. MRI is the diagnostic imaging of choice to visualize the spinal cord, ligaments, and nerve roots as well as the degree of compression. An X-ray may also be used to assess any degenerative changes. Conservative medical management is initially used and includes NSAIDs for pain and inflammation reduction, muscle relaxants for spasms contributing to pain, gabapentin or pregabalin for neuropathic pain, and epidural steroid injections to reduce inflammation around the nerves. Physical therapy is also recommended to strengthen back and abdominal muscles to support posture. A spinal brace or lumbar corset may also be used to provide stability and support. Activity modification and weight loss can reduce symptom exacerbations. If conservative interventions fail or neurological deficits are present, surgical intervention (e.g., decompressive laminectomy, spinal fusion, or microdiscectomy) may be necessary.

Spondylolisthesis

Spondylolisthesis occurs when one vertebra slides over the vertebra located below it (usually at L5-S1), which in turn causes back pain and nerve compression. There are five different types of spondylolisthesis: dysplastic, isthmic, degenerative, traumatic, and pathologic.

Dysplastic (congenital) spondylolisthesis occurs as a result of a congenital defect in the posterior elements of the vertebrae (pars interarticularis). It is most commonly seen in children and teenagers, but symptoms may not present until adulthood.

Isthmic spondylolisthesis occurs via a stress fracture or defect in the pars interarticularis due to repetitive stress in hyperextension, which is often seen in athletes like football players and gymnasts. This leads to the vertebrae slipping; as a result, isthmic spondylolisthesis is graded on the degree of slippage (e.g., Grade 1: up to twenty-five percent and Grade 4: greater than seventy-five percent).

Degenerative spondylolisthesis occurs most often in adults over fifty years of age, as degenerative changes to the intervertebral discs and facet joints cause prolonged wear and tear, less spinal stability, and the vertebrae to slip in an attempt to support the weakened structures.

Traumatic spondylolisthesis occurs from a fracture in the vertebral body, facet joint, or other spinal areas, which in turn causes the vertebrae to be displaced and slip.

Pathologic spondylolisthesis is caused by an underlying condition which weakens the vertebrae, such as osteomyelitis or Pott's disease. Common symptoms include back pain, radiculopathy, numbness, weakness, and improper gait. If severe compression is present on either the spinal cord or nerve root, the patient may also experience neurological deficits in addition to the prior listed symptoms.

During the physical assessment, it is important to visualize any postural changes like an uneven pelvis or lumbar lordosis. Tenderness may be present over the lumbar spine or other affected areas. A thorough neurological exam, including reflex, muscle strength, and sensation assessments, will help to determine nerve involvement. An X-ray is the diagnostic imaging option of choice as it helps to visualize the lumbar spine, measure or grade the slippage (Meyerding classification), and identify any degeneration present. An MRI may also be used to assess for any nerve root or spinal cord compression.

Medical management includes the use of NSAIDs for inflammation and pain management, with opioids for severe pain. Corticosteroid injections may be necessary to manage pain when nerve compression is present. Muscle relaxers like cyclobenzaprine may also be used if muscle spasms are present. Physical therapy is recommended to strengthen the core and surrounding spinal muscles. A lumbar brace may be needed (in the short-term, not recommended for long-term management) to help stabilize the spine while reducing spinal movement to aid in the healing process. Rest and activity limitations are also helpful for a conservative management plan. For those patients whose symptoms are unsuccessfully managed conservatively or who have significant and persistent symptoms (especially neurological symptoms like loss of bowel and/or bladder function), surgical intervention via a decompressive laminectomy, spinal fusion, or decompression and fusion may be necessary.

Spondylolysis

Spondylosis refers to the degenerative changes that occur to the intervertebral discs and facet joints within the spine. It is an umbrella term that includes other conditions like degenerative disc disease and facet joint osteoarthritis. Spondylosis is associated with the degeneration caused by aging and most commonly affects the cervical and lumbar regions. As individuals age, the intervertebral discs lose hydration and subsequently elasticity, causing less shock absorption and disc height decreases. This disc space narrowing leads to the discs either bulging or herniating, which causes nerve root compression (with coinciding numbness, weakness, and pain). The facet joint also ages over time, causing more damage to the cartilage, inflammation, and the development of osteophytes (with coinciding pain, stiffness, and decreased mobility). With this instability, the ligaments along the back of the spinal canal may also thicken, further causing the spinal canal to narrow and the nerves to compress. The most common symptoms include neck and/or back pain, spinal stiffness with bending and/or twisting, numbness, tingling, weakness, and radiculopathy or myelopathy.

During the physical assessment, diagnosis can be supported by visualizing the presence of forward head posture or lumbar lordosis. Tenderness may be present in the affected area. For lumbar spondylosis, a positive straight leg raise will be present, while in cervical spondylosis, a positive Spurling's test will be present. An x-ray is the diagnostic imaging option of choice to visualize any degeneration present, including narrowed disc space, presence of osteophytes, or arthritis in the facet joints. An MRI may also be used to visualize any bulging or herniated discs and identify the degree of nerve compression.

Conservative medical management includes the utilization of NSAIDs for pain and inflammation reduction, with corticosteroids being used for severe pain. Muscle relaxers may be used if muscle spasms are present. Neuropathic pain (when nerve compression is present) may be managed with gabapentin or pregabalin. Topical analgesics like lidocaine patches can be used for localized pain management. Physical therapy is recommended to strengthen the spinal muscles and improve posture. Weight loss, low-impact activities, and maintaining good posture can also aid in symptom management. For patients with severe and persistent symptoms even after conservative interventions have been implemented, surgical intervention via a laminectomy, foraminectomy, or spinal fusion may be necessary.

Torticollis

Torticollis, also called wry neck, is an abnormal neck posture caused by muscle imbalances or neurological dysfunction, where the head is tilted to one side and the chin in the opposite direction. Torticollis is characterized as muscular, neurological, or structural. Muscular torticollis is classified as either congenital (most common type in babies) or acquired. Congenital muscular torticollis occurs when the sternocleidomastoid muscle is tight or short, usually associated with trauma during birth, fetal positioning, or muscle fibrosis. Acquired muscular torticollis (most common type in adults) develops after a muscle strain, trauma, or infection occurs. The sternocleidomastoid muscle may spasm, which in turn causes the abnormal head positioning. It is most often associated with postural inefficiencies, certain sleeping positions, neck trauma, or long-term neck strain.

Neurological torticollis is also called cervical dystonia or spasmodic torticollis, as it is characterized by muscle spasms in the neck that lead to abnormal posture. The most common type is torticollis secondary to dystonia; however, the condition can also be caused by neurodegenerative disorders or brain injury. Structural torticollis is caused by abnormalities in the cervical spine, like malformations, fractures, or subluxation. Though rare, neoplasms and cervical/spine infections can also cause structural torticollis. The most common symptoms for all types of torticollis include the hallmark head tilt and neck rotation, as well as pain, stiffness, and decreased range of motion.

During the physical assessment, a palpable mass or tightness may be present in the sternocleidomastoid. An X-ray is the diagnostic imaging option of choice to rule out any structural causes, such as fractures or subluxations. Medical management includes the use of NSAIDs for pain and inflammation reduction, muscle relaxers if spasms are present, as well as heat and/or cold therapy to manage pain and muscle tightness. Physical therapy is also recommended to stretch and strengthen the neck muscles while working to improve posture. A soft collar may be necessary for patients with congenital muscular torticollis. Botox therapy can be used for cervical dystonia to paralyze the overactive muscles, which decreases the frequency and severity of the muscle spasms. Corticosteroids may also be used for acute management of inflammation or the presence of severe pain. For cases of torticollis that are unresponsive to other interventions or if symptoms are severe, surgical intervention (e.g., muscle release or rhizotomy) may be necessary.

Spinal Trauma

Spinal trauma is characterized as any injury to the spine or spinal cord, which can be caused by a myriad of events such as blunt force, falls, or motor vehicle accidents. Spinal trauma is an umbrella term encompassing injuries that range from sprains to spinal cord damage with subsequent paralysis. To prevent lasting damage and disability, prompt assessment and injury identification are necessary. Vertebral injuries include fractures and dislocations. Spinal cord injuries are characterized as complete (involving complete loss of motor and/or sensory function) or incomplete (partial loss of motor and/or sensory function).

A thorough physical assessment is imperative to identify the type and severity of the injury. Examination should include tests for motor and sensory function, reflexes and range of motion, strength assessment, pain and tenderness, numbness and weakness, additional injuries, and the presence of spinal shock (e.g., flaccid paralysis, areflexia, and hypotension). An MRI is the diagnostic imaging option of choice to visualize the spine, soft tissue, and the ligaments; additional uses include determining the severity of spinal cord damage as well as the presence of any herniated discs, inflammation, and edema. An x-ray may be used to visualize the spine for fractures or other injuries, while a CT scan may be used to assess complex fractures (e.g., burst fracture) as well as the presence of soft tissue injuries.

Acute medical management includes immobilizing the spine immediately via a cervical collar and backboard. The airway must be assessed for patency, especially in C1–C3 injuries; if the airway is compromised, intubation with ventilation support will be necessary. If hypotension is present, fluid resuscitation with normal saline or Lactated Ringer's will be necessary. Vasopressors may also be needed in severe cases. When spinal cord compression or a fracture dislocation is present, surgical intervention via a laminectomy, discectomy, or spinal fusion may be necessary. Pain can be managed with NSAIDs (or epidural analgesia for severe spinal injuries and pain), while muscle relaxers may be used for muscle spasms.

Traumatic Brain Injuries

Traumatic brain injuries (TBI) typically result from an acute incident to the brain and lead to a range of physical and cognitive effects. A brain does not heal like other injuries. There is a popular quote that says *recovery from a brain injury lasts a lifetime*, and it's also possible to never fully recover. The road to recovery can be vastly different even in the setting of similar injuries, and the onset of symptoms can range from immediate to delayed (e.g., days or weeks later). Symptoms may appear right away or may not be present for days or weeks after the injury. In these cases, as well as others, the patient with brain trauma does not realize that a brain injury has occurred. The TBI may either temporarily or permanently cause damage, depending on the severity of the blow to the head. TBIs occur during motor vehicle crashes, falls, or blows to the head, among many other potential causes.

An open TBI is one in which the scalp and skull are penetrated and the tissue beneath is exposed. A closed TBI occurs from violent shaking or blows to the head, but the skull is not penetrated. During both types of TBI, blood vessels can tear and leak and hematomas may form.

A TBI is also classified as either mild, moderate, or severe. Mild cases are those with a shorter duration of symptoms, including less than 30 minutes of loss of consciousness and less than 24 hours of confusion or disorientation. Moderate cases involve greater than 30 minutes of loss of consciousness, while the threshold for severe TBI is reached when loss of consciousness surpasses 24 hours. Although mild cases may not present with visible changes on MRI or CT scan, common symptoms include headaches, confusion, nausea, vomiting, and fatigue. Moderate and severe symptoms can be even more distressing, resulting in physical, sensory, and emotional changes or deficits.

The effects of a TBI can be profound. In severe cases, the devastating effects of the injury can result in long-term unresponsiveness and require extensive rehabilitation. Even with a mild TBI, changes in brain function can have a dramatic impact on memory, family, job, social and community interaction. Treatment depends upon the stage at which the TBI is discovered. Acute care, surgery, rehabilitation and supportive care are all options that are dependent upon the stage of recovery.

Epidural Hematoma

Epidural hematoma (EDH) is a life-threatening condition that is characterized by a collection of blood between the outer dura mater and the inner surface of the skull. EDH is typically caused by traumatic brain injury (TBI) but may also result from several non-traumatic modalities, including vascular abnormalities and hemorrhagic tumors. Young adult males are the highest risk population for EDH, partly due to the increased adherence of the dura mater to the skull over time, making EDH much less likely in older patients. Symptoms of EDH include a brief loss of consciousness following a traumatic event, such as motor vehicle accidents, falls, or assaults. This loss of consciousness is followed by a complete recovery, in which the patient is fully lucid for a period, which is then followed by a decline in cognition. This is the most likely presentation for EDH, although some patients may remain unconscious or experience no initial loss of consciousness before the cognitive deterioration. Additional symptoms may include nausea, vomiting, headaches, seizures, and ipsilateral pupillary dilation, which is caused by an increase in intracranial pressure (ICP). Hypertension, irregular respirations, and bradycardia (also known as Cushing's triad) may also be present, signifying brain stem compression, which requires rapid intervention to prevent death. Assessment and diagnosis involve laboratory studies including blood type and cross match, prothrombin time, platelet count, CBC, and activated partial thromboplastin time. Radiography may be used to assess the bleed, as well as a head CT scan, which is the first-line diagnostic tool for EDH. Brain MRI may also be used to assess EDH in the vertex area. Treatment involves neurosurgery as soon as possible to evacuate the clot and prevent further neurological decline or death. Massive transfusion may be necessary for continued hemorrhage and correction of coagulopathy.

Subdural Hematoma

A **subdural hematoma** forms when blood accumulates under the protective layer of the brain known as the dura mater. The brain is covered by three protective layers (known as **meninges**): the **dura** being the outermost layer, the **arachnoid mater** being the middle layer, and the **pia mater** being the inner layer closest to the brain. In a subdural hematoma, blood accumulates between the dura and the arachnoid layer, where there is rupture of the veins that bridge these three layers. Most commonly, subdural hematomas are caused by trauma, such as falls or motor vehicle accidents. As blood presses against the brain, this leads to damage to the tissues. Patients on blood thinners or with conditions that impair coagulation are at high risk for subdural hematoma with even mild injury to the head.

Symptoms include confusion, dizziness, nausea/vomiting, seizures, loss of consciousness, and changes to speech, vision, or balance. Diagnosis requires imaging, such as a CT scan of the head, to look for signs of bleeding. Blood tests to evaluate clotting factors and platelet levels may also be indicated. If patients are on blood thinners, have low platelets, or a high INR/PTT, reverse coagulopathy (e.g., platelet transfusion, fresh frozen plasma, or vitamin K) may be indicated.

The goal of treatment is to decrease pressure on the brain from the blood and stop the bleeding. To treat the bleeding, a **craniotomy** may be used to evacuate the blood. Alternatively, a **burr hole** may be drilled to allow the blood to drain. Nurses should monitor these sites to ensure there is no abnormal drainage or signs of infection.

Concussion

A **concussion**, or mild traumatic brain injury, occurs when normal brain function is disrupted by physical trauma to the head and/or neck. This in turn causes a disruption in the ion channels, affecting the release of neurotransmitters and leading to injury to the cells. As a result, the brain's energy demands increase, and the cells no longer have the capability to meet those increased needs. Neuroinflammation is also present after injury, which can impact the presence of symptoms and recovery time. The most common causes of concussion include sports injuries, falls, and motor vehicle accidents. Headache is the most common symptom; others include nausea and vomiting, dizziness, light sensitivity, blurred vision, confusion, slow reaction time, short-term memory problems, mood swings/irritability, anxiety, and emotional instability. Loss of consciousness (usually less than thirty minutes) may occur but is not required to make a concussion diagnosis.

Testing protocols for diagnosis include the **Glasgow Coma Scale** and the Sport Concussion Assessment Tool. Medical management in the acute stage includes rest (cognitive and physical), observation, and pain management with acetaminophen, since NSAIDs can impact platelet aggregation. A gradual return to play and normal activities plan should be made, with the goal of returning to full activity after the absence of symptoms for twenty-for to forty-eight hours. If symptoms last for more than seven to ten days, evaluation for post-concussion syndrome should be completed.

Post-concussion Syndrome

Post-concussion syndrome is defined as persistent concussion symptoms which may last for weeks to years after the initial concussion. It is unknown why some patients develop post-concussion syndrome, while others experience total recovery. However, a history of multiple and/or severe concussions, increased age, or presence of other mental health issues (e.g., anxiety, depression, PTSD) can increase the likelihood of post-concussion syndrome occurring. The symptoms are the same as a concussion but persist beyond seven to ten days at minimum. Medical management includes cognitive and physical rest, improving sleep hygiene, tricyclic antidepressants for chronic headaches, and acetaminophen for pain control due to the increased risk of bleeding with use of NSAIDs. Cognitive behavioral therapy may be used for mood disturbances, anxiety, and depression. Neurophysical and/or physical rehabilitation may be necessary to improve cognitive function, vestibular function, and for a gradual return to play protocol. Long-term risks, such as chronic traumatic encephalopathy, should also be evaluated and discussed with patients.

Non-accidental Trauma

Non-accidental trauma occurs when a child younger than five years sustains an injury to the skull or brain because of being shaken or struck by an adult. These types of injuries will often lead to skull fractures and subdural bleeds, among other injuries. Non-accidental trauma has the potential to cause death in children and infants, so patient education, monitoring, and reporting are vital to prevention and survival.

Behavioral and Psychosocial

Agitation

Agitation is an extreme form of arousal associated with increased verbal and motor activity. These symptoms are caused by a variety of etiologies, both medical and psychiatric. Patients with agitation may present not only to an emergency department or a psychiatric emergency service, but also to a clinic or acute care center that does not have the onsite medical resources of a physician or midlevel practitioner. A patient who acts nervous or anxious may be agitated. Agitation in a critically-ill patient, outside the range of normal, may be a sign of underlying mental disturbance.

The **Behavioral Activity Rating Scale** (**BARS**), which follows, should be used to assess the severity of agitation.

1. Cannot be roused easily
2. Sleeping, but responsive to verbal and physical contact in a normal fashion
3. Appears drowsy and sedated
4. Normal activity level (quiet and awake)
5. Calms with instructions and shows signs of overt physical or verbal activity
6. Does not require restraints but is continuously or very active
7. Requires restraint because of violence and aggression

Any patient with a BARS score of 1 requires immediate transfer to a medical ED. Patients with a score of 2, 3, or 7 should be transferred immediately to either a medical emergency department or a psychiatric facility with medical capability. For mild to moderate agitation, BARS 5 or 6, the patient may be calmed with verbal de-escalation techniques, and environmental modification. If this is successful, further evaluation at the clinic is acceptable. Oxygenation level and blood sugar level should be obtained if possible. The initial examination should be directed at identifying factors that could indicate serious, possibly life-threatening, conditions. Unless immediate intervention is indicated, de-escalation should be continued to gain patient cooperation.

Agitation can be due to a general medical condition, intoxication and withdrawal, or a decompensated psychiatric disease. Drug side effects, a mood disorder such as anxiety or depression, dementia, autism, or a neurological disorder should be ruled out. Finding out the underlying cause of the agitation is key to reversing it. If agitation is caused by a mental health disturbance, medication and behavioral therapy may be increased or adjusted to relieve the agitation.

If pharmacological agents are necessary for the treatment of agitation, one of the following three classes will likely be used. First-generation antipsychotics, such as Haldol, work by inhibiting dopamine transmission to the brain, which has a calming effect on the patient. Second-generation antipsychotics, formally called atypical antipsychotics, are serotonin-dopamine antagonists and less likely than first-generation antipsychotics to cause extrapyramidal motor control issues. Benzodiazepines act on GABA receptors to reduce anxiety, relax muscles, produce a sedative effect, and can be used as an anticonvulsant. A last resort for a severely agitated patient is the use of physical restraints which require a physician order and must meet strict hospital protocols.

Antisocial Behaviors, Aggression, and Violence

People with **antisocial personality disorders** (**ASPD**) show no signs of empathy. Awareness of feelings and perceptions concerning themselves or in interactions with others is limited. This can lead a spectrum of behaviors that range from social awkwardness to acts of cruelty and negligence. People with antisocial personality disorders (ASPD) show no signs of empathy. Awareness of feelings and perceptions concerning themselves or in interactions with others is limited. This can lead to a spectrum of behaviors that range from social awkwardness to acts of cruelty and negligence. In combination with lack of empathy for others, those with ASPD do not feel that typical societal norms and rules apply to them.

An aggressive history and a tendency to get into serious fights are an indicator of ASPD, and one that distinguishes it from psychopathy. There are two forms of **aggression**: reactive (threat response) and instrumental (for self-advancement). Reactive aggression occurs in connection to perceived threats, which may occur more frequently in the brain of ASPD individuals. According to one study in 2013, those with ASPD were more likely to have something called hostile intention bias, where they misinterpreted everything as a potential threat.

A study in 2009 found that people with ASPD have very strong rapid-response impulsivity but the same level of impulse control as non-sufferers when it came to future planning. There is a strong need to be independent and resist being controlled by others, who are usually held in contempt. There is a willingness to use untamed aggression to back up the need for control or independence. The antisocial personality usually presents in a friendly, sociable manner, but that friendliness is always accompanied by a baseline position of detachment. There is a total lack of investment in the comfort of others, a complete focus on their own feelings, and complete lack of remorse. It is very common that the person with ASPD is not the one who seeks help; often friends, families, or intimate partners attempt to get a diagnosis.

If the patient is officially diagnosed, they may be prescribed cognitive-behavioral therapy, mood stabilizers, and antidepressants. ASPD often comes with accompanying diagnoses of substance abuse disorder, borderline personality disorder, narcissistic personality disorder, and conduct disorder.

Restraints

When patients are acting violently or aggressively (whether due to ASPD or otherwise), they may require the use of restraints. **Restraints** can be defined as anything that is used, done, or said to intentionally limit a person's ability to move freely. Restraints, when applied properly, cannot be easily removed or controlled by the person. In addition to physical form, restraints can also be emotional, chemical, or environmental. Use of restraints is very controversial due to the ethical issue of personal freedom. These are a temporary solution to a problem and must always be used as a last resort. Restraints are used to limit a patient's movement to prevent injury to themselves or others and always require a physician's order.

Types of restraints include:

- Physical: vests, wrist restraints, straps, or anything that confines the body
- Emotional: verbal cues or emotions used to coerce the patient to act a certain way
- Environmental: side rails, locked doors, closed windows, or locked beds
- Chemical: any medication used to restrict a patient's movement

The medical doctor or practitioner is responsible for ordering the use of restraints. Nurses and caregivers are responsible for applying restraints safely and for the management of a patient with a restraint. After an order is given, the physician must visit the patient within 24 hours of placing the order to assess its further necessity.

Other methods must be tried before restraints. They include:

- Talking with the patient about being cooperative
- Using distractions such as television, music, knitting, and folding towels or cloths
- Placing the patient within view of a caregiver (i.e., near the main desk)
- Having someone sit with the patient
- Ensuring the patient's area is calming
- Ensuring that the patient's bathroom needs are being met
- Ensuring personal items are within reach

Each facility will have a specific protocol that must be followed for restraint use. Circumstances under which restraints could be used include:

- Signs of patient aggression toward self, staff, or other patients
- Interference with important medical devices, such as an IV or a catheter
- Patient movements that are potentially harmful to their health or may cause further injury
- Potential for a patient to interfere with a procedure

The following guidelines should be used whenever applying restraints:

- Always follow the facility's restraint policy.
- Obtain an order from a physician or medical practitioner.
- Obtain consent from the patient or their legal representative if the patient is not capable of understanding.
- Explain to the patient what is going to happen, even if the patient is unable to understand due to confusion or dementia.
- Always monitor the patient per facility policy, such as checking the positioning of the restraint every thirty minutes and removing every two hours for range of motion. Remember to reposition the patient and offer toileting every two hours.
- Explain the need for restraints and how long the restraints will be used.

Vest restraints have holes for the arms and the opening crosses in the back. The straps will be secured on either side of the bed or chair, depending on the patient's location. Tie it in a quick-release knot to a lower part of the bed that does not move. Make sure that two fingers fit underneath the vest on the patient's chest so that it is not too tight.

Wrist or ankle restraints are cloths that wrap around each wrist or ankle. They have a strap that is tied to a lower, immovable part of the bed or chair. Tie it in a quick-release knot. Ensure the restraints aren't too tight and that the patient's arms or legs aren't in an awkward position.

If restraints aren't used correctly or are used for the wrong reasons, the patient's family can take legal action against the facility. A patient in restraints becomes completely vulnerable and may feel helpless. They are at a greater risk of sexual abuse, elder abuse, psychological abuse, or violence from other patients.

Possible injuries from restraints can include:

- Broken bones
- Bruises
- Falls
- Skin tears or pressure sores
- Depression or fear due to lack of freedom
- Death from strangulation

Delirium

Delirium is a cognitive disorder which is marked by an abrupt change in one's mental state. The condition results in concerning symptoms (e.g., confusion, sleep disturbances, and problems with mood, memory, and focus) that are different from one's typical state of being. Triggered by a multitude of factors, delirium has been associated with stressors such as illness, hospitalization, drug/alcohol use, and nutritional imbalances. While the condition is most common in the elderly, delirium can be differentiated from dementia by the more abrupt nature of both its onset and potential for resolution. Yet, these two conditions (delirium and dementia) can also be risk factors for the development of the other.

There are three categories of delirium: hyperactive, hypoactive, and mixed. While hyperactive delirium causes symptoms of hyperactivity (e.g., restlessness), hypoactive delirium causes the opposite symptoms (e.g., lethargy). Mixed delirium presents as a combination of both types. This aligns with the often-inconsistent presentation that many cases of delirium are characterized by, varying greatly in nature among different individuals and at different times of day.

Diagnosis of delirium relies on history, physical exam, and behavioral observation. While laboratory testing does not diagnose the condition, it can be used to identify the underlying cause or rule out other reasons for behavioral changes. Examples include identification of infectious (e.g., CBC, blood cultures, urinalysis), hormonal (e.g., TSH), or nutritional (e.g., CMP) causes. Treatment of delirium is focused on resolution of any contributing factors along with supportive interventions to reduce stress levels, such as creating a calm environment, predictable routine, and interventions to ensure safety.

Medical Non-adherence

Medical non-adherence can refer to patients not taking their medication appropriately or not following the recommendations and prescribed treatments. Each individual patient case is different, and each case of non-adherence must be addressed based on patient circumstances and needs.

Medication nonadherence is widely recognized as a common and costly problem. Approximately 30% to 50% of US adults are not adherent to long-term medications. This leads to an estimated $100 billion in preventable costs in healthcare annually. Despite the widespread prevalence and cost of medication nonadherence, it is undetected and undertreated in a significant proportion of adults across care settings. The World Health Organization estimates that increasing the effectiveness of adherence may have a greater impact on the health of the population than any improvement in specific medical treatments.

One way to identify the population of at risk for medication non-adherence is to conduct screenings. However, most clinicians are not formally trained on screening for, and diagnosing, medication nonadherence, nor are they fully aware of how best to treat nonadherence if detected. One of the most common diagnostic assessments for medication nonadherence is simply asking patients if they have any problems taking the medication regimen as prescribed When no further questions are asked, potentially addressable medication issues are left unattended.

Mood Disorders/Depression

A **mood disorder** is a mental health classification for all of the disorders that alter or change a person's mood that are inconsistent with the situation they are experiencing (i.e., depression and bipolar). The following are the most common types of mood disorders:

1. **Major depression**: having a lack of interest in day-to-day activities, feelings of hopelessness, anxiety, anger, or having suicidal thoughts that last for 2 or more weeks.

2. **Dysthymia**: A low-grade feeling of depression that lasts for a minimum of two years

3. **Bipolar disorder**: a disordered characterized by periods of depression followed by periods of mania.

4. Mood disorder related to another health condition: having an acute or chronic medical illnesses can trigger symptoms of depression.

5. Substance-induced mood disorder: when depression is related to or caused by the use of drugs, alcohol, or other harmful substances.

Mood disorders may be caused by an imbalance of brain chemicals. Life events, abrupt changes in routine, and stress may also contribute to a depressed mood. Mood disorders also tend to run in families and are more intense and harder to manage than normal feelings of sadness. Children, teens, or adults who have a parent with a mood disorder have a greater chance of also having a mood disorder. Rates of depression are nearly twice as high as in women as they are in men. Once a person in the family has this diagnosis, their brothers, sisters, or children have a higher chance of the same diagnosis. Depending on age and the type of mood disorder, a person may have different symptoms of depression. The following are the most common symptoms of a mood disorder:

- Ongoing sad, anxious, or empty affect
- Feeling hopeless or helpless
- Having low self-esteem
- Feeling inadequate or worthless
- Excessive guilt
- Repeating thoughts of death or suicide
- Loss of interest in usual activities or activities that were once enjoyed, including sex
- Relationship problems
- Trouble sleeping or sleeping too much
- Changes in appetite and/or weight
- Decreased energy
- Trouble concentrating
- A decrease in the ability to make decisions
- Frequent physical complaints that don't get better with treatment
- Very sensitive to failure or rejection
- Irritability, hostility, or aggression

With a mood disorder, these feelings are more intense than what a person may feel occasionally. If these feelings continue over time, interfere with interest in family, friends, community, or work, or if there are thoughts of suicide, medical intervention is needed.

Antidepressant and mood stabilizing medicines, especially when combined with psychotherapy, have been shown to work very well in the treatment of depression. Treatment of bipolar disorder may include mood stabilizers such as lithium and carbamazepine, along with second-generation antipsychotics such as aripiprazole and risperidone. Psychotherapy is focused on changing the person's distorted views of self and the environment. It also helps to improve interpersonal relationship skills, identify stressors in the environment, and assist with avoiding them. Family therapy, electroconvulsive therapy, and transcranial stimulation may also be therapeutic.

Anxiety

Anxiety and panic attacks are characterized by extreme, sudden, and often unpredictable feelings of paralyzing fear, nervousness, and discomfort. These situations are often debilitating for the individual experiencing them, with some reporting symptoms such as chest pain, the inability to breathe, and feeling a sense of impending death. Other common symptoms include overwhelming dizziness, nausea, sweating, trembling, accelerated heart rate, and feelings of "checking out" from reality. For a true medical diagnosis, four or more of these symptoms must be present. Typically, these episodes can last anywhere from 10 minutes to over an hour. Individuals who experience an anxiety or panic attack for the first time may be unfamiliar with the event, and it can warrant a trip to the emergency department. Consequently, it is important for nurses to know how to address these situations to help the patient to receive proper, adequate, and cost-efficient treatment in the future. It is important to show support and compassion toward the patient's feelings, even if the patient's fears seem irrational.

For recurrent anxiety and panic attacks, medication and/or psychotherapy is often needed to support the patient's quality of life. Selective serotonin reuptake inhibitors (SSRIs) are often prescribed to help manage anxiety symptoms. Brand names include Prozac®, Zoloft®, Paxil®, and Lexapro®.

Post-Intensive Care Syndrome (PICS)

Post-Intensive Care Syndrome (**PICS**) are symptoms experienced by a patient who has received intensive care. These symptoms hinder the patient's well-being and can persist well after discharge. They include physical, mental, and emotional symptoms that are linked not only to the medical condition for which the patient received intensive care, but also due to emotional and mental stress from the general experience and from medications used in recovery. Symptoms can include cognitive dysfunction such as forgetfulness, difficulty completing routine tasks, and poor concentration.

Patients may also experience mental disturbances such as nightmares, anxiety, and depression. In addition, patients are likely to experience physical issues such as pain, fatigue, and general weakness from invasive procedures that are burdensome for the body. Furthermore, symptoms of PICS are reported in caregivers of the patient; caregivers are also likely to experience increased levels of stress and grief. Healthcare teams can support patients and caregivers by providing the lowest dose of medications needed, supporting physical movement, incorporating psychological and behavioral therapies, and encouraging general healthy lifestyle behaviors that support overall well-being.

Post-Traumatic Stress Disorder (PTSD)

PTSD is a disorder that arises in connection with the experience of a traumatic event (e.g., war situations, abuse, or serious accidents). The condition results in dysregulation of the individual's fight-or-flight response. While the fight-or-flight response is a typical reaction to stress meant to protect a person from harm, those with PTSD may experience these symptoms in a chronic state. Most people recover from initial symptoms naturally, but those who continue may be diagnosed with PTSD.

Symptoms usually begin within 3 months of the traumatic incident, but may occur later. Symptoms must last more than a month and be severe enough to interfere with relationships or work to be considered PTSD. The course of the illness varies, and it may become chronic. Some people recover within 6 months, while others have symptoms that last much longer. Re-experiencing symptoms may cause problems in a person's everyday routine. The symptoms can start from the person's own thoughts and feelings. Words, objects, or situations that are reminders of the event can also trigger re-experiencing symptoms.

To be diagnosed with PTSD, an adult must have all of the following for at least 1 month:

- At least one symptom related to reminders of the event
- At least one avoidance symptom
- At least two arousal and reactivity symptoms
- At least two cognition and mood symptoms
- Re-experiencing symptoms include:
    - Flashbacks, which may include physical symptoms like a racing heart or sweating
    - Bad dreams
    - Frightening thoughts

Avoidance symptoms typically present in relation to the setting that led to the initial development of PTSD. In order to prevent re-experiencing or additional trauma, one will often go to great lengths to avoid similar experiences that serve as reminders of the original event.

Arousal and reactivity symptoms involve generalized intense levels of awareness and emotional responses. These symptoms often occur in a continuous rather than episodic rhythm, resulting in significant disruption to one's daily activities and baseline stress levels.

Cognition and mood symptoms include: trouble remembering key features of the traumatic event, negative thoughts about self or the world, distorted feelings like guilt or blame, and loss of interest in enjoyable activities.

Cognition and mood symptoms result in diminished memory of the original triggering event as well as a baseline pessimistic viewpoint of oneself and others. The resulting numbness and negativity in one's frame of mind can lead to feelings of isolation.

While the greatest risk factor for PTSD lies in the severity and nature of the traumatic event itself, additional factors that increase risk include female gender, family history, and coexisting mental health conditions. Treatment is highly individualized and specific to the underlying causative event or circumstance. Both pharmacological (e.g., antidepressant medications) and psychological (e.g., cognitive-behavioral or exposure therapy) treatment options should be considered to enable the best possible quality of life for the patient.

A 2012 study of 395 military veterans with PTSD found a link between risk-taking behavior and the disorder. In addition to the above forms of riskiness, vets with PTSD have a propensity for firearms play, potentially endangering their lives. People with PTSD have already survived dangerous situations, and risk-taking behavior may give such individuals the feeling that they have more control over their present circumstances than those that led to them developing PTSD. Recognizing this propensity in their personality may help patients with risk-taking behavior, thus being the first step in remediating the problem. Behavioral and cognitive therapy, as well as psychological drugs such as antidepressants, may also aid in the treatment of this behavior.

Self-Harm

Suicidal ideation refers to having thought of suicide. It is often a component of another mental health diagnosis in an individual, such as depression. It can range from a spectrum of fleeting suicidal thoughts without a plan of action (also referred to as passive suicidal ideation) to suicidal thoughts with a plan of action (also referred to as active suicidal ideation). Suicidal ideation, like homicidal ideation, is an immediate cause for concern and emergency intervention. Risk factors for suicidal ideation include family history, above-average number of negative life experiences, chronically high levels of stress, inability to cope with or manage stressors, mental illness, guns in the home, domestic violence, and imprisonment. Men are more likely to experience suicidal ideation than women. Medical personnel should note patient symptoms associated with depression, comments made about death or dying, history of or visible marks from past suicide attempts, marks from self-harm, mood swings, extreme anxiety, and intense negative emotions. Suicide attempts that are not fatal can result in severe consequences, such as brain damage or falling into a long-term coma.

The nurse should assess patients for suicidal ideation using nonjudgmental, therapeutic methods that support the patient in being honest with the healthcare staff. This should include clear, direct questions related to plan, intent, and history of attempts. Euphemisms should not be used. If the patient is determined to be high risk, this should be communicated with the healthcare team, and the patient should not be left alone until further assessment by a social worker or psychiatry specialist can take place. Patient safety attendants are often utilized in hospitals for this purpose.

High-risk patients must be continually monitored, and their environment should be adapted for safety. In the hospital, this can mean removing cords, tubing, sharp items, and anything that could be used to cause harm. A patient's belongings should be checked for weapons and hoarded medications, which need to be removed if found. The nurse should work with the patient to create a safety plan and explain the precautions to the patient and the family. When administering medications, the nurse should ensure the medicine is taken promptly by the patient and not being stored for a future attempt. Social work should be involved, and discharge planning should include family and caregivers.

Substance Use Disorders

In 2013, the American Psychological Association (APA) released the fifth edition of the DSM. In this edition, the definitions revolving around addiction were changed. The APA threw away both "substance abuse" and "substance dependence" in favor of "**substance use disorder**." The difference between addiction and dependence can be difficult to understand. Differing as well as interchangeable use of the terms varies across organizations.

The term **dependence** usually refers to a physical dependence on a substance, characterized by tolerance and withdrawal. Although physical dependence and addiction do not always coincide, addiction can easily arise from dependence. Continued substance abuse causes a series of biochemical changes in the brain which can lead to the behavior changes associated with **addiction**. Substance use becomes the main priority of the addict, regardless of the harm they may cause to themselves or others.

An addiction causes people to act irrationally when they don't have the substance they are addicted to in their system. The effects of addiction are both mental and physical in nature.

Addiction is often present in the setting of mental and physical dependence. However, the main characteristic that distinguishes addiction from dependence is the combination of mental and physical dependence with uncontrollable behavior in obtaining and using a substance. The continuum of behavior between abuse and dependence can be defined by the time and degree of substance use. Essentially, abuse is like the early stage of dependence. As substance abuse becomes more frequent, the likelihood of developing a dependence disorder becomes greater.

Suicidal Ideation and/or Behaviors

It is important to take people seriously when they express having suicidal thoughts. Research has shown that about one-fifth of people who die by suicide had talked to their doctor or other healthcare professional about their decision. These types of thoughts may arise in people who feel completely hopeless or believe they can no longer cope with their life situation. **Suicidal ideation** can vary greatly from fleeting thoughts to preoccupation to detailed planning.

According to the Center for Disease Control (CDC), for every 25 attempts, there is one suicide death. Suicide is the tenth leading cause of death for all ages in the United States, and the third leading cause of death among 15- to 24-year-olds. Patients with borderline personality disorder face an extraordinarily high risk of suicidal ideation and suicide attempts. One study showed that 73% of patients with borderline personality disorder have attempted suicide, with the average patient having 3.4 attempts.

Warning signs may include hopelessness, racing thoughts, insomnia or oversleeping, mania, loss of appetite or overeating, loneliness, alcohol abuse, excessive fatigue, or low self-esteem. Research has found a variety of risk factors for suicidal ideation including the following:

- Mood and mental disorders
- Adverse life or family events (divorce, death of a loved one, job loss)
- Chronic illness or pain
- Previous suicide attempt
- Military experience
- Witnessing trauma
- Family violence
- Owning a gun
- Being the victim of abuse or bullying
- Unplanned pregnancy
- Drug or alcohol abuse

An act that is intended to cause injury to oneself, but not death, is called a **non-suicidal self-injury**. An example of this type of behavior is when patients cut themselves. It is a method of relieving psychological pain through physical pain. Men are more likely than women to commit suicide, as well as more likely to abuse alcohol and drugs concurrently. Men are less likely to seek help when they are depressed. Veterans have seen an increase in suicides in recent years. It is important to note that despite these risk factors for suicide, it can occur across a wide span of age groups, genders, and life circumstances.

Some patients who are more vocal about their suicidal ideation may be crying out for help and must be taken very seriously. Treatment should include psychotherapy and antidepressants. It should be noted, however, that antidepressants sometimes have the adverse side effect of worsened suicidal behavior. Caregivers should be instructed to be watchful for deepening of depression and thus an increased risk for suicide. Suicide hotlines are available to help suicidal patients in moments of crisis.

Practice Quiz

1. Which of the following manifestations is considered to be a late sign of increased ICP?
    a. Mental confusion related to time
    b. Blurred vision
    c. BP of 170/40
    d. HR of 94 bpm

2. The nurse is caring for the 25-year-old male patient with an acute spinal cord injury at the C3 to C4 level. Which of the following manifestations is consistent with this injury?
    a. Vital capacity 45 percent of normal, hemoglobin 10.4 g/dL, heart rate 96 beats per minute
    b. Loss of somatic and reflex function, BP 160/90, effective cough effort
    c. Coarse and fine crackles bilaterally, heart rate 56 beats per minute, core temperature 96.7 °F
    d. BP 104/60, urinary output 18 mL over the last 60 minutes, heart rate 120 beats per minute

3. The nurse is caring for a patient with an emerging ischemic stroke. The nurse prepares to administer which of the following fibrinolytic agents?
    a. Urokinase
    b. Streptokinase
    c. Alteplase
    d. Tenecteplase

4. Which of the following would the nurse expect to assess in a patient with Guillain-Barré syndrome who has cranial nerve involvement?
    a. Core muscle weakness
    b. Respiratory muscle weakness
    c. Limb weakness
    d. Eye muscle weakness

5. A patient has had three seizures lasting five to eight minutes over a 30-minute period. The nurse understands that the patient is experiencing which of the following conditions?
    a. Generalized seizures
    b. Focal seizures
    c. Status epilepticus
    d. Postictal state

See answers on the next page.

Answer Explanations

1. C: Cushing's triad of manifestations are late signs of increased ICP. Choice *C* is an example of widening pulse pressure: Normal pulse pressure is 40 to 60 mmHg, while the pulse pressure in Choice *C* is 130 mmHg, and thus is the correct choice. Choices *A, B,* and *D* are all early signs of increased ICP and, therefore, are incorrect.

2. C: Injuries above the T6 level are associated with neurogenic shock, due to alterations of the autonomic nervous system, resulting in the loss of vagal tone. This manifests as decreased vascular resistance and vasodilation. Injury at this level is also associated with alterations in respiratory function, which results in symptoms such as decreased vital capacity and the presence of adventitious breath sounds. In addition, hypothermia is common; therefore, Choice *C* is correct. A vital capacity level that equals 45 percent of normal is associated with injuries at the T1 level or below, and is an indication of hemorrhagic shock rather than neurogenic shock.

A hemoglobin level of 10.4 g/dL in a male patient is also associated with acute or occult blood loss rather than loss of vagal tone, and is indicative of hemorrhagic shock. The patient's level of injury is consistent with neurogenic shock, which is manifested by bradycardia, not tachycardia; therefore, Choice *A* is incorrect. Loss of somatic and reflex function is associated with spinal shock, and hypertension and an effective cough effort are inconsistent with the level of the patient's injury; therefore, Choice *B* is incorrect. The collective manifestations of hypotension, oliguria, and tachycardia are associated with hypovolemic shock rather than neurogenic shock; therefore, Choice *D* is incorrect.

3. C: Alteplase is the single fibrinolytic agent approved for the treatment of ischemic stroke because it is associated with fewer adverse effects than the remaining agents. Streptokinase and tenecteplase have been used effectively to treat patients with acute myocardial infarction; however, in patients with ischemic stroke, streptokinase has been associated with an increased risk of intracranial hemorrhage and death. Current evidence for the efficacy and safety of urokinase and tenecteplase does not support their use for the treatment of ischemic stroke. Therefore, Choices *A, B,* and *D* are incorrect.

4. D: The patient with Guillain-Barré syndrome with cranial nerve involvement may exhibit weakness or paralysis of the eye muscles, facial drooping, diplopia, dysphagia, and pupillary alterations.

5. C: Status epilepticus is prolonged seizure activity involving multiple seizures, each lasting five minutes or more, over a 30-minute period of time. A generalized seizure is a seizure that originates in two or more networks of the brain. A focal seizure is one that originates in a single area of the brain. The postictal state follows a seizure and is characterized by alterations in consciousness and awareness as well as increased oral secretions.

Multisystem

Acid-Base Imbalance

A person requires a homeostatic balance of acidic compounds and basic compounds within their body. This balance is regulated by the lungs, which remove carbon dioxide, and by hormones that regulate the kidneys in releasing compounds that are causing an acid-base imbalance. An **acid-base imbalance** occurs when a patient's blood becomes too acidic or too alkaline. A number of respiratory and renal conditions can cause acid-base imbalance, as these impact the respiratory and renal organs' ability to remove compounds contributing to the imbalance. These conditions include chronic lung disease, obesity, chronic kidney disease, alcoholism, uncontrolled Type 1 diabetes, and acute infections that cause dehydration. Symptoms of acidosis include difficulty breathing or rapid breath, fatigue, dizziness, and confusion. Symptoms of alkalosis include muscle spasms, nausea, and vomiting. Treatment includes administering electrolytes and fluids to correct the imbalance, oxygen or ventilation support, or treatment of any underlying infections that may be contributing.

Anoxic Injury

Hypoxic Ischemic Encephalopathy

Hypoxic-ischemic encephalopathy (**HIE**) occurs as a result of the brain having inadequate blood and oxygen supply to meet metabolic needs. In the United States, the most common cause is due to cardiac arrest, although other causes include shock, near-drowning, strangulation, and carbon monoxide poisoning.

HIE often results in an impaired level of consciousness, with many patients unable to follow verbal commands. Since patients often present in a coma, healthcare providers must rely on family or witnesses to produce relevant medical histories. It is important to obtain the circumstances around the brain injury to assess for associated injuries, such as cervical spine involvement, as well as inquire about comorbidities, prescription medications, drug use, or toxin exposures.

Diagnostic workup includes laboratory and radiological testing consisting of basic blood work, arterial blood gas, drug screen, and CT scan of the head without contrast. The CT scan will reveal structural impairments of the brain, such as lesions, skull fractures, or hydrocephalus. CT angiography may be performed to evaluate vascular injuries, while EEG may be used to evaluate seizure activity.

Treatment and management focus on treating the underlying cause and preventing further brain injury. For patients who are in a coma after cardiac arrest, **therapeutic hypothermia** is recommended. Mild hypothermia, where the body temperature is maintained between 32°C and 36°C, protects the brain by inhibiting cell death, lowering the metabolic rate to reduce oxygen consumption, and stabilizing the blood-brain barrier to decrease edema. Therapeutic hypothermia should begin within 6 hours of the brain injury and is typically maintained for 24 hours. In a hypothermic state, there will be impacts to regulation of glucose and electrolyte levels, renal function, clotting activity, heart rate, blood pressure, and drug metabolism. Measures should be taken to prevent shivering, which can lead to increased intracranial pressure and metabolic needs of the body; additionally, by attempting to warm the body, it can slow cooling. The following methods should be used to prevent and treat shivering: adequate analgesia and sedation; antipyretics and alpha-2 blockers; and counter-warming the hands, face, and upper chest.

Burns

A **burn injury** occurs when layers of the skin are destroyed by extreme heat, an electrical current, or exposure to harmful radiation or corrosive chemicals. Burns are classified by size and extent of tissue damage. The severity of tissue damage directly correlates with the amount of time the area is exposed to the harmful agent and the agent's intensity. How quickly a burn heals is contingent upon how expeditiously treatment is rendered.

Types of Burns

- First-degree (superficial thickness) burns affect only the top layer of the skin, cause localized redness and pain, and typically heal within three to six days.

- Second-degree (superficial partial thickness) burns are deeper (e.g., a sunburn) and consist of skin bubbling, a weepy surface, and eventual peeling away of damaged skin; these usually heal between ten days and three weeks with no scarring.

- Second-degree (deep partial thickness) burns are deeper still, affecting more than one skin layer and resulting in scarring and possible skin grafting. This type of burn may heal anywhere from three to six weeks, but this depends on treatment and patient compliance with medical recommendations.

- Third-degree (full thickness) burns result when injury and destruction of deeper layers of skin is so severe that the wound will not heal by itself. Eschar (dead tissue) will form over the damaged area and must peel or be scrubbed off for the burn to begin the healing process. Nerve damage and decreased blood supply cause reduced or absent sensation. Depending on the patient's preexisting comorbidities, healing may take weeks to months.

- Fourth degree (deep full thickness) burns are the deepest burns and extend through all skin layers to muscles, tendons, and bone; there is no pain because nerve endings have been irrevocably damaged.

Complications resulting from a burn injury largely depend on the burn location. Burns of the upper body (head, neck, and chest) are associated with pulmonary issues. Burns involving the extremities require immediate therapy to prevent immobility caused by contractures (shortening and hardening of muscles and tendons, leading to extremity inflexibility and disfigurement), which may occur further into the healing process. Any burn in the perineal area is at an increased risk to develop infection from urine and feces.

Nursing considerations when caring for a patient with any type of burn injury must focus on the following phases: emergent, acute, and resuscitative/rehabilitative. In the emergent phase, hypovolemic shock is a concern, as well as impaired cognition or altered mental status as a result of severe pain. Thorough patient assessment and rapid response are essential in this phase to prevent potential complications. The nurse must assess adequacy of air exchange, monitor fluid loss, administer pain medication, and thoroughly cleanse and dress the wound.

During the acute phase of the burn, wounds form eschar (partial-thickness burn), and re-epithelialization, or wound healing, presents as the beginning of pinkish scar tissue. In this phase, wound infection is very likely, and prophylactic antibiotic treatment should be initiated. The main interventions during this phase consist of rigorous wound care, pain management, infection prevention, and psychosocial care.

While in the rehabilitative phase, a patient may experience more mature repair of the injury with the formation of new, short scar tissue and healing itching. The nurse should encourage the patient and caregiver to actively participate in the plan of care and treatment goals; this is imperative in the facilitation of the healing process. Topical ointments and lotions should be used and applied to affected areas to promote healing and keep skin moisturized, as well as to reduce itching. The patient is encouraged to remain compliant in continuing physical and occupational therapies.

Education revolves around explanation of the burn process, phases of healing, and expected outcomes related to burn management. Infection control (i.e., handwashing, keeping the affected area clean and dry, and performing necessary dressing changes) must be discussed with the patient and caregiver upon discharge from the facility. The patient should be able to recognize signs and symptoms of infection so that treatment may begin immediately. Nurses should be able to refer to the appropriate mental/emotional health providers in the community, and referrals to family and support groups will assist in long-term emotional management, manage self-esteem issues, and setting reasonable expectations.

Comorbidity in Patients with Transplant History

It is common to have some medical problems after transplant. Many transplant recipients manage two or more diseases at the same time. Some of the most common are: Cancer, diabetes, hypertension, kidney disease, and cardiovascular disease.

Cancer is more common in transplant patients than the general population. Research has shown that it is likely for patients who live for at least 10 years after a transplant to develop some type of cancer, including skin cancer. The main risk factor contributing to an increased incidence of cancer is due to suppression of the immune system, including the duration and intensity of immunosuppression. All types of immunosuppressant medications can increase the risk for certain types of cancer.

The best option for improving outcomes in transplant recipients is to stabilize and improve any existing comorbidities as much as possible before performing the operation. This will, in turn, improve the probability of the transplant tissue being accepted. Obesity is one example of a comorbidity that often complicates outcomes, including transplant tissue acceptance or rejection. Improving diet and maintaining regular exercise programs, as well as correcting obesity-related behaviors such as binge-eating, may improve the probability of transplant acceptance.

Graft-vs-host disease (GVHD) may occur as a comorbidity of transplantation. This may manifest itself as fever, rash, hepatitis, vomiting, diarrhea, and abdominal pain. Patients who are unrelated to the tissue donor or are of older age may be at greater risk for developing GVHD, which may be acute or chronic. Prevention of GVHD includes more accurate screening methods for matching donor and recipient. Treatment of GVHD may include methylprednisolone IV as an immunosuppressant while the transplant tissue heals.

Palliative Care

Palliative care is comprehensive care provided for symptoms and illness exacerbated by a chronic condition, including cancer, liver failure, end-stage renal disease (ESRD), dementia, and chronic obstructive pulmonary disease (COPD). Palliative care is delivered by a multidisciplinary team of physicians, nurses, nutritionists, pharmacists, social workers, case managers, and several specialists in a collaborative manner.

The characteristics that distinguish palliative care from hospice care are the timing of services and the continuation of curative care in palliative care. Progressive care nurses may advocate for palliative care to be administered at any stage of an illness or at any age. Ideally, palliative care should be initiated upon diagnosis for conditions like cancer and continue for the duration of therapy, follow-up care, and end-of-life care, as indicated. **Hospice care** is typically administered as a component of end-of-life care to those who are suffering from terminal illness with less than six months to live.

Palliative care can improve one's quality of life, addressing physical, behavioral, spiritual, and practical needs. Palliative care delivers a variety of options to patients that go far beyond pain assessments and management.

Palliative care may be delivered in the patient's home if they are under the supervision of a physician, or it may be a component of hospice or provided in a facility. It is typically covered by health insurance and in some instances may be covered by Medicare and Medicaid, while hospice care is always a covered benefit for Original Medicare recipients. Those who do not qualify for palliative care by any of the identified entities may need further assistance from their progressive care nurse and/or social worker to identify potential resources that can provide the necessary support.

End-of-Life Care

Nurses provide comprehensive and compassionate **end-of-life care**. This includes recognizing when death is near and conveying that information to families. Nurses should collaborate with other members of the healthcare team to ensure optimal symptom management and to provide support for the patient and family.

Nurses and other healthcare providers have a responsibility to establish decision-making processes that reflect physiologic realities, patient preferences, and the recognition of what, clinically, may or may not be accomplished. Establishing goals of care for this patient at this time may provide a framework for discussion about what care should be provided. This process often involves collaboration with experts in decision-making, such as ethics committees or palliative care teams. Decision-making for the end of a patient's life should occur over years rather than just in the minutes or days before a patient's death. Nurses can be a resource and support for patients and families at the end of a patient's life and in the decision-making process that precedes it. Nurses are often ideally positioned to contribute to conversations about end-of-life care and decisions, including maintaining a focus on patient preferences, and to establish mechanisms to respect the patient's autonomy.

There are times when the preferences of the family do not represent, or are in conflict with, the preferences of the patient. In those cases, the nurse's primary responsibility is to provide care and support to the patient and to respect the patient's autonomy while continuing to support the family as they struggle to adjust to the impending reality of the patient's death. Standards for excellent care for patients at the end of life should be evidence based, and should integrate national and international standards of care.

Nursing care includes not only disease management but also attention to physical comfort, and the recognition that patient well-being also includes psychological, interpersonal, and spiritual dimensions. Nurses have the knowledge and skills to manage pain and other distressing symptoms for patients with serious or life-limiting illness, and to work with patients and their families in palliative and end-of-life care decision-making.

Advance directives are an expression of the patient's preferences for medical care that are based on a person's values and beliefs. Advance directives come into play when that person is unable to, or chooses not to make decisions. Advance directives include identification of a surrogate, someone who will represent the patient's preferences in decision-making. Examples of advance directives include durable powers of attorney for healthcare, do not resuscitate order, and medical/physician orders for life-sustaining therapy (MOLST, POLST).

The loved ones of the dying patient need support as well. Educating them on what to expect when their loved one passes will help them be ready for the moment. The patient will likely lose consciousness and the ability to speak in the final days and hours. When the patient does pass, bereavement services should be made available to the surviving loved ones. Cultural preferences should be honored. Quiet time alone with the body may be desired and this request should be respected. Many hospitals have designated rooms and floors for end-of-life care, and spaces for the bereaved to mourn. Proper, dignified end-of-life care by the nurse and the healthcare team will aid in the healing process for the loved ones who remain.

Failure to Thrive

Failure to thrive in adults is a condition that encompasses a wide variety of motor and cognitive symptoms that lead to an overall decline in patient condition. Failure to thrive is typically the result of comorbidities, which may include mental and physical ailments such as malnutrition, chronic infection or inflammation, isolation, depression, pharmacotherapy, and malignancy. This condition typically occurs in older adults, although it may arise in median age groups in patients with severe comorbidities. Malnutrition is the leading cause of failure to thrive in adults, which then leads to physical and psychological issues. Symptoms include weight loss, gastrointestinal changes, and mental and physical deterioration, which lead to an increased risk of mortality. Diagnosis follows assessment of nutrition, height, weight, comorbidities, pharmacotherapies, and psychological status. Treatment includes addressing the underlying cause of the condition as well as supporting diet, nutrition, and mental health.

Fluid and Electrolyte Imbalances

One of the kidney's most important jobs is to maintain a healthy balance of fluid and electrolytes in the body. Imbalances in these substances, such as potassium, sodium, magnesium, and calcium, can be life-threatening and need emergent medical intervention.

When potassium levels exceed normal, it is called **hyperkalemia**. There are different grades of hyperkalemia. An amount greater than 5.0 mEq/L is considered mildly hyperkalemic, while moderate hyperkalemia is 6.0 mEq/L to 7.0 mEq/L, and severe hyperkalemia is greater than 7.0 mEq/L. Hyperkalemia will manifest itself on the ECG as tented T waves, widening QRS waves and deep S waves. The patient may go into cardiac arrest as a result of a toxic level of potassium running through their veins. If hyperkalemia is suspected, any potassium the patient is receiving must be immediately stopped. If it is a severe case of hyperkalemia, potassium needs to be immediately shifted back into the cells using one or a combination of the following therapies: glucose plus insulin, sodium bicarbonate, calcium chloride, and/or nebulized albuterol.

Low potassium, called **hypokalemia**, is defined as a potassium level of less than 3.5 mEq/L. This can be caused by diarrhea or massive fluid volume loss from the kidneys. A patient with hypokalemia may exhibit weakness, polyuria, cardiac cells that are hyperexcitable, and muscle cramping. Potassium must be replaced, whether orally or via IV infusions, depending on the severity of the case. The critical care nurse must monitor for over-supplementation that turns into hyperkalemia, especially in patients with ESRD whose kidneys cannot properly metabolize and regulate potassium.

Healthcare-Associated Infections

Due to the invasive nature of caring for a patient, there is almost always a risk for infection when a patient enters the healthcare environment. From IV lines and urinary catheters to ventilators, there are many different ways that the immune system can become compromised.

VAP (Ventilator-Associated Event or VAE)

Patients who are on mechanical ventilation are at risk of developing a lung infection related to being intubated, referred to as **ventilator-associated pneumonia** or **VAP**. The endotracheal tube used in mechanical ventilation is a foreign body in the airway, one that poses risk of infection. Microorganisms can easily use the tube as a route of entry to the patient's lungs; thus, special care must be given to prevent these types of infections.

The first and foremost way VAP may be prevented is limiting the amount of time the patient is on mechanical ventilation. The sooner that foreign object can be removed from the airway, the better. Hand hygiene for general care and sterile technique for invasive procedures are vital prevention techniques. Raising the head of the patient's bed to at least 45 degrees may aid in preventing bacteria from traveling down the tube and into the patient's lungs. Some hospitals use antiseptic mouthwashes such as chlorhexidine to keep the patient's oral cavity clean, thus preventing bacterial and other infectious growths from occurring.

Catheter-Associated Urinary Tract Infection (CAUTI)

Patients admitted to the critical care unit will often have urinary catheters for collecting, measuring, and observing urine output. Some patients may be at risk for skin breakdown that is aggravated by urinary incontinence and have a catheter for that reason. Whatever the reason for the urinary catheter, the nurse must be aware of its potential for causing infection and take steps to prevent such infections. Hand hygiene before and after caring for the patient is always one of the best ways to prevent the spread of infection. The nurse must ensure that aseptic technique is practiced when placing the urinary catheter. As with the central line, the urinary catheter must be removed as soon as it is no longer needed. Most hospitals have strict policies and procedures in place to prevent catheter-associated urinary tract infections (CAUTIs). They usually have checklists that must be addressed before placing the catheter, and daily while the patient has it. When the patient no longer meets criteria for having a catheter, the catheter must be removed to prevent infection.

Central Line-Associated Bloodstream Infections (CLABSI)

Many patients who are critically ill will need a central venous catheter. These central lines are often placed in the neck, groin, or chest of the patient for access to large blood vessels. The larger the vessel, the more medications, fluid, and blood transfusions can be administered to quickly stabilize critically ill patients. The problem with these lines, as with any other route into a body that does not naturally occur, is that they are prone to infection. Infection not only complicates the patient's care, but it also worsens the patient's chance of making a fast and full recovery from the original illness.

The critical care nurse must be extremely cautious when placing, caring for, and removing central lines, to prevent infectious agents from entering the patient's body. Hand hygiene is the first line of defense. When assisting with the placement of the central line, the nurse must don sterile gloves, gown, cap, mask, and utilize proper sterile draping. After placement, the nurse must strictly follow maintenance practices such as dressing changes as outlined by the facility. To prevent infection, the central line must be removed as soon as it is no longer needed.

Central line-associated bloodstream infection (CLABSI) and catheter-associated urinary tract infection (CAUTI) are costly and morbid. Despite evidence-based guidelines, some ICUs continue to have elevated infection rates.

Infectious Diseases

Influenza

Influenza is a type of virus that causes an upper respiratory infection of three types (A, B, and C). Some infections are mistakenly called the "flu," but are not actually caused by the influenza virus, resulting in a bit of confusion. A nasal swab can differentiate between influenza and other organisms. Symptoms of the flu include cough, coryza, fever, headache, and a generalized malaise. Flu season differs around the world, occurring in the coldest months of the year when the flu virus thrives. In the US, the accepted season is October through March. The number of influenza infections in a geographic region sometimes escalates rapidly, turning into an epidemic.

Everyone over 6 months of age should be vaccinated against the flu annually, at the beginning of their respective flu season. Patients at high risk of developing a severe case of influenza infection may be given antivirals. Those at lower risk may be treated for symptoms alone, allowing the virus to run its course naturally.

When influenza occurs at the pandemic level, it may be severe enough to cause even healthy, young patients to die. For this reason, vaccination of the population is vital.

Multidrug-Resistant Organisms

Over time, due to overuse of antibiotics, some organisms have become resistant to treatments that used to work. They have mutated in such a way that they can no longer be killed with previously effective antibiotics. **Methicillin-resistant staphylococcus aureus** (**MRSA**) is one such organism. Sometimes called a super bug, it is highly resistant to common antibiotic treatments. Discovered in the 1960s when it was resistant only to methicillin, it is now resistant to amoxicillin, penicillin, and oxacillin. MRSA infections spread by contact and are common in those with weakened immune systems who are admitted to healthcare facilities. Catheters, central lines, and surgical wounds are common sites for MRSA infections.

Vancomycin-resistant enterococci (**VRE**) and **carbapenem-resistant Enterobacteriaceae** (**CRE**) follow the same pattern as MRSA. VRE and CRE have become resistant to vancomycin and carbapenem, respectively, and are increasingly difficult to treat, as they continue to mutate. Both VRE and CRE are like MRSA in that they most commonly affect patients with weakened immune systems in healthcare settings. All three occur around central lines, ventilators, and urinary catheters.

Treating drug-resistant organisms can be tough, but not impossible. An intensive regimen of antibiotics that will kill the specific infection is necessary. Prevention is always the best intervention; practice meticulous handwashing, contact precautions, and remove lines as early as possible held reduce the spread of drug-resistant infections.

Life-Threatening Maternal/Fetal Complications

Preeclampsia

Preeclampsia is characterized by the onset of hypertension and proteinuria after twenty weeks of gestation and may persist for four to six weeks postpartum. The cause is unknown; however, there is evidence of alterations in the endothelium of the vasculature accompanied by vasospasm. Risk factors include nulliparity, maternal age over forty years old, family history, chronic renal disease, obesity, hypertension, and diabetes. Early manifestations include visual disturbances, altered mental state, dyspnea, facial edema, and possible upper right quadrant pain. Severe manifestations include hypertension on bedrest, increasing liver enzymes with increased pain, progressive renal dysfunction, pulmonary edema, and thrombocytopenia. Routine labs, fetal nonstress testing, and corticosteroids for lung maturation are done prior to delivery, which is the only known cure.

Eclampsia

Eclampsia is the life-threatening complication of severe preeclampsia that is manifested by the onset of seizure activity and/or the development of coma and is associated with hypertension, proteinuria, intrauterine fetal growth delay, and diminished amniotic fluid. There are no specific diagnostic tests, and while the specific etiology is unknown, there are indications that the condition results from the interchange of maternal and fetal tissue or allografts. Magnesium sulfate is recommended for short-term use for 24 to 48 hours to stabilize the patient for delivery, which is the only curative measure.

HELLP Syndrome

HELLP syndrome is also associated with significant maternal and fetal mortality, resulting from liver rupture and strokes due to cerebral edema or hemorrhage. The syndrome is characterized by hemolysis of RBCs, elevated liver enzymes, and low platelet levels (HELLP). Some authorities consider HELLP syndrome to be a severe form of preeclampsia, while others view it as a separate entity. The coagulation defects and liver dysfunction are the result of microvascular changes in the endothelium in the presence of hypertension; however, the cause is unknown. Risk factors are similar to risk factors for preeclampsia. Manifestations include elevated liver enzymes, coagulation defects including thrombocytopenia and hemolytic anemia, and right upper quadrant pain, and there are classification systems that assess the condition according to the extent of hepatic dysfunction. The treatment involves stabilization of the patient and prompt delivery with attention to correction of the coagulation defects and liver dysfunction. The emergency care of all of these life-threatening conditions is focused on treating hypertension, safe delivery of the fetus, and prevention of associated complications.

Maternal/Fetal Transfusion

Maternal/fetal transfusion is characterized by fetal blood entering the maternal circulation, which may occur during pregnancy or delivery. Less than 0.1 percent of fetal blood is commonly found in the maternal system and is not cause for intervention. Conversely, fetal hemorrhage is characterized by the presence of greater than 150mL of fetal blood in maternal circulation, leading to an increased risk of fetal mortality. Symptoms include reduced fetal movement or activity typical for near-term pregnancies. Assessment should involve fetal heart monitoring, which may display decelerations in heart rate. The **Keilhauer-Betke test** (KB test) is used to determine the percentage of fetal blood in the mother's circulation to determine the extent of maternal/fetal transfusion. Alpha-fetoprotein (AFP) is also an indicator of fetal blood in the maternal system. Potential causes of maternal/fetal transfusion may include blunt trauma, amniocentesis, external cephalic version (ECV), and placental abruption. Fetal hemorrhage may lead to fetal anemia, which can then result in non-immune hydrops fetalis. Hydrops is characterized by edema in the subcutaneous tissues as well as pericardial or pleural effusions.

Treatment involves cesarean section for viable pregnancies, typically after 20 weeks of gestation. Additional support, such as fluid management and transfusion, may be required for the fetus post-delivery.

Placental Abruption

Placental abruption refers to the premature separation of the placenta from the uterine wall and is the most significant cause of hemorrhage in the third trimester. Descriptive terms for the condition include the identification of the degree of separation (either partial or complete), or the location of the separation (either marginal or central). Clinically, Class 0 indicates only the identification of a blood clot in the expelled placenta, while the manifestations in Classes 1, 2, and 3 progress from mild vaginal bleeding to hemorrhage, from mild uterine pain to tetanic or continuous contractions, from normal vital signs to maternal shock, from absent fetal distress to fetal demise, and from normal clotting to fibrinogen deficiency and hemorrhage. The exact cause is not known. However, there are several common risk factors, including maternal hypertension, which occurs in 40 percent of the cases of abruptio placenta; smoking; trauma in the form of car accidents, falls, or assaults; cocaine or alcohol abuse; maternal age greater than thirty-five or less than twenty years old; and previous history of abruptio placenta.

Depending on the patient's presenting manifestations, diagnostic studies include CBC, coagulation tests, type and screen, Kleihauer-Betke test in Rh-negative mothers to identify fetal-to-maternal transfer of blood, a nonstress test, fetal monitoring, and the possible use of ultrasonography; however, ultrasounds have a low sensitivity for identifying the separation of the placenta. The emergency care of the patient starts with fetal monitoring, initiation of IV access for fluid resuscitation with crystalloids and colloids, assessment and correction of any coagulopathy, administration of RhoGAM as needed, consideration of steroids for fetal lung maturity in preterm newborns, and preparation for delivery of the newborn.

Placenta Previa

Placenta previa is defined as the abnormal placement of the placenta with either complete coverage of the internal cervical os (complete) by the placenta, or location of the placenta within two centimeters of the internal cervical os (marginal). The condition generally presents with painless vaginal bleeding during the third trimester of pregnancy and is associated with the possibility of hemorrhage at the onset of labor, due to cervical dilation and the relative inability of the lower uterine segment to effectively contract the vessels of the exposed maternal implantation site. Risk factors for this condition include maternal age greater than thirty-five years, infertility treatments, increased number of previous pregnancies, multiple births, previous C-sections, previous abortions, previous placenta previa, and smoking or cocaine use.

Once the condition is identified, the patient can be safely observed as long as the maternal and fetal monitoring parameters remain stable. Betamethasone therapy is indicated for the maturation of the fetal lungs if the pregnancy duration is less than thirty-four weeks. At the first sign of bleeding, immediate surgery is necessary. The care of the patient who presents with hemorrhage without prior identification of the placenta previa will trigger the agency protocol for obstetrical emergencies, which will include the transvaginal ultrasound confirmation of the condition and preparations for emergency surgery, including coagulation studies and type and cross match for six units of blood. Depending on the cause of the placenta previa, surgical removal of the uterus may be the only alternative surgical approach.

Postpartum Hemorrhage

Postpartum hemorrhage is commonly defined as the loss of more than 500 milliliters following a vaginal delivery or 1000 milliliters after a Caesarean section (C-section) in a pregnancy that has progressed for at least twenty weeks. Less substantial losses can result in alterations in fluid volume status in patients with comorbidities such as anemia, cardiac disease, dehydration, or preeclampsia, which means that postpartum hemorrhage is the loss of any amount of blood that results in altered hemodynamic status. There are multiple contributing factors; however, the most common precipitating pathophysiology for hemorrhage is uterine atony. These factors are related to tone, tissue, trauma, or thrombosis. Alterations in tone may be due to uterine atony resulting from distention of the uterine muscles in prolonged labor or with a large-for-gestational-age (LGA) newborn. Tissue alterations include retained placental tissue or placenta accreta. Trauma may result from manipulation of the fetus during delivery, history of previous C-section, prolonged labor, and internal version and extraction of a second twin. Alterations in coagulation may be due to preexisting coagulopathies.

The diagnosis depends on the presenting manifestations of postpartum vaginal bleeding and deteriorating hemodynamic status. Commonly, the emergency care of postpartum hemorrhage includes notification of obstetrical, anesthesia, and surgical suite providers; type and cross match for six units of packed red blood cells (PRBCs); assignment of data recording to one provider; aggressive fluid management, including appropriate blood products; assessment of the placenta for missing fragments of tissue; baseline lab studies, including CBC, coagulation studies, renal function tests, and electrolytes; and oxygen by mask. The goal of treatment is to reverse the coagulopathy, resolve the underlying defect, and maintain close surveillance of the contractility of the uterus, or surgical intervention in the event of massive hemorrhage.

Amniotic Embolism

Amniotic embolisms are a risk in pregnant and postpartum individuals. Amniotic embolisms can occur when amniotic fluid or other fetal cells enter the parent's bloodstream; this results in an inflammatory immune response that causes the parent to experience extreme blood clotting and internal bleeding. Symptoms are sudden and rapid; they are primarily seen in the parent. Symptoms include difficulty breathing, a drop in blood pressure, bleeding (usually from the uterus or incision sites), significant mood shifts, and seizures. More severe complications include heart failure and a positive feedback loop of blood clotting and clot breakdown, which leads to internal hemorrhage. In some cases, the fetus or newborn may also show signs of distress.

Multi-Organ Dysfunction Syndrome (MODS)

The incremental process by which multiple organs start shutting down individually is called **multiple organ dysfunction syndrome** (**MODS**). It is a process rather than a single event and may take place slowly over the course of days to weeks. Alteration in organ function can vary widely from a mild degree of organ dysfunction to completely irreversible organ failure. The degree of organ dysfunction has a major clinical impact. The Sequential Organ Failure Assessment (SOFA) scoring tool can be used to measure the level of dysfunction across each body system, with higher scores representing a greater risk of mortality.

Events that can lead to the eventual development of MODS include sepsis, trauma, myocardial infarction, and toxic exposures. These events trigger a series of inflammatory reactions and organ damage throughout the body, with the respiratory system often being impacted first. Prevention of MODS centers on avoidance of the initial events associated with the condition. When MODS is suspected, prompt awareness and intervention are key to improving the chance of survival. Treatment of the condition is focused on resolution of the precipitating event and interventions to support the impacted body systems (e.g., respiratory support, blood transfusion, dialysis) as required by the individual clinical presentation.

Obesity-Related Complications

Obesity is a complex condition characterized by excessive body fat, often resulting from a combination of genetic, environmental, and behavioral factors. It is typically diagnosed using the **Body Mass Index** (BMI), a measurement calculated from a person's weight and height. A BMI of thirty or higher indicates obesity. Individuals with obesity will have an increase in body weight, a high waist circumference, and associated health issues such as fatigue, joint pain, and sleep apnea. Obesity significantly raises the risk for numerous health conditions, including type 2 diabetes, cardiovascular disease, certain cancers, and mental health disorders. The patient's medications should be evaluated for those that may be contributing to weight gain, such as gabapentin, antidepressants, or mood stabilizers.

A multidisciplinary approach is required for obesity treatment, often including a primary care provider and dietician as well as physical therapy and mental health counselling. Lifestyle modifications such as a balanced, calorie-controlled diet and regular physical activity are essential first steps, and behavioral therapy may help patients develop healthier habits as well as improve their mental well-being. Prescription medications or weight-loss surgery may be recommended for individuals with severe obesity or for those who have not succeeded using lifestyle changes alone. Regular follow up and support are crucial for long-term success in managing obesity and its associated health risks.

Acute and Chronic Pain

Pain has been called the fifth vital sign and is an important clue as to how well the patient is doing. Pain is the most frequent reason patients seek medical care. Pain has sensory and emotional components and is classified as acute or chronic. **Acute pain** is frequently associated with anxiety and hyperactivity of the sympathetic nervous system (tachycardia, increased respiratory rate and BP, diaphoresis, dilated pupils). **Chronic pain** does not involve sympathetic hyperactivity, but may be associated with vegetative signs and depressed mood.

People vary considerably in their tolerance for pain. However, the severity of tissue injury does not always predict the severity of chronic or acute pain. Chronic pain may also result from ongoing damage to or dysfunction of the peripheral or central nervous system, which then causes neuropathic pain.

Somatic pain receptors are located in skin, subcutaneous tissues, fascia, other connective tissues, periosteum, endosteum, and joint capsules. Stimulation of these receptors usually produces sharp or dull localized pain, but burning is not uncommon if the skin or subcutaneous tissues are involved. Visceral pain receptors are located in most viscera and the surrounding connective tissue. Visceral pain due to obstruction of a hollow organ is poorly localized, deep, and cramping and may be referred to remote cutaneous sites. Visceral pain due to injury of organs or other deep connective tissues may be more localized and feel sharp.

Thoughts and emotions have an important role in the perception of pain. Many patients who have chronic pain also have psychologic distress, especially depression and anxiety. Because certain syndromes characterized as psychiatric are defined by self-reported pain, patients with poorly explained pain are often mischaracterized as having a psychiatric disorder and are thus deprived of appropriate care. Pain impairs attention, memory, concentration, and content of thought.

The common measure of pain is the pain scale, rated one to ten. The nurse assess pain by asking the patient what aggravates the pain, alleviates it, the location, quality, and onset. The nurse should ask about when exacerbations occur, what signs and symptoms accompany an exacerbation, how the pain affects overall functioning ability, how intense it becomes, and its temporal characteristics.

A simple tool to determine what type of medication is helpful for different pain levels is the World Health Organization ladder:

Step 1. Mild pain (intensity 1 to 3): acetaminophen; NSAIDS; adjuvant medications, such as tricyclic antidepressants and muscle relaxants

Step 2. Moderate pain (4 to 6 intensity): combination opioids, such as hydrocodone and acetaminophen or oxycodone and acetaminophen, plus continued adjuvant drugs

Step 3. Severe pain (7 to 10 intensity): opioids, such as morphine and hydromorphone, plus continued adjuvant drugs.

Rhabdomyolysis

A breakdown of the skeletal muscle that causes the release of muscle contents into the bloodstream is called **rhabdomyolysis**. Myoglobin is the skeletal muscle content that is leaked and can be detected in elevated levels in the urine. Diagnosis is made based on symptoms and urinalysis. Rhabdomyolysis may occur for many different reasons, any of which include an insult to the muscle tissue that causes its breakdown. Among the common reasons for the development of rhabdomyolysis are crush injuries, severe burns, cocaine use with hyperthermia, extreme physical activity such as heavy eccentric weight training or marathon training, drug and/or alcohol intoxication, a prolonged comatose state, falls in the elderly followed by prolonged lying on the ground, and prolonged seizures.

A patient with rhabdomyolysis may be asymptomatic. If symptoms do present, they may include muscle pain or myalgia, stiffness, and weakness. The patient's urine may become a dark amber, resembling the color of cola. Rhabdomyolysis may progress quickly to kidney failure. The kidneys have trouble processing myoglobin and begin to shut down as a result. Rhabdomyolysis may also lead to compartment syndrome, where muscle swelling and rising pressure within a confined space compromises the blood circulation to the area. The lower leg is often the site of compartment syndrome.

Treatment of rhabdomyolysis depends on the underlying cause. IV fluid resuscitation will likely be used to flush out the toxic muscle contents and prevent further damage. Electrolytes may be replaced if they are imbalanced. If there is underlying muscle disease, this must be treated. The case is much more complicated if kidney failure has occurred, making early detection crucial to preventing damage to the kidneys.

The Sepsis Continuum

In the case of **systemic inflammatory response syndrome**, or **SIRS**, two or more criteria must be met: a temperature of greater than 38 degrees Celsius or less than 36 degrees Celsius; a pulse of greater than 90 beats per minute; a respiratory rate of greater than 20 breaths per minute; or a white blood cell count of greater than 12,000. Two or more of these criteria being met in a critically ill patient would suggest that a systemic inflammatory response has begun, and potential complications may be ahead. SIRS is the first step in a continuum of worsening illness.

The next stage after SIRS is **sepsis**, in which criteria for SIRS has been met and there is a known source of infection. Severe sepsis follows when sepsis is present along with organ dysfunction and/or hypotensive crisis. **Septic shock** occurs when severe sepsis is present, hypotension is unresponsive to fluid resuscitation, and hypoperfusion abnormalities are present. Lactic acidosis, oliguria, and altered mental status are examples of hypoperfusion abnormalities. Multiple organ dysfunction syndrome, or MODS, is the final step in the continuum, with evidence of more than two organs failing. Treatment of the continuum of SIRS to MODS includes fluid resuscitation, blood cultures to identify the source of infection, empirical antibiotics to fight infection, vasopressors for hypotensive support, lactate level measurements, and central venous pressure measurement.

The Sepsis Continuum

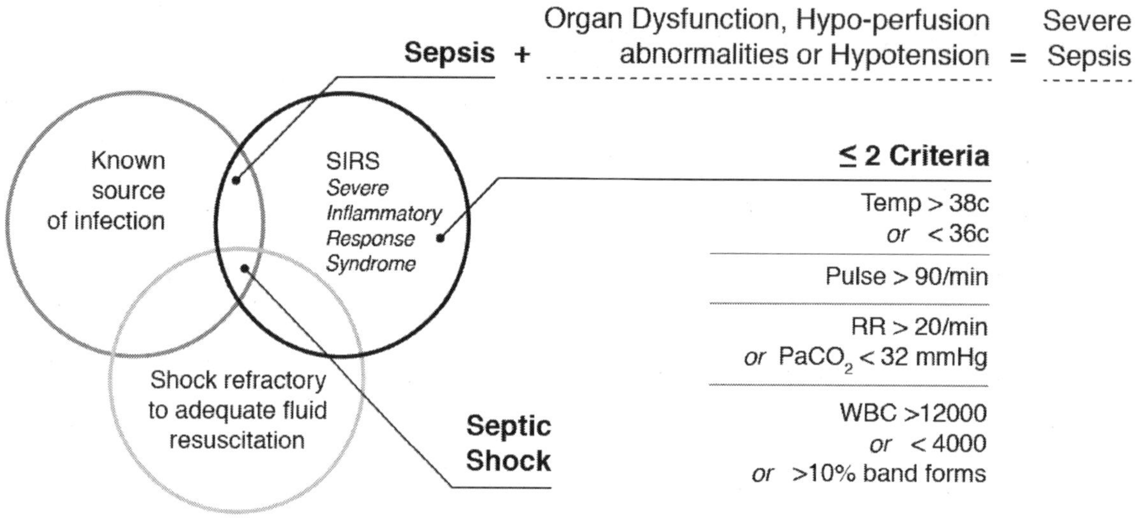

Shock States

Shock occurs in the body when the blood pressure suddenly falls, and perfusion is lost to the vital organs. Shock patients will often present with tachycardia, tachypnea, hypotension, altered mental status, and oliguria.

Distributive

Distributive shock is a type of hypotensive crisis in which the vascular smooth muscle is no longer vasoconstricting but massively vasodilating, resulting in dropped pressures systemically. The vascular bed is not responsive to vasoconstrictive agents. Fluid resuscitation may be occurring, but hypotension persists with mixed venous oxygen saturations. This type of shock may occur because of an anaphylactic response in the body after exposure to an allergen. An injury to the brain or spinal cord may also result in distributive shock, referred to as neurogenic.

To treat distributive shock, an ICU admission is necessary. Constant hemodynamic monitoring, measurement of intake and output, respiratory support, and possible endotracheal intubation are all types of intervention for stabilizing the patient. Discovering the underlying cause of distributive shock and reversing it is a priority.

Hypovolemic

Patients who are dehydrated or have lost massive amounts of blood from injury may progress into **hypovolemic shock**. If bleeding is the cause, it must be stopped as soon as possible. Concurrent with efforts to stop hemorrhaging, fluid resuscitation is performed to raise the patient's blood pressure and bring vital oxygen to the organs and tissues of the body.

Losing more than twenty percent of the body's total blood volume is considered life-threatening and will likely throw the body into hypovolemic shock. Organ failure will follow profound hypotension as the heart struggles to compensate for the blood loss. Conditions that may dehydrate the body and cause a significant loss of blood volume include severe burns, prolonged diarrhea, excessive vomiting, and excessive sweating. Treatment for hypovolemic shock will be correction of underlying cause, vasoactive drugs, and most importantly, fluid resuscitation.

Sleep Disruptions

Poor sleep is a common issue among all patients in the hospital, with those admitted in ICU care being no exception. The physical challenges of pain and discomfort stemming from a patient's serious condition and treatment interventions make it difficult to achieve quality sleep. Additionally, the environment of the ICU often involves bright lights, beeping alarms, and frequent assessments that disrupt the patient's ability to rest. Not only does this impact their ability to physically heal from illness or injury, the mental and emotional effects of poor sleep can lead to the development of anxiety and delirium. While some interruptions to sleep are unavoidable, healthcare workers in the ICU can work to support a restorative environment when possible. Members of the interdisciplinary care team can be encouraged to round together to both improve communication between providers and decrease interruptions for the patient. Specific interventions that can foster a quality sleep environment include dimming lights when appropriate, limiting extraneous noise near the patient's room, implementing quiet times when visiting hours are restricted, and bundling of care interventions to minimize the number of disruptions.

Submersion Injuries (Near-Drowning)

Submersion is defined as the condition of being placed under the surface of a fluid medium. A **near-drowning** experience is one that results in the survival of a living organism for at least 24 hours after submersion under water or other liquid. Hypoxemia and asphyxiation are main concerns, as these result in widespread cell and organ damage. Brain cells sustain permanent impairment after four to six minutes of submersion, and cardiac arrest is another complication that is considered a direct consequence of hypoxemia. Aspiration pneumonia, although rare, is nevertheless an outcome when the submersion occurs in stagnant and warm fresh water. Uncommon bacteria that reside in these types of waters may cause the pneumonia as well as other categories of infections in the lungs, sinuses, and CNS. Hypothermia is another issue to consider if submersion was prolonged and occurred in water that was below freezing temperatures.

Infants and very young children are at increased susceptibility to near-drownings and actual drownings, as their muscle strength is still developing, and they often cannot hold themselves or their heads up and out of water. Babies have been known to drown in an inch or less of water; this usually occurs in the bathtub when a caregiver has left the room for just a matter of seconds.

The prognosis after a near-drowning is primarily based on the length of time an individual was submerged, the age of the individual, the degree of contamination in the fluid medium, the temperature of the medium, the symptoms displayed after the submersion, and any underlying comorbidities. Other factors include the timing of the resuscitative efforts and the physical and mental response of the victim to those efforts. The outcome may be hopeful if the submersion was five minutes or less and the person shows positive neurological responsiveness, reactive pupils, and normal cardiac rhythm. An individual, especially a child, who has been submerged for 10 minutes or more and does not respond to cardiopulmonary resuscitation (CPR) within a half hour after submersion has an extremely unfortunate prognosis, consisting of either severe neurological damage, death, or both.

A patient presenting to the emergency department who is symptomatic after a submersion injury will demonstrate altered vital signs (decreased core body temperature, tachycardia, or bradycardia), altered level of consciousness, anxiety, wheezing, and coughing. Medical interventions for an individual who has suffered a submersion injury focus on immediate adequate ventilation, as the primary target organ of submersion is the lungs (endotracheal intubation and mechanical ventilation may be necessary), circulatory support, temperature management, and close and continual assessment of neurological condition while awaiting a bed in the intensive care unit (ICU). If the individual does not exhibit unprompted, purposeful extremity mobility and normal brain stem function 24 hours after the incident, it is highly likely he or she has sustained serious neurological sequelae. Tests including ABGs, CBC, electrolyte levels, and renal function will be done to determine the level of multisystem organ involvement, as well as chest x-rays, CT, and ECG for a patient who has a significant cardiac history.

Outpatient care is determined by the characteristics and level of residual functional neurological impairment. Rehabilitative attention for one who has suffered severe neurological injury after submersion will revolve around frequent physical, occupational, and speech therapies. Neurosurgical and orthopedic consultation will most likely be necessary for those patients suffering significant head or neck damage. After initial recuperation, an individual may experience non-pulmonary issues, such as osteomyelitis and brain abscesses. Surgical consultation may be required for such conditions, as they sometimes don't respond to antibiotic or antimicrobial therapy alone. Medication therapy that is effective after recovery may include an inhaled beta-agonist bronchodilator, such as albuterol, which relaxes smooth muscles in the bronchi of the lungs.

Thermoregulation

The body maintains a healthy temperature through a process called **thermoregulation**. Homeostatic adjustments involved in thermoregulation include sweating to stay cool and shivering to stay warm. Healthy human temperature is somewhere near 98 degrees Fahrenheit or 37 degrees Celsius, though this may vary by a degree or so from individual to individual.

Colder than normal body temperature is called hypothermia and warmer than normal body temperature is called hyperthermia or fever. Either condition, if prolonged, may lead to death if left uncorrected. Drug and alcohol use, and hypothyroidism may lead to hypothermia, while digestion, fever, and exercise may cause hyperthermia. Exposure to extreme heat or cold in the environment can lead to hypo- or hyperthermia.

Toxic Ingestion and Inhalations

Any chemical that can cause harm to the body when ingested or inhaled is considered toxic. Exhaust fumes from cars, lead in drinking water, asbestos in old buildings, and pesticides on plants can all cause harm to the body if ingested or inhaled. Ingestion occurs through eating or swallowing the substance, which then travels through the body's GI tract and is absorbed into the circulatory system from the small intestine. Short-term effects produce symptoms such as headaches and vomiting, while long-term effects could include cancer and other disease states. Substances that are inhaled travel through the airways, into the lungs, and are absorbed into the circulation through the pulmonary capillary beds.

Treatment of toxic ingestions depends on the toxic substance ingested. Stomach pumping and administration of activated charcoal may be necessary to rid the body of the toxin. Activated charcoal works by absorbing the toxin before the body gets a chance to, decreasing its toxic effects.

Overdose

The definition of an **overdose**, in simplest terms, involves consumption of a dangerously high amount of something. Drug overdoses may be through accidental overuse or intentional misuse. Illicit drugs, which are used to achieve or maintain a euphoric state, may be used hazardously when the body's metabolism cannot detoxify the substance rapidly enough to avoid unplanned side effects.

Accidental overdoses normally occur either with very young children or elderly adults. Young children, as discussed previously, are curious and at a developmental stage when everything goes into their mouths. The elderly are usually coping with failing vision and memory impairment, so they may misread the directions on a bottle or retake something they've already taken. Adolescents and adults are most likely to overdose on one or more substances, either illicit or prescribed, for the purpose of intentionally harming themselves.

Drug overdose symptoms vary with the type of drug taken, but typically they reflect a heightened level of the therapeutic effects seen with prescribed use. In an overdose, the anticipated side effects are more distinct, and other effects that would not normally occur with recommended usage will appear. Vital signs will be erratic (pulse, respirations), mental state will most likely be altered (confusion, intense sleepiness, stupor), angina (chest pain) is possible if overdose caused heart or lung damage, and GI symptoms, such as nausea and vomiting, may be apparent.

Some commonly-abused drugs include (but are not limited to) the following:

- Barbiturates: Sedatives like Nembutal® and Seconal®, which are usually prescribed to manage anxiety, panic attacks, and insomnia
- Benzodiazepines: Sedatives such as Valium® and Xanax®, used to manage anxiety and panic attacks
- Sleep medications: Ambien®, Lunesta®, Sonata®
- Opioids: Pain management drugs such as codeine, morphine, Oxycontin®, Percocet®, and Percodan®
- Opioids plus acetaminophen for pain management: Vicodin®, Lortab®, Lorcet®
- Amphetamines: Stimulants like Adderall® and Dexedrine®; also known as *speed*
- Dextromethorphan (DXM): Common ingredient in OTC medications normally used for cough and other cold symptoms; effective when administered in the correct dosage, but too much causes a euphoric state and hallucinations.
- Pseudoephedrine: Common ingredient in OTC decongestants; it is also a main component of methamphetamine ("meth") and, for this reason, is stored behind the pharmacist's counter.

Illicit drug (marijuana, cocaine, heroin) use is at an all-time high, and abuse of one or more of these can lead to detrimental, if not fatal, effects. The youth of America seem especially vulnerable to the risk of overdose of illegal substances, as they are still physically and psychologically developing. Marijuana continues to be the most commonplace prohibited drug used by young people, while cocaine and heroin overdose-related events seem to be chiefly among adults in their mid-to-late thirties.

Practice Quiz

1. The nurse in the perioperative unit is caring for a 26-year-old female patient with abnormal uterine bleeding. Which of the following tests does the nurse anticipate will be obtained first?
   a. Pap smear
   b. Uterine biopsy
   c. Pelvic ultrasonography
   d. Pregnancy test

2. While completing an assessment on a patient with a gastrointestinal illness that has caused several days of diarrhea, which acid-base imbalance secondary to changes in electrolyte status does the medical-surgical nurse expect to note on the laboratory results?
   a. Metabolic Alkalosis
   b. Metabolic Acidosis
   c. Respiratory Alkalosis
   d. Respiratory Acidosis

3. When assessing a pregnant woman at 24 weeks gestation, which early manifestation would alert the nurse to a possible diagnosis of preeclampsia?
   a. Hypertension on bedrest
   b. Facial edema
   c. Increasing liver enzymes
   d. Thrombocytopenia

4. The nurse is caring for a patient with pneumonia that she believes may be starting to show symptoms of septic shock. What findings support a septic shock diagnosis? Select all that apply.
   a. Metabolic acidosis
   b. Respiratory alkalosis
   c. Narrowing pulse pressure
   d. Increased cardiac output
   e. Hypertension

5. A patient overdosed on acetaminophen after retrieving it from their visitor's purse during visiting hours. While providing emergent care with the code response team, which medication should the nurse administer to counteract the effects of this poisoning?
   a. Atropine
   b. Acetylcysteine
   c. Naloxone
   d. Flumazenil

See answers on the next page.

Answer Explanations

1. D: A pregnancy test is performed first to determine if the patient is pregnant. A Pap smear, uterine biopsy, and pelvic ultrasound may be performed, based on the patient's history and physical findings, but they would not be the first test performed, making *A*, *B*, and *C* incorrect answers.

2. B: Choice *B* is often assessed in the patient who has been experiencing diarrhea. Metabolic acidosis can also be witnessed in renal failure, diabetic ketoacidosis, and aspirin overdose. Choice *A* is seen with vomiting and the overuse of antacids. Choice *C* is observed with hypoxia, fever, and hyperventilation. Choice *D* is witnessed secondary to airway obstruction and pulmonary edema.

3. B: Early manifestations of preeclampsia include hypertension, facial edema, visual disturbances, altered mental state, dyspnea, and possible right upper quadrant pain. Severe manifestations include seizure activity, increasing liver enzymes with increased pain, thrombocytopenia, progressive renal dysfunction, and pulmonary edema, making Choices *A*, *C*, and *D* incorrect answers.

4. A, B: During septic shock, metabolic acidosis and respiratory alkalosis are expected findings, along with a symptom presentation of shortness of breath, temperature changes, confusion, and diaphoresis. Thus, Choices *A* and *B* are correct. Choice *C* is incorrect, as the patient would likely experience a widening pulse pressure, not one that is narrowing. Choice *D* is incorrect, as the patient would display a decreased cardiac output. Choice *E* is incorrect, as the patient would typically present with hypotension in this case.

5. B: Choice *B* should be administered to the patient to counteract the effects of the acetaminophen overdose. Choices *A*, *C*, and *D*, while all antidotes for a variety of medications, would not prove effective in reversing the progression of acetaminophen poisoning.

Professional Caring & Ethical Practice

Ethical principles are the basis for personal and professional behavior. While generally moral behavior based on ethical principles is required from all individuals in a society, nurses are held to a more stringent standard for professional practice. Professionally, nurses are responsible for applying ethical principles to the care of patients and to the support of novice nurses as they develop their own professional identity.

Advocacy/Moral Agency

The American Nurses Association (ANA) provides this definition of nursing practice: "The protection, promotion, and optimization of health and abilities; prevention of illness and injury; facilitation of healing; alleviation of suffering through the diagnosis and treatment of human response; and advocacy in the care of individuals, families, communities, and populations." The ANA also addresses the importance of advocacy in its Code of Ethics, specifically in Provision 3: "The nurse promotes, advocates for, and protects the rights, health, and safety of the patient." The ANA Code of Ethics further states: nurses must advocate "with compassion and respect for the inherent dignity, worth, and uniqueness of every individual, unrestricted by considerations of social or economic status, personal attributes, or the nature of health problems."

Advocacy is a key component of nursing practice. An **advocate** is one who pleads the cause of another; and the nurse is an advocate for patient rights. Preserving human dignity, patient equality, and freedom from suffering are the basis of nursing advocacy. Nurses hold a significant role that gives them the opportunity to care for patients in every way: meeting their needs, addressing concerns, and working to achieve positive outcomes. Additionally, they aid in communicating with physicians while and serve as a guide through the complexities of the medical system. Nurses educate the patient about tests and procedures, while maintaining awareness of how culture and ethnicity affect the patient's experience. Throughout the process, nurses strictly adhere to all privacy laws.

Advocacy is the promotion of the common good, especially as it applies to at-risk populations. It involves speaking out in support of policies and decisions that affect the lives of individuals who do not otherwise have a voice. Nurses meet this standard of practice by actively participating in the politics of healthcare accessibility and delivery. They are educationally and professionally prepared to evaluate and comment on the needs of patients at the local, state, and national level. This participation requires an understanding of the legislative process, the ability to negotiate with public officials, and a willingness to provide expert testimony in support of policy decisions. The advocacy role of nurses has the potential to address the needs of the individual patient, society, and members of the nursing profession.

In clinical practice, nurses represent the patient's interests through active participation in the development of the plan of care and subsequent care decisions. Advocacy, in this sense, is related to patient autonomy and the patient's right to informed consent and self-determination. Nurses provide the appropriate information, assess the patient's comprehension of the implications of the care decisions, and act as patient advocates by supporting the patient's decisions. In the critical care environment, patient advocacy requires the nurse to represent the patient's decisions even though those decisions may be opposed to those of the healthcare providers and family members.

Professionally, nurses advocate for policies that support and promote the practice of all nurses regarding access to education, role identity, workplace conditions, and compensation. The responsibility for professional advocacy requires nurses to provide leadership in the development of the professional nursing role in all practice settings that may include acute care facilities, colleges and universities, or community agencies. Leadership roles in acute care settings involve participation in professional practice and shared governance committees, providing support for basic nursing education by facilitating clinical and preceptorship experiences, and mentoring novice graduate nurses to the professional nursing role. In the academic setting, nurses work to ensure the diversity of the student population by participating in the governance structure of the institution, conducting and publishing research that supports the positive impact of professional nursing care on patient outcomes, and serving as an advocate to individual nursing students to promote their academic success. In the community, nurses may collaborate with government officials to meet the needs that are specific to that location.

The nurse must function as a **moral agent**. This means that the nurse must be morally accountable and responsible for personal judgment and actions. **Moral agency** is defined as the ability to identify right and wrong actions based on widely accepted moral criteria. The performance of nurses as moral agents is dependent on life experiences, advanced education, and clinical experience in healthcare agencies. Moral agency can often be difficult to decipher when managing complex patient situations. When ethical dilemmas arise, such as handling end-of-life and refusal of treatment cases, the care team must work together to make the best care decisions possible with the patient in mind.

The role of moral agent requires nurses to have a strong sense of self and a clear understanding of the definition of right and wrong; however, nurses must also be aware that these perceptions of right and wrong will be challenged every day. The nurse can expect to encounter difficult situations where the moral action related to the patient's right to self-determination is opposed to the moral action with respect to competent patient care.

Caring Practices

The introduction of nursing processes in the 1970s led to the development of nursing models in the 1990s. Generally, there are three components to a **nursing model**: a set of core beliefs and values, a statement of the goals the nurse is trying to achieve, and the knowledge and skills the nurse needs to practice (Pearson et al, 1996). In 1995 Fawcett explained that all nursing models have four central concepts: Person (the recipient of all nursing actions); Environment (the recipient's specific surroundings); Health (wellness or illness state of the recipient); and Nursing (actions taken by nurses on behalf of or in conjunction with a recipient).

On the following page are a few of the more recent, and perhaps best known, nursing models.

The 5 C's of Caring

The **5 C's of caring** is a concept developed by Sister Simone Roach in 2002. Roach stated that nurses consistently applying the five C's in the workplace can lead to improved work relationships, improved patient relationships, and increased likelihood of career advancement.

1. Commitment: dedicated to going above and beyond normally expected behaviors; pledging to uphold the values; and commitment to pursuing life-long career learning that will enhance the level of care delivered to patients.

2. Conscience: a sense of moral responsibility resulting from a strong conscience; working consistently on another's behalf and representing the concerns of the patient; continued focus on empathy and putting oneself in the patient's shoes.

3. Competence: consistently arriving to work on time; presenting a professional manner; holding self to a high standard of excellence when fulfilling daily tasks; asking for help or clarification when there is uncertainty about a specific duty or method; continually improving skills to develop competence.

4. Compassion: empathize with patients; provide kind and considerate treatment at all times. In return, nurses may receive an inspirational sense of human connection and confirmation of the meaning of their work.

5. Confidence: confidence ties the other 4 of the 5 C's together. It takes confidence in skills and knowledge to act with commitment, follow conscience, constantly act in a competent manner, and express compassion, even in the most challenging circumstances. A confident nurse can assist others who are dealing with difficult news. A strong sense of self will summon positive change in patient care.

Family-Focused Care (Shelton and Stepanek, 1994)

1. Recognizing that the family is the constant in the patient's life while the service systems and personnel within those systems fluctuate

2. Being aware of family strengths and individuality and having respect for different methods of coping

3. Encouraging and facilitating family-to-family support and networking

4. Sharing complete and unbiased information about the patient's care with family members on a continuing basis in a supportive manner

5. Designing accessible healthcare delivery systems that are flexible, culturally competent, and responsive to family needs

The Needs of the Critical Care Family (Molter, 1997)

1. To have questions answered honestly

2. To know specific facts regarding what is wrong with the patient and their progress

3. To know the prognosis/outcome/chance of recovery

4. To be called at home about changes

5. To receive information once a day

6. To receive information and understandable explanations

7. To believe the hospital personnel care about the patient

8. To have hope

9. To know exactly what and why things are being done to the patient

10. To have reassurance that the best possible care is being given to the patient

The Synergy Model for Patient Care

The American Association of Critical-Care Nurses developed their Synergy Model for Patient Care in 1996 as a new framework for AACN's certification programs. The **Synergy Model** shifted the assessment of nursing skills from the then-prevalent body systems/medical model, which didn't consistently match actual practice, to a "nurse competencies" framework. The central idea of the model is that synergy results when the needs and characteristics of a patient, clinical unit, or system are matched with a nurse's competencies. A patient's needs drive the nurse competencies required for patient care.

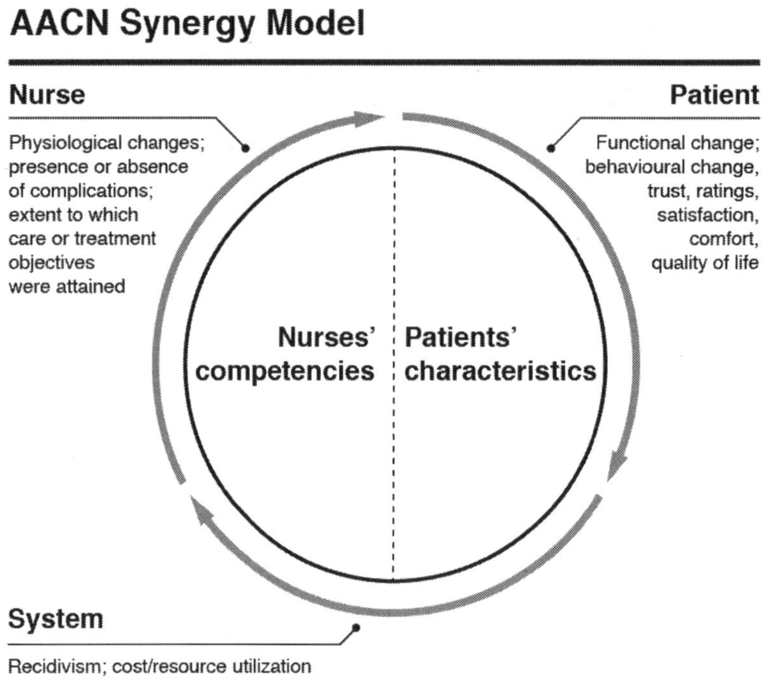

There are five assumptions that guide the AACN Synergy Model of Nursing:

1. Patients are biological, psychological, social, and spiritual entities who present at a particular developmental stage. The whole patient must be considered.

2. The patient, family, and community all contribute to providing a context for the nurse-patient relationship.

3. Patients can be described by a number of characteristics, and all characteristics are connected and contribute to each other. Characteristics cannot be looked at in isolation.

4. Nurses can be described on a number of dimensions, and the interrelated dimensions create a profile of the nurse.

5. A goal of nursing is to restore a patient to an optimal level of wellness as defined by the patient. Death can be an acceptable outcome, in which the goal of nursing is to move the patient toward a peaceful death.

The Synergy Model also identifies the following 8 patient characteristics and 8 nurse competencies. Each of these can be evaluated on a continuum of 1-5.

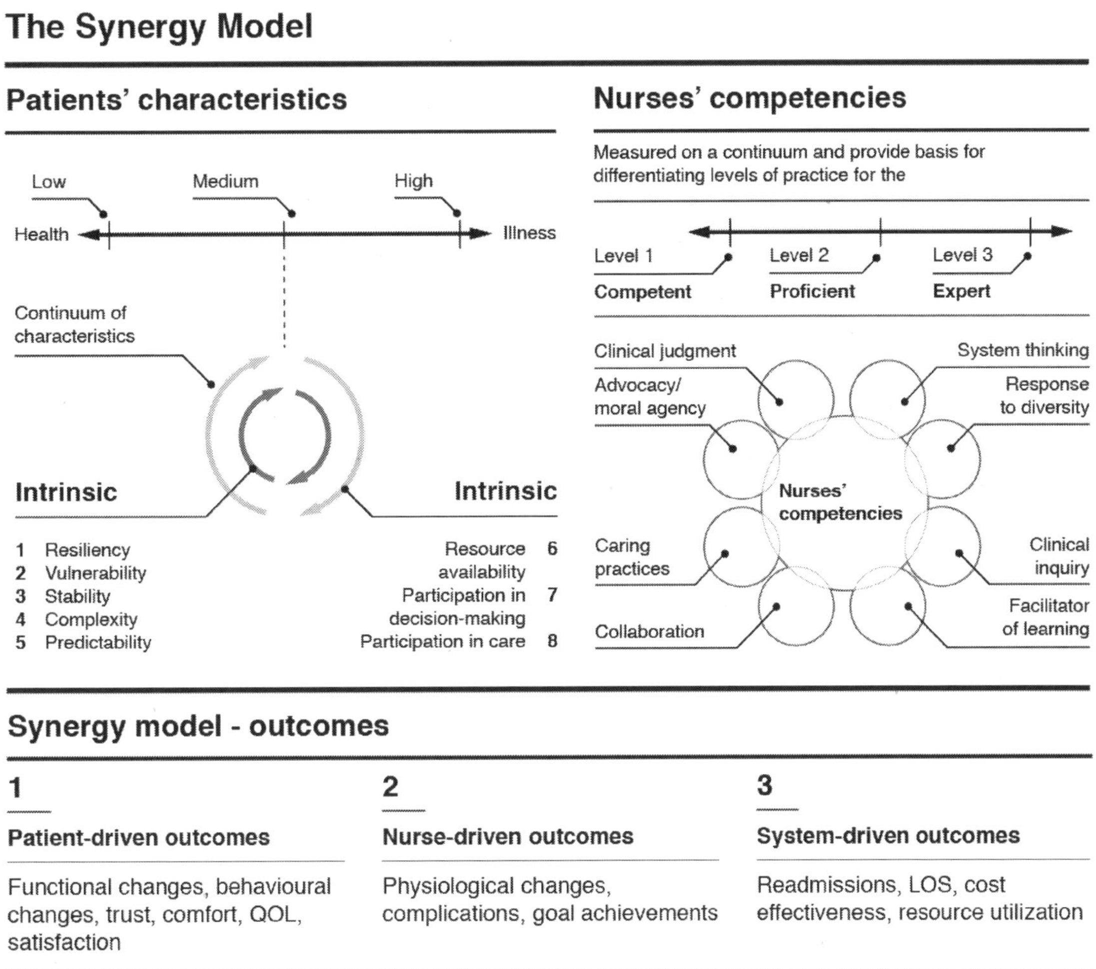

The American Hospital Association's Patient Care Partnership Document

Although not a nursing care model, **The American Hospital Association's Patient Care Partnership Document** produced in 2005 mandated a decision-making partnership between the healthcare system and the patient, facilitating patients' efforts to determine their own future. This decision-making partnership highlighted the responsibilities of the healthcare system to fully communicate treatment options and the plan of care, mandating a change in care patterns and nursing practices.

The model identifies vigilance and engagement as essential elements. Vigilance as a caring skill is viewed on a continuum according to the ability of nurses to recognize and respond to patient needs. Novice nurses are capable of responding to usual and predictable changes in the patient's condition; however, responding to more subtle cues requires an increased level of clinical competence, and preventing any potential hazards requires even greater nursing skill. Engagement in the nurse-patient relationship refers to the degree to which nurses commit to the relationship. Researchers note that favorable patient outcomes are associated with the degree of caregiver engagement; however, there is also evidence that the incidence of burnout in experienced nurses is related to the degree of their engagement in patient care. The third attribute of the caring practices is responsiveness, which means that the reaction of the patient's family, the healthcare institution, and the nursing staff will all have an effect on the patient's progress.

Clinical Inquiry

Clinical inquiry is an ongoing process that evaluates and challenges clinical practice in order to propose the needed change. Clinical inquiry has several components or attributes, including critical thinking, clinical reasoning, clinical judgment, critical reasoning and judgment, and creative thinking. The process is viewed as the critical structure for the establishment of evidence-based practice and quality improvement efforts. In the Synergy Model, professional nurses employ clinical inquiry to innovate and facilitate interventions that are appropriate to patient care needs. Clinical inquiry is a rigorous process that requires attention to the rules of nursing research, such as attention to sample size, and a correct match among the data, the study design, and the statistical measures.

When used to implement evidenced based practice, clinical inquiry can result in replacing an outdated, even counter-productive nursing intervention with an intervention that effectively addresses the needs of the patient. Nurses who are involved in this form of clinical inquiry are viewed as evaluators and innovators in the Synergy Model. Matching patient needs with nursing competencies means that professional nurses are responsible for challenging all nursing interventions to be sure that they represent current best practice standards. As innovators, nurses are in the best position to research, implement, and evaluate alternative care practices.

Nurses acquire clinical inquiry skills on a continuum that is based on education and clinical experience. As is the case with the other nursing competencies included in the Synergy Model, this progressive development is consistent with **Benner's Novice to Expert model** that views the development of nursing expertise as a progressive process that requires ongoing education and clinical experience. Novice nurses are able to implement clinical innovations developed by others, identify their own learning needs, and enlist the aid of other nurses to identify critical needs of the patient.

Experienced nurses are able to question the adequacy of interventions and challenge the "we have always done it this way" philosophy that is the most common rationale for many nursing interventions. They are also able to assess the utility of alternative interventions. The Synergy Model views the practice of expert nurses as the point at which clinical inquiry and clinical reasoning become inseparable elements of clinical practice. Expert nurses are able to predict changes in the patient's condition that require revision of the plan of care, and they are also able to develop and implement alternative approaches to address those changes.

Public funds are the most common source of research funding, which means that researchers are obligated to design studies that provide valid results that are applicable to some form of patient care and to disseminate the results appropriately. Common barriers to nursing research efforts include inadequate funding, limited access to appropriate patient populations, and lack of institutional support for research initiatives. The rapid expansion of new knowledge from multiple sources can also inhibit the assimilation and application of new care interventions by expert nurses. In addition, the final step of the clinical inquiry process, knowledge translation or dissemination, may be the most important step.

Knowledge translation refers to the complex process of synthesizing the research findings, disseminating those findings to others, and integrating the findings into clinical practice. Barriers to this process include lack of rigor in the original research design with respect to sample size, data interpretation, and the applicability of the research findings. The failure of nursing researchers to access all possible modes of the dissemination of study results has also been identified as a significant barrier to the application of new interventions. All of these system-wide and individual barriers potentially limit the use of innovative patient care interventions.

Collaboration

The integration of physical and mental healthcare is an important aspect of the Medical Home, also known as the Medicaid health home model. The model shows collaborative care programs as an approach to integration in which primary care providers, care managers, and psychiatric consultants work together to provide care and monitor patient progress. These programs have been shown to be both clinically-effective and cost-effective for a variety of mental health conditions, in a variety of settings, using several different payment mechanisms.

Some of the benefits of collaboration include improved patient outcomes, decreased healthcare costs, decreased length of stay, improved patient and nurse satisfaction, and improved teamwork. Collaboration related to patient care has been widely studied and is considered as both a process and an outcome, which occurs when no single individual is able to solve a patient problem. **Collaboration** as a process is defined as a synthesis of diverse opinions and skills that is employed to solve complex problems. As an outcome, collaboration is defined as a complex solution to a problem that requires the expertise of more than one individual. This view of collaboration characterizes the process as a series of actions by more than one individual, which creates a solution to a complex problem.

Initially, all members of the collaborative team must identify their own biases and acknowledge the effect of these mental models on the decision-making process. In addition, members must also be aware that the complexity of the problem will be matched by the complexity of the mental models of the collaborative team members, which will influence the decision-making process. It is also essential for team members to recognize the elements of diversity in the group. For instance, while stereotyping is obviously to be avoided, there are gender differences that should be considered.

Research indicates that men tend to be more task oriented, and women tend to be more relationship oriented in the problem-solving process; this means that consideration of both points of view is necessary for genuine collaboration. Another requisite skill of the collaborative team is the development and usage of conflict resolution skills, which are required to counteract this common barrier to effective collaboration. Team members are required to separate the task from the emotions in the discussion. Effective collaboration also requires that members of the team display a cooperative effort that works to create a win/win situation, while recognizing that collaboration is a series of activities that require time and patience for satisfactory completion.

Common barriers to effective collaboration include conflicting professional opinions, ineffective communication related to the conflict, and incomplete assessment of the required elements of the care plan. Research indicates that physicians tend to stress cure-related activities while nurses tend to encourage care-related activities. This means that some resolution of these differences is required for effective communication. Although the Synergy Model defines collaboration as a necessary part of the process that matches the patient needs with the appropriate nursing competencies, it is also possible that the end product may be the best solution for the patient and at the same time be totally unacceptable to the patient. Collaborative team members should also be aware that while successful collaboration improves patient outcomes, research indicates that genuine collaborative efforts are rarely noted in patient care, often because the group is unable to integrate the diverse mental models of the group members.

Facilitation of Learning

Facilitation of learning refers to the process of assessing the learning needs of the patient and family, the nursing staff, and caregivers in the community, and creating, implementing, and evaluating formal and informal educational programs to address those needs. Novice nurses often view patient care and patient education as separate entities; however, experienced nurses are able to integrate the patient's educational needs into the plan of care. Nurses are aware that the patient often requires continued reinforcement of the educational plan after discharge, which necessitates coordination with home care services.

As facilitators of learning, nurses may be involved in a large-scale effort to educate all patients over 65 years of age about the need for both Prevnar 13 and Pneumovax 23 vaccinations to prevent pneumonia. In contrast, nurses may provide one-on-one instruction for a patient recently diagnosed with diabetes. The first step of any teaching-learning initiative is the assessment of the learning needs of the participants. Specific needs that influence the design and content of the educational offering include the language preference and reading level of the participants. Nurses must also consider the effect of certain characteristics, identified in the Synergy Model, on the patient's capacity to process information. Diminished resiliency or stability, as well as extreme complexity, are examples of characteristics that must be considered in the development of the educational plan. Nurses are also responsible for creating a bridge between teaching and learning in the acute care setting and the home environment. A detailed discharge plan, close coordination with outpatient providers, and follow-up phone calls to the patient may be used to reinforce the patient's knowledge of the plan of care.

Successful learning plans for staff members and colleagues also consider the motivation of the participants to engage in the process. Successful facilitators include a variety of teaching strategies to develop the content and evaluate learning, in order to address adult learning needs and preferences, such as preferred language and reading level. Research indicates that when adults do not have a vested interest in the outcomes of the teaching/learning process, they may not participate as active learners.

The remaining element of successful facilitation of learning is the availability and quality of learning resources. There is evidence that individuals with different learning styles respond differently to various learning devices. The minimum requirements for successful facilitation of learning include the skilled staff to develop the educational materials, paper, a copy machine, and staff to interact with the patient in the learning session.

Barriers to the facilitation of learning must be anticipated and accommodated. Changes in the patient's condition commonly require reduction in the time spent in each learning session due to fatigue. Cognitive impairment can impede comprehension and retention of the information and will require appropriate teaching aids. The learning abilities of the patient's family members must also be assessed. Adequate instruction time might be the greatest barrier. Learning needs are assessed, and discharge planning is begun on the day of admission; however, shortened inpatient stays require evaluation of the patient's comprehension of the plan of care.

Response to Diversity

National League for Nursing believes that diversity and quality healthcare are inseparable and together they create a path to increased access, improved health, and elimination of health disparities. **Diversity** signifies that each individual is unique and recognizes individual differences such as race, ethnicity, gender, sexual orientation, gender identity, socio-economic status, age, physical abilities, and religious and/or political beliefs. The result is self-awareness and respect for all persons, embracing and celebrating the richness of each individual. It also encompasses organizational, institutional, and system-wide behaviors in nursing, nursing education, and healthcare.

The Agency for Healthcare Research and Quality (AHRQ) states that healthcare quality remains suboptimal for diverse populations in the United States because some individuals do not receive quality care or believe that their values are honored or respected. The Patient Protection and Affordable Care Act (ACA) of 2010 expanded coverage and improved access to the nation's healthcare system. ACA's creation of subsidies made insurance more affordable and benefited immigrant citizens. The sheer numbers of immigrants coming into the healthcare system create enormous opportunities to provide culturally competent care.

Culture can be defined as the beliefs, values, and social ways of a particular group. These beliefs are generally passed down from generation to generation and can hold influence over one's thoughts and actions. Culture can be the lens that the person uses to view the world, including health and the need for care. Cultural competence of the healthcare workforce and the healthcare delivery system is increasingly tied to improved client outcomes and quality of care provided. **Cultural competence** is the ability to provide effective care for patients who come from different cultures. It requires sensitivity and effective communication in both verbal and non-verbal communication. Financial reimbursement for care provided to clients can be negatively affected if there is not a system in place to support the culturally competent delivery of care.

A culturally-competent clinical nurse will develop an awareness of, and sensitivity to, their own cultural heritage and recognize how their own values and biases may affect patients. The nurse is expected to do the following:

- Demonstrate comfort with cultural differences
- Know specifics about the cultural groups they work with
- Respect and be aware of the unique needs of specific women, men and children
- Understand that diversity exists within and between cultures
- Try to understand other points of view
- Demonstrate flexibility and tolerance, be nonjudgmental
- Maintain a sense of humor
- Demonstrate a willingness to relinquish control
- Promote cultural practices that are potentially helpful

Nurses are aware that unmet cultural or diversity needs and preferences can adversely affect patient outcomes in much the same way that somatic illness affects outcomes. Therefore, cultural sensitivity is an essential nurse competency. The development of cultural sensitivity and demonstrated appreciation of diversity by nurses is also viewed as a continuum in the Synergy Model. Novice nurses, who are learning to negotiate the institutional environment, may assess the patient's preferences but often continue to provide care that is consistent with their own belief system.

As competent nurses gain life and clinical experience, they actively question patients to learn about and accommodate the traditions and customs of a diverse population, while helping the patient and family to understand the culture of the institution. Expert nurses are able to anticipate the needs of the patient and family by integrating cultural differences into the plan of care whenever possible. All of these nursing interventions work to alleviate the stress related to the acute care environment.

Research indicates that diversity in the workplace strengthens the workgroup by allowing consideration of multiple worldviews and a better understanding of the patient population served by the institution. Multiple viewpoints can also be an advantage in conflict resolution, especially when the conflict is related to diversity issues. The Synergy Model suggests that nurses become more sensitive to diversity issues with experience and that this sensitivity is applicable to the work environment as well as direct patient care. Attention to diversity issues also, however, requires institutional support for resource allocation and management. Depending on the specific needs of the patient population, services such as foreign language interpreters, appropriate food service, counseling services, and accommodation for religious observances must be considered. To optimize patient care, expert nurses assess the needs of the patient and family and provide access to the appropriate institutional resources.

Attention to diversity issues requires that providers proceed on the assumption that ethnocentrism is a universal human characteristic that must be addressed by the provision of appropriate information and instruction. In addition to understanding their own cultural views, nurses must be aware that many patients have preconceived views of western cultural norms, which may or may not be accurate, but can potentially affect the nurse-patient relationship. The resolution of ethnocentrism in a caring relationship requires acknowledgment of its existence and education as to the meaning of the traditions and practices.

Systems Thinking

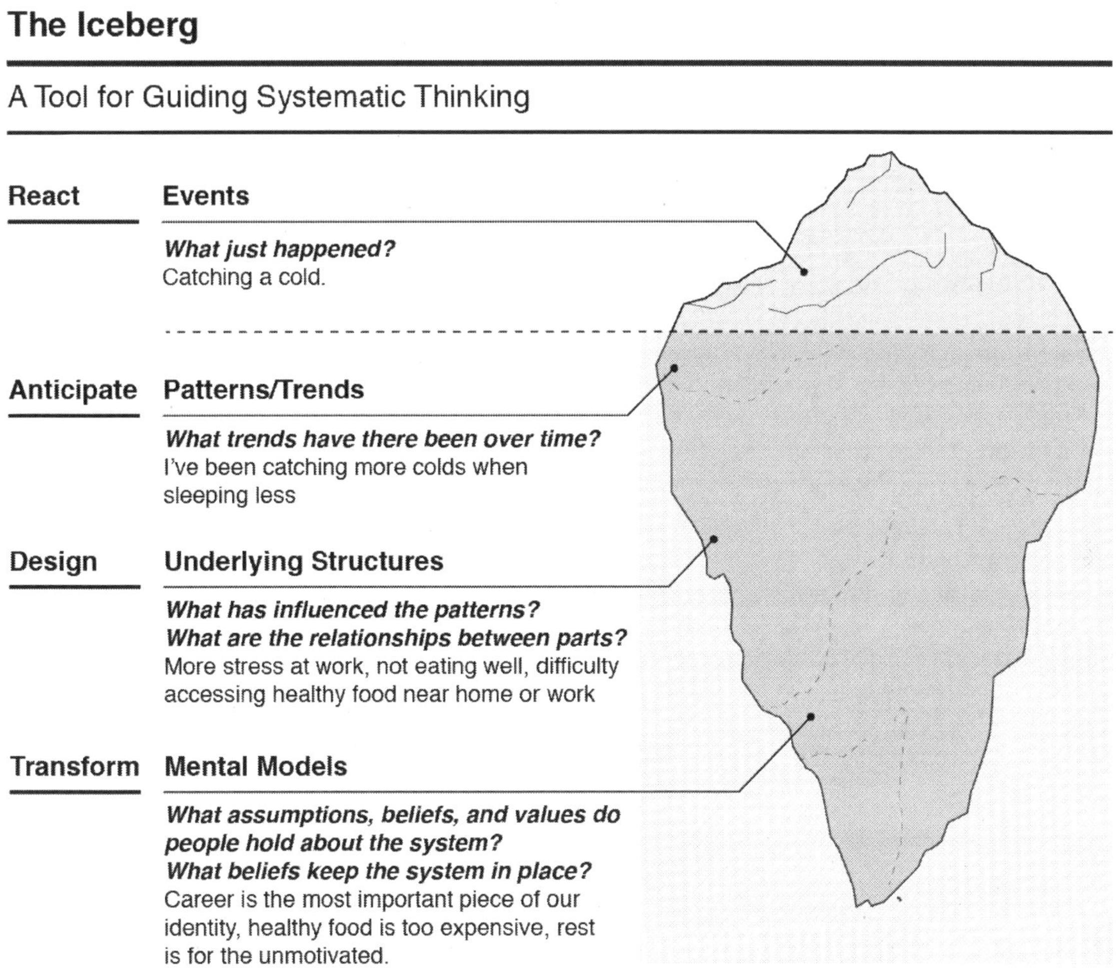

Systems thinking is defined as a link between individuals and their environment. For nurses, this refers to their ability to understand the influence of the healthcare environment on patient outcomes. Systems thinking is identified as the goal of all of the **Quality and Safety Education for Nurses (QESN) competencies**, which are acquired by nurses on a continuum that ranges from the care of the individual patient to the care of the entire patient population.

The QESN competencies were originally identified to improve patient outcomes in response to extensive research that identified a significant difference between the care of patients and the improvement in patient outcomes resulting from that care. The nursing competencies include patient-centered care, evidence-based practice, teamwork and collaboration, safety, quality and improvement, and informatics. Successful interventions associated with each of these criteria for professional nursing practice require the ability to apply the systems thinking approach to care.

Competency related to systems thinking requires appropriate education and clinical experience, and is also identified as one of the nursing competencies in the Synergy Model. In that model, novice nurses view the patient and family as isolated in the nursing unit rather than being influenced by the healthcare system, while experienced nurses are able to integrate all of the resources in the healthcare system to improve patient outcomes. Several of the learning activities designed to improve nurses' ability to acquire systems thinking include creation of a grid that identifies the nursing competencies across the continuum from isolated, individual care to the level of care associated with systems thinking. There are assessment models that apply this exercise to specialty care units such as emergency care, long-term care, and outpatient care, which identify specific systems needs for these areas. Other exercises include tracking unit statistics for the QESN competencies followed by the creation, implementation, and evaluation of a plan that applies systems thinking to address that competency. All of these activities help nurses integrate patient needs with all available resources in order to improve outcomes.

Root cause analysis can also be used as a learning exercise for systems theory because this process, which is commonly used to investigate errors, looks at all elements of an institution's relationship with the error. Case studies and reflection are also recommended as useful learning aids for systems thinking. In addition, there are valid assessment instruments that can be used to assess systems thinking skills acquired through these learning activities.

A **cause-and-effect diagram** examines why something happened or might happen by organizing potential causes into smaller categories. It can also be useful for showing relationships between contributing factors. One of the seven basic tools of quality, it is referred to as a **fishbone diagram** or **Ishikawa diagram**. Although it was originally developed as a quality control tool, the diagram is used in the healthcare setting to discover the root cause of a problem, uncover bottlenecks in a process, or identify where and why a process isn't working. This is called a root cause analysis or a cause-and-effect analysis.

Example of a Root Cause Analysis

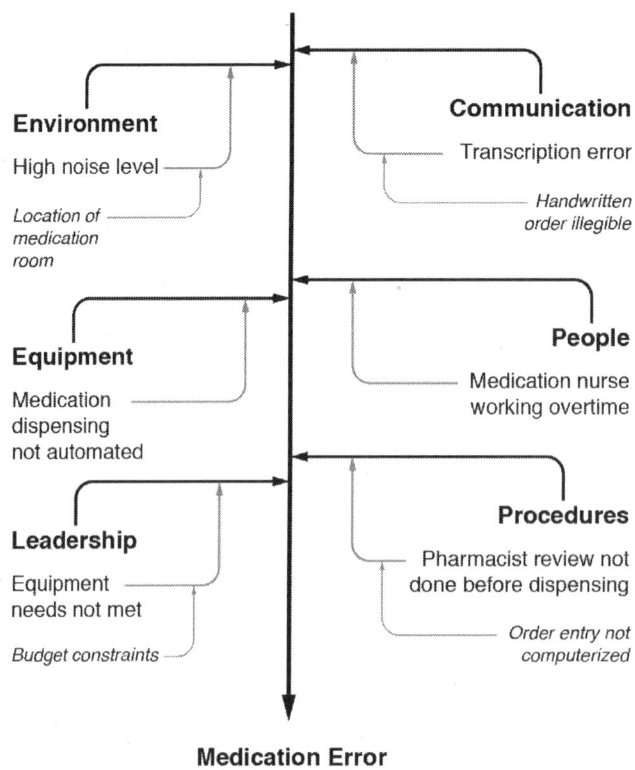

The root cause analysis (RCA) is used when there is an adverse event, a sentinel event, or close call in the medical setting. It can also be used when there is a concern about a process due to repeated errors, when there is a possibility of serious errors, and when there are high-cost errors. The RCA answers the following critical questions:

- What happened or is still happening?
- How did it happen?
- Why did it happen?
- How can we prevent it from happening again?
- What can we learn from this?

Practice Quiz

1. Which of the following is an example of a healthcare provider showing cultural consideration to a patient?
   a. A healthcare provider does not allow a patient's same-sex spouse to visit in the recovery room due to the healthcare provider's religious beliefs.
   b. A healthcare provider allows a patient of the Islamic faith to keep her headscarf on during a physical exam.
   c. A healthcare provider tells a person who identifies as Asian on his intake form that she does not like Chinese food.
   d. A healthcare provider tells an older patient that unless he or she enrolls in the online patient portal, the provider will not provide treatment.

2. When healthcare providers see patients who are unconscious or not of a sound state of mind, what principle is utilized in order to provide treatment?
   a. Assumption
   b. Risky consent
   c. Informed consent
   d. Implied consent

3. Nurses are responsible for which of the following elements of informed consent?
   a. Identification of alternatives to the planned procedure
   b. Description of associated risks and benefits
   c. Explanation of the planned procedure or diagnostic test
   d. Assessment of the patient's understanding of the information that is provided

4. While explaining discharge instructions, the nurse finds that the Japanese American patient frequently nods their head. How should the nurse understand this behavior?
   a. The patient agrees to the discharge plan.
   b. The patient is nervous and unsure of the plan.
   c. The patient is producing normal cultural conduct.
   d. The patient is encouraging the nurse to finish their sentence.

5. Which ethical principle guides the nurse's actions while guaranteeing that the patient with the most critical condition receives priority treatment?
   a. Hedonism
   b. Virtue ethics
   c. Act deontology
   d. Utilitarianism

See the answers on the next page.

Answers Explanations

1. B: In this case, the healthcare provider considered religious and cultural beliefs of the patient to make her feel comfortable during the exam. Effective cultural considerations improve patient satisfaction scores. In the other options listed, the healthcare providers act inconsiderately, insultingly, and make assumptions about the patient's culture.

2. D: When patients are physically or psychologically unable to provide verbal or written consent to treatment, healthcare providers rely on implied consent, acting on the belief that the patient would like the best treatment to benefit their life.

3. D: While the physician is legally responsible for satisfying all elements of informed consent, nurses are ethically responsible for assessing the patient's ability to process and understand the implications of informed consent. Nurses protect the patient's autonomy by raising these questions and concerns. The remaining elements of informed consent are required of the physician, rather than the nurses.

4. C: Choice *C* indicates a thorough understanding of cultural considerations to care as this behavior represents normal cultural conduct. Choices *A*, *B*, and *D* are inappropriate as this behavior does not insinuate anything more than cultural norms regarding the patient's level of understanding, agreement, or pace of discussion.

5. D: Choice *D* includes bringing about the greatest good for the greatest number of people, which is what the nurse does when prioritizing patient care. Choices *A*, *B*, and *C*, while all ethical considerations, do not align with the nurse's actions at this time.

Adult CCRN Practice Test #1

1. A 29-year-old female presents with severe pain in her knee joint with papules, redness, and tenderness surrounding. What type of organism does the nurse suspect has caused this acute infectious arthritis?
   a. *Neisseria gonorrhoeae*
   b. *Staphylococcus aureus*
   c. *Streptococcus pyogenes*
   d. *Candida*

2. Which of the following statements is consistent with clinical inquiry in the Synergy Model?
   a. Novice nurses begin to compare and contrast alternative solutions to patient problems.
   b. Changes in clinical practice result from clinical experience and applying research findings.
   c. Clinical inquiry is critical to the care of the vulnerable patient.
   d. The model identifies clinical inquiry as identical to clinical reasoning.

3. Which item in the family history assessment performed by the critical care nurse is a red flag for hypertrophic cardiomyopathy and should be investigated further?
   a. Heart disease of the father
   b. Diabetes mellitus of the mother
   c. Sudden death of a grandmother
   d. Stroke of a grandfather

4. Common barriers to effective collaboration include which of the following?
   a. Incomplete care
   b. Cure vs care activities
   c. Conflicting professional opinions
   d. All the above

5. According to the Frank-Starling law of the heart, a patient with heart failure will respond to an increase in preload in which of the following ways?
   a. Increased contractility
   b. Decreased cardiac output
   c. Change in rhythm
   d. Increased heart rate

6. Which of the following is/are true regarding advance directives?
   a. They are an expression of the patient's preferences.
   b. They based on a person's values and beliefs.
   c. They include identification of a surrogate.
   d. All of the above

7. "The protection, promotion, and optimization of health and abilities; prevention of illness and injury; facilitation of healing; alleviation of suffering through the diagnosis and treatment of human response; and advocacy in the care of individuals, families, communities, and populations." This statement is best described as which of the following?

a. The ANA Code of Ethics
b. The AACN definition of clinical care
c. The ANA definition of nursing practice
d. The five assumptions of the Synergy Model

8. Which of the following statements is consistent with the QESN competencies?

a. Using systems thinking increases collaboration.
b. Systems thinking is the goal of all nursing competencies.
c. Successful application of all QESN nursing competencies will improve patient safety.
d. The ability to use systems thinking is dictated by the nurse's level of basic nursing education.

9. Which of the following statements is true?

a. Ninety-five percent of the patients diagnosed with multiple sclerosis will potentially advance to a non-remitting disease pattern.
b. The clinically isolated incident is a definitive precursor of active MS.
c. The primary-progressive form of MS is the most common presenting form of the disease.
d. Prednisone is the medication of choice to slow progression in all forms of MS.

10. Which of the following word pairs identifies the C's of caring practices that are most closely associated with the critical care certification in nursing?

a. Compassion and curiosity
b. Confidence and collaboration
c. Conscience and creativity
d. Commitment and competence

11. Which of the following descriptions does NOT describe a patient diagnosed with antisocial personality disorder (ASPD)?

a. Aggressive
b. Reclusive
c. Disrespectful
d. Violent

12. Which of the following terms refers to severe bronchoconstriction with wheezing that does not respond to the usual bronchodilation treatment?

a. *Delirium tremens*
b. *Status asthmaticus*
c. *Pulsus paradoxus*
d. *Febre rubra*

13. Which of the following are true regarding encephalopathy?

I. It is complication of a primary problem.
II. It is brain damage.
III. It is an altered mental state.
IV. It is caused by a lack of oxygen to the brain.

a. Choices I, II, and III
b. Choices I, II, and IV
c. Choices II, III, and IV
d. All of the above

14. Which of the following is an example of a neurosurgery performed on the peripheral nervous system?
a. Lumbar laminectomy
b. Aneurysm clipping
c. Conventional open surgery
d. Carpal tunnel correction

15. The nurse is caring for a patient with cirrhosis who is complaining of increasing abdominal distention. The nurse assesses the presence of ascites. Which of the following statements correctly describes the pathogenesis of ascites?
a. Epinephrine and norepinephrine levels are decreased.
b. Plasma albumin levels are decreased.
c. Portal hypotension is the initial defect.
d. Plasma oncotic levels are increased.

16. When administering activated charcoal to a patient who has ingested a toxic substance, only give it with which of the following substances?
a. Water
b. Milk
c. Sherbet
d. Ice cream

17. In planning care for a patient with acute renal failure, what imbalance does the critical care nurse expect to manage?
a. Elevated GFR
b. Decreased BUN
c. Elevated calcium
d. Decreased sodium

18. A patient in the critical care unit tells the nurse that his pain is in his abdomen, just below the rib cage and to the right of his stomach. Which component of pain assessment has the patient reported?
a. Location
b. Exacerbation
c. Alleviation
d. Aggravation

19. The patient in the ICU is having trouble sleeping due to sensory overload. The ICU nurse may do all the following interventions except:
   a. Limit visitors wherever possible
   b. Limit conversations with co-workers outside the patient's room
   c. Turn off the lights in the patient's room when they are not needed
   d. None; all of the above are appropriate interventions

20. Which of the following is not a common cause of air-leak syndromes?
   a. Obstruction of blood vessels
   b. Blunt force trauma
   c. Chemical injury
   d. Overdistention of lungs

21. When is root cause analysis used?
   a. When anything goes wrong in the medical setting
   b. When there are adverse events or close calls
   c. When the doctor orders one
   d. Only when a patient death or serious injury occurs

22. The best way to prevent catheter-associated urinary tract infections is to do which of the following?
   a. Measure strict intake and output while the catheter is in place
   b. Monitor the urethra for signs of infection
   c. Remove the catheter as soon as possible
   d. Follow protocol before placing the catheter

23. A 9-month-old baby is in the ER, and shaken baby syndrome is suspected. This falls under what category of traumatic brain injury?
   a. Closed
   b. Developing
   c. Open
   d. Insidious

24. According to the Synergy Model, at what level of nursing competence do the nursing competencies of clinical inquiry and clinical reasoning become inseparable in the research process?
   a. The experienced nurse
   b. The novice nurse
   c. The expert nurse
   d. The two competencies are linked in all levels of competency.

25. The nurse is caring for a patient with endoscopic evidence of esophageal varices. Which of the following statements correctly identifies the interventions associated with primary prevention of hemorrhage for this condition?
   a. Sclerotherapy ablation of the esophageal arteries
   b. Vasopressors to maintain the hepatic venous pressure gradient above 20 mmHG
   c. Transjugular intrahepatic portosystemic shunt implantation
   d. Endoscopic band ligation

26. Which of the following statements is consistent with the concept of moral agency?
    a. The patient's decisions will always be honored.
    b. Nurses assume accountability for their decisions.
    c. Institutions rarely act as moral agents.
    d. Advocacy and moral agency are interchangeable concepts.

27. The nurse is caring for a thirty-eight-year-old male who presents with marked left-sided scrotal swelling and distention of the abdomen. The nurse understands that which of the following is NOT an expected finding in this patient?
    a. Diarrhea
    b. Tachycardia
    c. Rebound tenderness
    d. BUN 27

28. A patient with idiopathic thrombocytopenia purpura presents with the classic purpura on the skin. Which of the following statements explains how to differentiate between the signs and symptoms of a thrombocytopenia?
    a. Purpura are larger than petechiae, but smaller than ecchymoses
    b. Purpura are larger than both petechiae and ecchymoses
    c. Purpura are smaller than both petechiae and ecchymoses
    d. Purpura are smaller than petechiae, but larger than ecchymoses

29. Psychosis is a common side effect of which of the following?

    I. Schizophrenia
    II. Methamphetamine, cocaine, or LSD use
    III. Bipolar Disorder
    IV. HIV antiviral medications

    a. Choices II and IV
    b. Choices I and II
    c. Choices I, II, and III
    d. All of the above

30. High blood sugar stimulates the kidneys to do which of the following?
    a. Produce less urine
    b. Concentrate the urine
    c. Retain more sodium
    d. Produce more urine

31. Nursing practice is based on the principles of ethical behavior. Which of the following correctly identifies the moral principle that may require knowledge of the legislative process?
    a. Fidelity
    b. Autonomy
    c. Advocacy
    d. Beneficence

32. Which body system will exhibit the most obvious effects of a state of hyperosmolar hyperglycemic nonketotic syndrome (HHNK)?
   a. Neurologic
   b. Cardiac
   c. Endocrine
   d. Pulmonary

33. What is the most common cause of edema caused by venous insufficiency?
   a. Deep vein thrombosis (DVT)
   b. Obesity
   c. Pregnancy
   d. Old age

34. When used to implement evidenced-based practice, clinical inquiry can result in which of the following?
   a. Replacing an outdated nursing intervention
   b. The nurse becoming an innovator
   c. Matching patient needs with nursing competencies
   d. All the above

35. Which of the following procedures confirms a diagnosis of pulmonary hypertension?
   a. Transesophageal echocardiography
   b. Right cardiac catheterization
   c. Left cardiac catherization
   d. Lung transplantation

36. Which term is used interchangeably with leukopenia, a condition in which the white blood cell count is lower than normal?
   a. Thrombocytopenia
   b. Lymphocytopenia
   c. Neutropenia
   d. Monocytopenia

37. Which of the following is/are true regarding the Medical Home model?
   a. It is the model Medicaid uses.
   b. It incorporates collaborative care.
   c. It has been proven cost-effective in mental healthcare.
   d. All of the above

38. How long must symptoms last for an episode of neurological deficits to be considered a transient ischemic attack (TIA) rather than a cerebrovascular accident (CVA)?
   a. More than 1 hour but less than 2 hours
   b. More than 5 minutes but less than 1 hour
   c. More than 24 hours
   d. More than 2 hours but less than 3 hours

39. A 35-year-old male presents with headaches, memory loss, and periods of disorientation. The nurse discovers that he played professional football for many years and is now retired. The nurse suspects which type of encephalopathy will be diagnosed?
   a. Chronic traumatic encephalopathy
   b. Hepatic encephalopathy
   c. Hashimoto's encephalopathy
   d. Toxic-metabolic encephalopathy

40. Joel is in a car accident where his left foot and lower leg are crushed upon impact. However, he remains conscious and waits for emergency services to arrive. He notices the outside of his calf is visibly swollen and becoming noticeably more painful. By the time emergency services arrive, the pain is excruciating. What is Joel likely experiencing?
   a. Acute compartment syndrome affecting his lateral gastrocnemius
   b. Shock and hallucination from the trauma
   c. Deep vein thrombosis in his leg
   d. Sciatic nerve damage

41. A 39-year-old female has been admitted with acute tubular necrosis (ATN) and is receiving IV medications to rebalance fluid and electrolyte abnormalities. Which of the following precipitating events likely led to her developing kidney failure?
   a. Hypertensive crisis
   b. Acetaminophen overdose
   c. Upper respiratory tract infection
   d. Hypotensive crisis

42. Over what area of the heart will the nurse auscultate a holosystolic murmur accompanied by a thrill when there is a mitral regurgitation caused by papillary muscle rupture following an MI?
   a. Aortic
   b. Tricuspid
   c. Pulmonic
   d. Apical

43. If dopamine does not do an adequate job of maintaining blood pressure in a patient experiencing cardiogenic shock, which potent vasoconstrictor will be considered to raise the blood pressure?
   a. Dobutamine
   b. Norepinephrine
   c. Milrinone
   d. Nitroglycerin

44. Which of the following has NOT been identified as a barrier to the application of nursing research findings to clinical practice?
   a. Inadequate funding
   b. Insufficient translation
   c. Lack of qualified nursing staff
   d. Limited patient populations

45. The drug Mannitol is used to treat which of the following?
   a. Cancers
   b. Status epilepticus
   c. Seizures
   d. Brain herniation

46. Which of the following groups of symptoms are indicative of cauda equina syndrome, a condition that requires immediate treatment?
   a. An inability to stay awake, with excessive drooling from the mouth, occurring for at least ten minutes
   b. A loss of feeling along the cervical column and limited mobility along the shoulders and arms
   c. An inability to control bowel and bladder movements, and a sudden loss of strength in the lower body
   d. A history of horseback riding injury and a slipped sacroiliac joint

47. A 64-year-old Caucasian male enters the emergency department with a burn to his left forearm. You notice that the top layer of skin is discolored and darkened and has started to peel off. He is also complaining of "not being able to feel my arm." You know, based on the initial physical assessment and his complaints, that he is suffering from which of the following?
   a. A second-degree burn
   b. A third-degree burn
   c. A first-degree burn
   d. A fourth-degree burn

48. Patients on the cusp of respiratory failure may exhibit which of the following early signs and symptoms?
   a. Decreased respiratory rate
   b. Unconsciousness
   c. Cyanosis
   d. Agitation

49. Which of the following interventions will NOT help prevent a pressure ulcer from occurring in a bedridden patient?
   a. Turning the patient every two hours
   b. Encouraging early mobility
   c. Removing the pillows from the bed
   d. Proper nutrition

50. The American Hospital Association's Patient Care Partnership mandates which of the following?
   a. How hospitals communicate with families
   b. Responsibility for caring for terminal patients
   c. A decision-making partnership between patients and healthcare system
   d. Access to affordable insurance for everyone

51. Which of the following is NOT a toxic effect of nicotine inhaled during cigarette smoking?
   a. Plaque buildup
   b. Inflammation of endothelium
   c. Vasoconstriction of blood vessels
   d. Hypertension

52. The nurse taking care of a patient with an MRSA infection knows that multidrug-resistant organisms arise from which of the following causes?
  a. Overuse of antivirals
  b. Underuse of antivirals
  c. Underuse of antibiotics
  d. Overuse of antibiotics

53. A 60-year-old male with a history of alcohol abuse and IV drug abuse presents to the emergency department with encephalopathy, ascites, and jaundice. Which organ of the abdomen does the nurse suspect is in failure?
  a. Kidney
  b. Liver
  c. Stomach
  d. Spleen

54. Goals of care conversations are used at the end of life to do which of the following?
  a. Collaborate with experts.
  b. Keep the focus on what the patient wants.
  c. Support families during a difficult time.
  d. Get the patient into palliative care.

55. A 29-year-old veteran of the Marine Corps experiences a recurrent nightmare that revisits his combat experience. Last week at a Fourth of July celebration in his town, he experienced a dissociative state of mind after hearing the popping of the fireworks. The nurse recognized he may have what psychological disorder?
  a. Antisocial behavior disorder
  b. Panic attack disorder
  c. Bipolar disorder
  d. Post-traumatic stress disorder

56. Which of the following is not a result of emphysema?
  a. Blebs
  b. Air trapping
  c. Air space enlargement
  d. Bronchoconstriction

57. The nurse is caring for a patient with diabetic ketoacidosis. Which of the following statements is consistent with the cause of this disorder?
  a. This condition results from having excess insulin in the body.
  b. Poor management of diabetes can cause this disorder.
  c. Reduced glucose ingestion can lead to this disorder.
  d. Taking too much oral anti-diabetic medication can cause this disorder.

58. Which of the following statements about the cardiac catheterization procedure is true?
  a. The brachial artery is a common access site.
  b. The thin tube threaded into the patient's heart has a camera called a scope on the end for visualization of heart structures.
  c. Angioplasty and stent placement are commonly performed to open occluded coronary vessels.
  d. The patient is put under general anesthesia for the procedure.

59. Where should nurses assess for pallor in a patient with dark skin who is suspected to be anemic?
   a. Forearms
   b. Cheeks
   c. Conjunctiva
   d. Scalp

60. A 68-year-old woman with a history of gallstones is in the same-day surgery unit today for a cholecystectomy. This procedure will likely be performed using which technique that involves small incisions and minimal invasion?
   a. Laparoscopic
   b. Endoscopic
   c. Bronchoscopic
   d. Laparotomy

61. During the emergent phase of a burn injury, which of the following might a nurse expect to see?
   a. Decreased blood pressure
   b. Increased urine output
   c. Decreased heart rate
   d. Pink skin

62. Which of the following is a common symptom of COPD?
   a. Dry cough
   b. Morning headache
   c. Narrow chest
   d. Weight gain

63. A patient experiencing itching related to an allergic reaction likely has the substance histamine being secreted by which type of white blood cell?
   a. Lymphocytes
   b. Basophils
   c. Neutrophils
   d. Monocytes

64. Which of the following choices is most consistent with nurses' responsibilities for advocacy?
   a. Notify the nursing supervisor of any conflict to assure resolution of the patient issue.
   b. Consider the patient's point of view and be prepared to support and explain the point of view as needed.
   c. Provide comprehensive documentation of the patient's care in the EHR.
   d. Understand all relevant laws associated with the nursing care of the patient.

65. Which of the following is NOT a usual sign that a patient is in shock?
   a. Increased urine output
   b. Distant heart sounds
   c. Bluish tinted skin
   d. Faint and rapid pulse

66. A 49 -year-old patient experiencing severe alcohol withdrawal exhibits vestibular disturbance by reporting which of the following symptoms?
   a. "I have a terrible headache."
   b. "The room is spinning!"
   c. "My hands won't stop shaking!"
   d. "I am nauseated."

67. The nurse is caring for a patient with suspected HELLP syndrome. The patient asks the nurse to explain the complications associated with this diagnosis. Which of the following statements correctly identifies the complications of this syndrome?
   a. The syndrome creates a state of hypercoagulation that can result in infarction of the hepatic vasculature.
   b. Liver dysfunction is reversible with correction of the coagulation defects.
   c. Cerebrovascular effects are rare.
   d. The "complete" form of HELLP is manifested by red cell hemolysis, elevated liver enzyme levels, and low platelet levels.

68. Which of the following potentially provides the most comprehensive view of the institution?
   a. Root cause analysis
   b. Competency grids
   c. Process diagrams
   d. Case studies

69. Which of the following is NOT a way in which mechanical ventilation benefits the patient?
   a. Creates alkalotic state of the blood
   b. Decreases the work of breathing
   c. Increases cardiac output
   d. Creates positive end-expiratory pressure (PEEP)

70. Which of the following drugs is often used for treatment of acute seizure activity?
   a. Memantine HCl
   b. Phenytoin
   c. Pregabalin
   d. Rifaximin

71. Which of the following nursing interventions is most consistent with the competencies of caring practices, advocacy, and moral agency?
   a. Developing cultural awareness of care team members
   b. Mentoring novice nurses in the use of research findings
   c. Facilitating the patient's transition from one level of care to another on the health continuum
   d. Refining educational programs for patients and families

72. The critical care nurse caring for a patient on a mechanical ventilator performs all except which of the following interventions to prevent ventilator-associated pneumonia?
   a. Lays the head of the bed flat while the patient is sleeping
   b. Keeps the bed at 45-90 degrees at all times
   c. Removes the endotracheal tube as soon as the patient can tolerate breathing on their own
   d. Performs regular oral hygiene interventions

73. A patient who has experienced an ischemic stroke will likely be put on which type of drug therapy to prevent future clots from occurring?
   a. Beta blockers
   b. Statins
   c. Platelet antiaggregants
   d. Antihypertensives

74. A 33-year-old female presents to the emergency room complaining of vomiting blood. Which description of the hematemesis indicates an active upper GI bleed?
   a. Coffee ground
   b. Bright red
   c. Large amount
   d. Small amount

75. What is the most common and deadly heart rhythm detected in patients experiencing cardiac arrest?
   a. Atrial fibrillation
   b. Ventricular tachycardia
   c. Ventricular fibrillation
   d. Supraventricular tachycardia

76. Which of the following metabolic components involved in diabetic ketoacidosis is responsible for the "fruity" smell that a person with DKA gives off when they breathe?
   a. Alanine
   b. Triglycerides
   c. Acetone
   d. Glycerol

77. Which of the following is not a usual drug of choice when providing analgesia to the mechanically ventilated patient?
   a. Morphine
   b. Dopamine
   c. Fentanyl
   d. Propofol

78. Which psychological disorder often precedes a dementia diagnosis?
   a. Bipolar disorder
   b. Panic disorder
   c. Depressive disorder
   d. Schizophrenia

79. Which of the following statements is most accurate concerning assent and informed consent?
   a. *Assent* refers to the conversation, while *informed consent* refers to the signed document.
   b. Unemancipated minor clients can provide *informed consent* but cannot *assent.*
   c. Mandated clients can *assent* but cannot provide *informed consent.*
   d. Unemancipated minor clients who cannot provide *informed consent* can still *assent.*

80. Apnea and loss of normal oxygenation during a spontaneous breathing trial are signs that what should occur?
   a. Sedation should be increased.
   b. The breathing trial should continue for a few more minutes.
   c. An antidote for respiratory distress should be administered.
   d. Mechanical ventilation should continue.

81. Which of the following ethical principles is MOST closely related to advocacy?
   a. Distributive justice
   b. Beneficence
   c. Nonmaleficence
   d. Fidelity

82. Which category of pulmonary embolism entails impairment of right ventricular function as well as severe hypotension?
   a. Small
   b. Submassive
   c. Massive
   d. Grand

83. Why did the AACN develop their Synergy Model?
   a. To match nursing practice to competencies
   b. To shift from the care model
   c. To standardize accreditation
   d. All the above

84. What type of drug therapy coupled with antithrombotic therapy is often used post-endarterectomy?
   a. Antiplatelet
   b. Beta-blocker
   c. Angiotensin-converting enzyme
   d. Angiotensin II receptor blockers

85. What risk does high blood pressure pose in the postoperative period following an endarterectomy?
   a. Bleeding
   b. Infection
   c. Pulmonary edema
   d. Stroke

86. Which of the following is not a congenital heart defect found in the tetralogy of Fallot?
   a. Pulmonary valve stenosis
   b. Ventricular septal defect
   c. Atrial septal defect
   d. Hypertrophic right ventricle

87. A 19-year-old patient diagnosed with bipolar disorder has been admitted to the psychiatric unit following a spending spree, several instances of risky and promiscuous sex with strangers, and finally being caught shoplifting several hundred dollars' worth of clothes from a local Target. The nurse concludes that the patient was in which portion of the bipolar cycle?

a. Anxious
b. Depressive
c. Mania
d. Panic

88. A 73-year-old male has developed urinary incontinence related to cognitive impairments as a result of a stroke. Which of the following drugs may be prescribed to increase urinary sphincter tone and prevent incontinence?

a. Furosemide
b. Duloxetine
c. Doxazosin
d. Finasteride

89. Which of the following causes of thrombocytopenia is considered an immunological cause?

a. Folate deficiency
b. Drug side effects
c. Acute respiratory distress syndrome
d. Viral infection

90. Research indicates which of the following regarding diversity in the workplace?

a. It requires more money.
b. It encourages competition.
c. It strengthens the workgroup.
d. It must be led by management.

91. A novice nurse is caring for a patient who requires a blood transfusion. The patient, however, has refused the transfusion due to a religious objection to the therapy. The nurse says, "I don't understand why the patient's sister can't donate the blood. No one should object to receiving blood from a family member when you need it." Which of the following statements correctly identifies the critical issue in this situation?

a. The nurse is displaying an ethnocentric attitude.
b. The nurse thinks that the patient is concerned about contracting an infectious disease.
c. The nurse thinks that the patient doesn't understand the necessity of the blood transfusion.
d. The nurse believes that blood donation from family members is safe.

92. A 55-year-old male is undergoing an endoscopy to discover the source of his hematemesis. The gastroenterologist encounters an active, bleeding lesion. What procedure using the application of heat to seal the lesion will probably be used next?

a. Banding
b. Biopsy
c. Angioplasty
d. Cauterization

93. What amount of blood loss is considered life-threatening and will throw a patient into hypovolemic shock?
   a. 1/8
   b. 1/7
   c. 1/5
   d. 1/10

94. Which technique is most appropriate when inserting a urinary catheter into a patient to help in the prevention of CAUTIs?
   a. Sterile
   b. Clean
   c. Sanitary
   d. Aseptic

95. Which of the following is NOT an example of an air-leak syndrome?
   a. Emphysema
   b. Pneumothorax
   c. Subcutaneous emphysema
   d. Flail chest

96. The nurse is looking at a patient's ECG and notices tented T waves, a widening QRS wave, and deepened S waves. She suspects which life-threatening imbalance is occurring?
   a. Hyperkalemia
   b. Hypernatremia
   c. Hypokalemia
   d. Hyponatremia

97. A 52-year-old male is admitted with symptoms of severe abdominal pain centered around the epigastric region of the abdomen and has a history of alcohol abuse and cigarette smoking. The nurse suspects which of the following conditions will be diagnosed?
   a. Gastritis
   b. Hepatitis
   c. Pancreatitis
   d. Kidney failure

98. How might an institution best support diversity?
   a. By requiring all employees to speak a second language
   b. By providing mandatory cultural sensitivity training for all managers
   c. By offering alternative food services
   d. By providing alternative solutions to all patient requests

99. The critical care nurse is admitting a patient fresh out of the surgical suite following repair of multiple tears and lacerations after being stabbed several times during a gang fight. Which of the following signs signals an improvement in the patient's condition?
   a. Rise in heart rate
   b. Stabilization of blood pressure
   c. Development of fever
   d. Low urine output

100. What other condition may mimic the symptoms of a heart attack?
   a. Cirrhosis of the liver
   b. Kidney failure
   c. Acid reflux
   d. Pneumonia

101. Which structure of the brain is responsible for producing cerebrospinal fluid?
   a. Pons
   b. Ventricles
   c. Thalamus
   d. Corpus callosum

102. There is a 3 percent loss of muscle mass within the thigh muscles within 7 days of bedrest, and contractures begin within 3 weeks. This is an example of which of the following?
   a. Immobility
   b. Decompression syndrome
   c. Deconditioning
   d. Debilitation

103. Which of the following is most likely to cause an abscess?
   a. Human papillomavirus
   b. Low estrogen levels
   c. Acne inversa
   d. Staphylococcal bacteria

104. What serological marker indicates, with high specificity, that cardiac muscle tissue has been damaged and cell contents are being released into the bloodstream?
   a. Creatinine
   b. BUN
   c. Creatine kinase
   d. Troponin

105. What is one way a woman may present differently than a man when experiencing a heart attack?
   a. Symptoms beginning days to weeks before actual attack
   b. Profuse sweating
   c. Crushing chest pain
   d. Elevated serological markers

106. Which of the following actions by a patient with COPD creates its own positive end-expiratory pressure?
   a. Tripod posing
   b. Wide open-mouth breathing
   c. Pursed-lip breathing
   d. Frequent coughing

107. Which side effect of chronic kidney disease indicates a decrease in the release of erythropoietin?
   a. Anemia
   b. Leukemia
   c. Hypovolemia
   d. Hypocalcemia

108. Which process is the first intervention for someone experiencing a maxillofacial injury?
   a. Airway management
   b. Splinting bone fractures
   c. Diagnostic x-rays
   d. Removing foreign objects and other debris

109. A STEMI, in which the full thickness of the heart wall has been damaged, results in which of the following ECG changes?
   a. T-wave inversion
   b. ST-segment elevation
   c. QT prolongation
   d. U-wave elevation

110. What are the four steps of systems thinking in order?
   a. Anticipate, design, transform, react
   b. React, anticipate, design, transform
   c. Design, anticipate, react, transform
   d. Transform, react, anticipate, design

111. What differentiating factor would let a nurse know that a lower extremity ulcer is arterial rather than venous?
   a. Color of wound
   b. Culture taken from wound
   c. Depth of wound
   d. Measurement of wound

112. Which of the following is an example of toxic substance ingestion?
   a. A child eating a Tide pod
   b. Breathing exhaust fumes
   c. Sniffing glue
   d. All of the above

113. According to the Synergy Model, which of the following choices is associated with the patient's vulnerability?
   a. The patient is financially stable.
   b. The patient smoked cigarettes for thirty years prior to quitting five years ago.
   c. The patient is married.
   d. The patient actively participates in decisions related to the plan of care.

114. A 22-year-old male comes in with a gunshot wound to the right upper quadrant of his abdomen. The bleeding has been controlled, the wound was closed, and he has been hemodynamically stabilized. What solid organ of the abdomen does the nurse suspect might have been hit by the gunshot?

a. Stomach
b. Small intestine
c. Liver
d. Colon

115. What myocardial conduction defect is hereditary, may result in syncope or sudden death, and often occurs in healthy adults or children?

a. Third-degree heart block
b. First-degree heart block
c. Bundle branch block
d. Long QT syndrome

116. Perioperative inoculation of bacteria into the joint describes which of the following?

a. A post-op infection
b. A prosthetic joint infection
c. Infectious arthritis
d. All of the above

117. What test is often used to determine if a patient has peripheral arterial disease?

a. Echocardiography
b. CT scan of the leg
c. Electrocardiogram
d. Ankle-brachial BP index

118. Pulmonary hypertension will likely be treated with all but which of the following drug therapies?

a. Sildenafil
b. Amlodipine
c. Epoprostenol
d. Diazepam

119. The balloon pump inflates during diastole for what purpose in a patient experiencing cardiogenic shock?

a. To allow more space in the aorta
b. To push more blood flow out into the peripheral circulation
c. To raise blood pressure in hypotensive states
d. To encourage perfusion of coronary arteries and diastolic filling of the heart

120. In the continuum of worsening illness, sepsis is an infection paired with what factor?

a. Organ dysfunction
b. Systemic inflammatory response syndrome (SIRS)
c. Hypotensive crisis
d. Lactic acidosis

121. Which of the following statements is consistent with the Synergy Model?
   a. Family participation in patient care improves outcomes.
   b. The model is based on the condition of patients and the function of the nursing staff.
   c. The model only relates to critical care environments.
   d. Synergy exists when the environment and nursing competencies are consistent with the needs of the patient and the patient's family.

122. The Synergy Model views the practice of expert nurses as which of the following?
   a. Being able to anticipate the patient needs
   b. Being able to address change
   c. The point where clinical reasoning and clinical inquiry are inseparable
   d. Being able to incorporate research findings

123. When assessing a patient's wound, reddening, malodor, and pus discharge are sign of what?
   a. Healing
   b. Surgery
   c. Trauma
   d. Infection

124. A morbidly obese 25-year-old male has elected to undergo a bariatric surgery in which the stomach and duodenum will be bypassed and rerouted from a stomach pouch directly to the jejunum. Which type of bariatric procedure is this?
   a. Adjustable gastric banding
   b. Gastrectomy
   c. Liposuction
   d. Roux-en-Y gastric bypass

125. What is the main concern faced when using an artificial graft to bypass an occluded artery in the fem-pop bypass procedure?
   a. Localized infection
   b. Narrowing leading to reocclusion
   c. Lower extremity edema
   d. Tissue rejection

126. Which of the following statements about thyroid conditions is correct?
   a. T4 deficiency is an example of a hyperthyroidism disease, while T3 deficiency is an example of a hypothyroidism disease.
   b. Grave's disease is an example of a hyperthyroidism disease, while Hashimoto's disease is an example of a hypothyroidism disease.
   c. Goiter is an example of a hyperthyroidism disease, while gout is an example of a hypothyroidism disease.
   d. Cancer is an example of a hyperthyroidism disease, while gestational diabetes is an example of a hypothyroidism disease.

127. Which of the following would NOT indicate arterial insufficiency?
   a. Cyanosis of lower extremities
   b. Loss of hair in legs
   c. Sores that will not heal
   d. Pooling of blood and edema

128. The nurse is caring for a 30-year-old male patient with a ventriculoperitoneal shunt who is being assessed for shunt failure. The shunt was inserted four years ago when the patient developed hydrocephalus after a severe closed-head injury, and the patient has exhibited satisfactory control of ICP until 12 hours ago, when the patient complained of a headache, nausea, and tiredness. The patient's vital signs are BP 130/70, HR 82, RR 24, T 98.6 °F, PaO_2 97 percent. Which of the following complications is most likely responsible for the patient's condition?

a. Choroid ingrowth of the proximal catheter
b. Migration of the distal catheter to an area that impedes absorption of the CSF
c. Disconnection of the distal reservoir from the distal catheter tip
d. Infection of the proximal catheter

129. A patient who is silently aspirating may exhibit which of the following signs and symptoms?

a. Flat, red rash on the thoracic region
b. Constant clearing of the throat
c. Swollen lymph nodes on the neck
d. Trouble remembering person, place, and time

130. An 8-month-pregnant woman presents to the ED with eclampsia. Which IV medication will be given to prevent seizures?

a. Magnesium sulfate
b. Sodium chloride
c. Dextrose in water
d. Potassium supplement

131. A patient with a history of depression and suicidal ideation demonstrates a non-suicidal self-injury (NSSI) by doing which of the following?

a. Taking an entire bottle of aspirin all at one time
b. Telling a friend that she's thought about killing herself
c. Cutting her inner arms with a razor
d. Intentionally crashing their vehicle

132. A decreased amount of vasopressin in the body will likely produce which of the following conditions?

a. SIADH
b. Diabetes type I
c. Central diabetes insipidus
d. Diabetes type II

133. To correct the hyponatremia associated with syndrome of inappropriate antidiuretic hormone (SIADH), which of the following solutions is used?

a. Normal saline
b. Hypertonic saline
c. Hypotonic saline
d. Lactated ringer's solution

134. Which of the following answers is true about pain?
   a. Pain can always be controlled by opioids
   b. Pain always causes depression
   c. Pain can slow thought processes and impair memory
   d. All of the above

135. Which of the following is NOT an example of a drug that may cause respiratory failure in higher doses or in sensitive patients?
   a. Morphine
   b. Hydrocodone
   c. Naloxone
   d. Alprazolam

136. The nurse has a 16-year-old girl as a patient who is pale, fatigued, underweight, and refusing to eat, with a history of psychological issues. With what diagnosis will this girl likely be admitted to the hospital?
   a. Overnutrition
   b. Malabsorption
   c. Gastritis
   d. Anorexia

137. A 22-year-old male diagnosed with schizophrenia is acting out on the psych unit. He is verbally assaulting other patients, pacing nervously, and says his heart feels like it is "beating out of control!" The nurse sees that the patient is agitated and knows which intervention will be the last resort in assisting this patient?
   a. First-generation antipsychotics
   b. Second-generation antipsychotics
   c. Verbal de-escalation
   d. Physical restraints

138. A nurse is caring for a patient who had a colectomy two days ago. While assisting the patient back to bed, the nurse notes that the patient's heart rate and respiratory rate are slightly elevated, and the patient states, "I can feel my pulse." The nurse assesses the patient for additional signs of heart failure. This intervention is an example of which of the following caring practices according to the Synergy Model?
   a. Engagement by a novice nurse
   b. Vigilance by an experienced nurse
   c. An expected response to predictable changes by the novice nurse
   d. Collaboration by an experienced nurse

139. A nurse is working in an outpatient clinic giving flu shots at the beginning of the flu season. While educating a patient on the importance of the flu vaccine, she advises that the patient get the flu vaccine administered how often?
   a. Once per lifetime
   b. Every six months
   c. Annually
   d. Every two years

140. The nurse is assessing a 19-year-old college student who presents with sudden onset of headache that is associated with neck stiffness and fever. In caring for the patient with meningitis, the nurse understands that which of the following observations is correct?

a. The presence of a skin rash eliminates the diagnosis of viral meningitis.
b. Brain herniation after lumbar puncture is more common in immunosuppressed patients.
c. The CSF protein level is decreased in bacterial meningitis.
d. The MCV4 vaccine has dramatically decreased the incidence of meningitis in patients in long-term care facilities.

141. The nurse notices the site around the patient's peripheral IV has become puffy, cold, and tight. She suspects what has occurred?

a. Infection
b. IV infiltration
c. Allergic reaction
d. Nothing, this is a normal assessment of peripheral IV

142. In an attempt to diagnose a PE in a patient with renal failure, which type of scan will likely be performed?

a. Transesophageal echocardiography
b. CT scan with contrast
c. MRI of the thoracic cage
d. V/Q scan

143. Which of the following correctly identifies a critical distinction between the two concepts of advocacy and moral agency?

a. Advocacy is legally binding.
b. Moral agency requires accountability for right and wrong decisions.
c. Advocacy is implied in the paternalistic view of patient care.
d. Moral agency only refers to support for at-risk populations.

144. A nurse is developing a plan of care for a patient population that is culturally diverse. Which statement correctly identifies the appropriate nursing actions?

a. The nurse follows the standard protocol for the predominant culture of the community.
b. The nurse focuses on the cultural needs of the largest group in the population.
c. The nurse Identifies and acknowledges self-biases and addresses the needs of the patient.
d. The nurse meets the needs of the group according to personal values and beliefs.

145. Which of the following words describes delirium and differentiates it from dementia?

a. Slow onset
b. Irreversible
c. Chronic
d. Transient

146. A patient enters the emergency department with myalgia, stiffness, and weakness. Myoglobin is discovered in the urine and a diagnosis of rhabdomyolysis is made. The nurse would expect to see what color urine coming from the patient?

a. Clear
b. Light yellow
c. Dark amber
d. Tinged with blood

147. A patient at a clinic with a Behavior Activity Rating Scale (BARS) score of 1 requires which of the following?

a. Verbal de-escalation techniques
b. Further evaluation at the clinic
c. Immediate transfer to a medical ED
d. Environmental modification

148. Which of the following is cited as the MOST common source of funding for nursing research?

a. Pharmaceutical companies
b. Public funds
c. Non-profit organizations
d. Private institutions

149. Which category of pneumonia is more likely to occur in a patient who is undergoing chemotherapy for a metastatic lung cancer?

a. Community acquired
b. Hospital acquired
c. Immunocompromised
d. Healthcare associated

150. What is the most common bacterial cause of pneumonias in patients?

a. *Streptococcus pneumoniae*
b. *Klebsiella pneumoniae*
c. *Chlamydophila pneumoniae*
d. *Mycoplasma pneumoniae*

Answer Explanations #1

1. A: *Neisseria gonorrhoeae* is a common cause of acute infection of a joint. *Staphylococcus aureus* is a common infectious agent in osteomyelitis. *Streptococcus pyogenes* is the causative bacterial organism in strep throat. *Candida* is a type of yeast that can cause fungal infections; acute infectious arthritis is often caused by a bacterial infection.

2. B: The Synergy model identifies clinical inquiry as a nursing competency that develops as a result of clinical experience and enables nurses to apply research findings to clinical practice. Novice nurses in the model are able to identify changes in the patient's condition, but do not have the skill to identify alternative interventions. Nursing competencies that are identified as critical to the care of vulnerable patients include advocacy, moral agency, collaboration, and systems thinking. Clinical inquiry and clinical reasoning are not identical; they are two distinct competencies.

3. C: The sudden death of a grandmother needs to be probed for if a cause was determined. If she passed away suddenly because of hypertrophic cardiomyopathy that had been previously undiagnosed before autopsy, the patient should be screened for this condition as well, as it often may be asymptomatic until syncope or sudden death occurs. The other three items listed are of value, but do not point toward hypertrophic cardiomyopathy specifically.

4. D: Common barriers to effective collaboration include conflicting professional opinions, ineffective communication related to the conflict, and incomplete assessment of the required elements of the care plan. Research indicates that physicians tend to stress "cure" related activities while nurses tend to encourage "care" related activities, which means that some resolution of these differences is required for effective communication.

5. B: A patient with heart failure will not be able to respond to increased preload as a normal, healthy patient would, resulting in decreased cardiac output. Contractility is not increased as well as in a healthy heart. Changes in rhythm and rate are not significant as far as patients with heart failure and their response to preload.

6. D: The patient's preferences, values, and beliefs, as well as indication of a surrogate decision maker, are all included in advance directives.

7. C: The statement provided in the question is ANA definition of nursing practice: "The protection, promotion, and optimization of health and abilities; prevention of illness and injury; facilitation of healing; alleviation of suffering through the diagnosis and treatment of human response; and advocacy in the care of individuals, families, communities, and populations."

8. C: The QESN competencies were originally identified to improve patient safety in response to research that indicated that nearly 100,000 people died each year as a result of provider errors. The QESN competencies refer to nursing activities and are often used as the basis for undergraduate nursing curricula. Systems thinking is the process by which nurses meet the competencies, and attainment of this ability is an incremental process based on nurses' continuing education and clinical experiences. Although systems thinking is associated with the QESN competencies, and the use of systems thinking has improved patient outcomes, the basic assumption of the QESN competencies was improved patient safety as a result of expert nursing care.

9. A: Ten percent of MS patients are initially diagnosed with the primary-progressive form of MS, which means that the disease is always active without periods of remission. The relapsing-remitting form of MS accounts for 85 percent of the patients diagnosed with MS, which means that they will eventually progress to the secondary-progressive form; this means that the disease is always active. The potential progression of an isolated incident to MS depends on the presence or absence of plaque formation on MRI scans. The presence of alterations in the myelin sheath is strongly predictive of eventual progression. However, the absence of those lesions does not rule out the possibility of subsequent progression to MS; therefore, Choice *B* is incorrect. Only 10 percent of MS patients present with the primary-progressive form; therefore, Choice *C* is incorrect. Disease-modifying drugs are the preferred agents to treat MS. However, prednisone may be used if a patient is unable to tolerate the DMDs; therefore, Choice *D* is incorrect.

10. D: The nurse demonstrates professional competence as a result of a commitment to lifelong learning that is required for all areas of nursing. The other choices each contain only a single element of the five elements of caring: commitment, conscience, competence, compassion, and confidence.

11. B: A reclusive person may have agoraphobia and social anxiety, but not antisocial personality disorder (ASPD). A person with ASPD acts out in a way that is aggressive and disrespectful toward people they are around, making them antisocial in that way; this can include violent behaviors.

12. B: *Status asthmaticus* is the Latin term for a severe asthma attack, characterized by wheezing and bronchoconstriction, that is unresponsive to the usual therapy of bronchodilators. *Delirium tremens* is the set of symptoms experienced by an alcoholic in withdrawal, making Choice *A* incorrect. *Pulsus paradoxus* is defined as a drop in the systolic blood pressure by ten points and a decrease in the amplitude of pulse waves during inspiration. This phenomenon can be observed during cardiac tamponade, making Choice *C* incorrect. Choice *D* is incorrect, as *febre rubra* is the Latin term for scarlet fever.

13. A: Encephalopathy is a general term that means brain disease, damage, or malfunction, with the major symptom being an altered mental state. It is not always caused by a lack of oxygen to the brain; that is anoxic encephalopathy. However, there are other possible causes. For example, hepatic encephalopathy is caused by liver disease. Encephalopathy is often considered a complication of a primary problem.

14. D: Correction of carpal tunnel syndrome would require a type of neurosurgery affecting the peripheral nervous system. Lumbar laminectomy affects the lumbar region of the spine and not the peripheral nervous system. Clipping of aneurysms usually occurs in the brain or other centralized regions of the nervous system. Conventional open surgery is the general term for a surgery where a large incision is made to view and access internal organs or tissues; it is not the name of a surgical procedure itself.

15. B: Hypoalbuminemia is an essential element in the development of ascites. Decreased oncotic pressure resulting from deficient plasma proteins allows the movement of fluid from the vasculature into the extracellular fluid where it accumulates as ascites. Cirrhosis can result in increased levels of nitric oxide, which leads to vasodilation. The renal response to this abnormal condition is sodium retention and the secretion of increased epinephrine and norepinephrine due to stimulation of the sympathetic nervous system. Therefore, Choice *A* is incorrect. The development of ascites is a complication of portal hypertension, not hypotension. Portal hypertension is defined as the blockage of blood flow through the vasculature of the liver due to fibrotic changes resulting from cirrhosis or hepatitis; therefore, Choice *C* is incorrect. Plasma oncotic levels are decreased, rather than increased, because the diseased liver is not able to synthesize albumin; therefore, Choice *D* is incorrect.

16. A: Activated charcoal will work best if it is administered with water only. Milk, sherbet, and ice cream all have the potential to diminish its absorptive qualities, decreasing its effectiveness against the toxic substance ingested.

17. D: Choice *D* is a likely imbalance that presents in a patient with acute renal failure and will require diligent management. Choices *A*, *B*, and *C* are unlikely as the patient is at risk for a decreased GFR, increased BUN, and decreased calcium level. Acute renal failure involves poor filtering ability and a buildup of waste in the blood.

18. A: The patient has reported the location of his pain. Alleviation (Choice *C*) refers to an action that makes the pain better. Aggravation (Choice *D*) refers to an action that makes the pain worse. Exacerbation (Choice *B*) is a particularly intense flare-up of a chronic pain issue.

19. D: All of the choices represent ways the nurse can limit the patient's sensory input so that they can get neurologic rest.

20. A: Obstruction of blood vessels causes ischemia in tissues, not alveolar rupture, which leads to air-leak syndromes. Common causes of air-leak syndromes include blunt force trauma, chemical injury, overdistention of lungs, or uneven ventilation. They can also arise spontaneously, called idiopathic.

21. B: The root cause analysis is used when there is an adverse event, a sentinel event, or a close call in the medical setting. It can also be used when there is a concern about a process due to repeated errors, when there is a possibility of serious errors, and when there are high-cost errors.

22. C: The urinary catheter must be removed as soon as possible to prevent infection from developing. Never placing the catheter in the first place would be the absolute best way to prevent infection, but that is not an option, nor is it realistic in the acute care setting. Monitoring the urethra for infection will not prevent infection. Recording intake and output does not affect infection. Following protocol before placing the catheter will help prevent careless and needless placements of catheters, but may not affect preventing infection if the catheter is not removed in a timely manner.

23. A: Shaken baby syndrome in this case falls under the category of closed traumatic brain injury (TBI), as there is no open wound that is bleeding. A TBI that includes an open skull wound is called an open TBI. The other two terms listed do not refer to TBI and are thus not appropriate for this scenario.

24. C: The Synergy Model identifies expert nursing practice as the level of nursing competency in which clinical reasoning becomes an integrated element in the process of clinical inquiry. According to the model, prior to that point, nurses are capable of performing at some level of clinical inquiry and may be able to use clinical reasoning in patient care, but the total integration of the two does not occur until the expert level of nursing practice.

25. D: Endoscopic band ligation should be implemented for all varices that are 5 millimeters or more in diameter or are associated with red wales, because these characteristics are associated with a greater risk for hemorrhage. Band ligation decreases this potential but may be associated with stricture formation and obstruction of the esophageal lumen. This procedure may need to be repeated as the liver failure progresses. Therefore, Choice *D* is correct. Sclerotherapy of the esophageal veins is considered as a form of secondary prevention by many because beta-blocker therapy is readily available, well tolerated, and equally effective as compared to sclerotherapy.

In the event of hemorrhage due to ruptured esophageal varices, sclerotherapy can be used to decrease the blood loss; therefore, Choice *A* is incorrect. The recommended use of nonselective beta-blockers as primary prevention is intended to decrease the hepatic venous pressure gradient (HVPG) to less than or equal to 12 mmHg. An increase of this measurement would result in enlargement and possible rupture of the varices; therefore, Choice *B* is incorrect. The transjugular intrahepatic portosystemic shunt (TIPS) connects the portal and systemic circulations to decrease portal hypertension. The TIPS is appropriate to the care of the patient with active hemorrhage of esophageal varices and is not currently recommended as primary prevention of hemorrhage; therefore, Choice *C* is incorrect.

26. B: When nurses act as moral agents, they are required to also assume responsibility for their decisions. The patient's opinions will be identified and accommodated whenever possible; however, there may be conflict between the patient's opinions and the recommended plan of care, making Choice *A* incorrect. The institution may act as the moral agent for patients without any social support, making Choice *C* incorrect. The difference between moral agency and advocacy is the element of accountability. Moral agents are required to take responsibility for their decisions, making Choice *D* incorrect.

27. A: The patient's manifestations are consistent with an incarcerated or strangulated hernia that is progressing to a small-bowel obstruction as evidenced by the abdominal distention. This complication is associated with decreased peristalsis and eventual absence of bowel activity, which means that diarrhea would be an uncommon manifestation. Tachycardia and a BUN of 27 are related to fluid volume losses resulting from the accumulation of fluid proximal to the obstruction in the small bowel; therefore, choices *B* and *D* are incorrect. Rebound tenderness is also an expected finding in a bowel obstruction due to the trapped gas and fluid proximal to the obstruction; therefore, Choice *C* is incorrect.

28. A: It is true that purpura are larger than petechiae and smaller than ecchymoses or bruises. Bruises are the largest lesion of thrombocytopenia, characterized by a large pooling of blood beneath the skin. Petechiae are the smallest lesion of thrombocytopenia, characterized as tiny, pinpoint, red, flat dots on the skin. Purpura fall between ecchymoses and petechiae in size.

29. C: Schizophrenia and bipolar disorder are mental disorders in which hallucinations and delusion (key components of psychosis) are common. These characteristics can also result from mind-altering drugs, specifically methamphetamines, cocaine, and LSD. Antiviral medications used to treat HIV do not normally cause psychosis.

30. D: Massive urine production, or polyuria, is the result of a hyperglycemic state in the body and a hallmark sign of any diabetic condition. Urine is not concentrated, but rather diluted. Sodium, potassium, and other electrolyte imbalances may occur as a result of polyuria but are not a direct effect of hyperglycemia.

31. C: Advocacy involves supporting appropriate programs and actions for marginalized or at-risk populations. At the community level, the role of advocate for the nurse may require knowledge of the legislative process to bring about change. In direct patient care, the nurse will be the advocate for the patient by providing the information necessary for informed choices and supporting those choices in the development of the plan of care. Fidelity refers to trust. Autonomy refers to the right to self-determination. Beneficence refers to acting in the best interest of other individuals in society.

32. A: The most obvious effects of the super-concentrated blood that are characteristic of HHNK will appear neurologically. Confusion, seizures, coma, stroke-like syndromes, dizziness, and drowsiness are all neurological symptoms that appear in HHNK. The other systems of the body, such as cardiac, endocrine, and pulmonary may be affected but are not directly associated with the usual symptomology of HHNK.

33. A: DVT is the most common cause of edema caused by venous insufficiency. The other three factors are also potential causes, but are not as common as DVT.

34. D: When used to implement evidenced based practice, clinical inquiry can result in replacing an outdated, even counter-productive nursing intervention with an intervention that effectively addresses the needs of the patient. Matching patient needs with nursing competencies means that professional nurses are responsible for challenging all nursing interventions to be sure that they represent current best practice standards. As innovators, nurses are in the best position to research, implement, and evaluate alternative care practices.

35. B: Right cardiac catheterization is a procedure that will confirm a diagnosis of pulmonary hypertension. Transesophageal echocardiography is useful in visualizing the back side of the heart but does not fit with this specific scenario, making Choice *A* incorrect. Left cardiac catheterization enters the opposite side of the heart and is not helpful in confirming diagnosis, making Choice *C* incorrect. Lung transplantation is a surgical procedure used to treat severe cases of pulmonary hypertension, making Choice *D* incorrect.

36. C: Neutrophils are the most numerous of the white blood cells, which is the reason why the general term leukopenia is often used interchangeably with the slightly more specific term neutropenia. Monocytopenia and lymphocytopenia both refer to lower than normal levels of two other types of white blood cells. Thrombocytopenia is unrelated to the white blood cells, but rather refers to a lowered platelet count, a different component of the blood.

37. D: The integration of physical and mental healthcare is an important aspect of the Medical Home, also known as the Medicaid health home model. The model shows collaborative care programs as an approach to integration in which primary care providers, care managers, and psychiatric consultants work together to provide care and monitor patient progress. These programs have been shown to be both clinically-effective and cost-effective for a variety of mental health conditions, in a variety of settings, using several different payment mechanisms.

38. B: For a neurologic attack to be considered transient, as in a transient ischemic attack (TIA), the stroke-like symptoms must last less than one hour, though most symptoms resolve within five minutes. Greater than an hour will likely result in and/or indicate a cerebrovascular accident, in which brain tissue is damaged due to an ischemic event. The other three answers do not fall in line with this parameter.

39. A: Based on the history of playing football and the presenting symptoms, the patient likely has chronic traumatic encephalopathy (CTE). Hepatic encephalopathy results from liver dysfunction. Hashimoto's encephalopathy is a subacute condition associated with Hashimoto's thyroiditis. Toxic-metabolic encephalopathy is related to metabolic disorders and is unrelated to head trauma.

40. A: Acute compartment syndrome, characterized by swelling and pain from fluid buildup in a section of muscle and fascia, is common after crushing injuries. Shock would not cause the calf to swell or cause the patient to hallucinate an injury. Deep vein thrombosis normally occurs from inactivity and poor circulation, not from injury. The sciatic nerve is not located in the calf and injuries to it do not cause localized swelling.

41. D: A hypotensive crisis could definitely lead to necrosis of the tubular cells of the kidney due to lack of perfusion. Hypoperfusion can lead to kidney failure. A hypertensive crisis would not have the same effect on the kidney cells, though hypertension over the long term can cause kidney damage. Acetaminophen overdose primarily affects the liver, though severe and long-term cases can cause kidney damage. An upper respiratory infection would likely have no effect on the kidneys. Nephrotoxic drugs include ibuprofen and are damaging to the kidneys in high doses.

42. D: An apical holosystolic murmur accompanied by a thrill may be noted when a patient has experienced papillary muscle rupture following an MI. The aortic, tricuspid, and pulmonic auscultation points will not bring out the same auscultated sounds, as they are not as close to the mitral valve that has been affected by the event.

43. B: Norepinephrine is a potent vasoconstrictor that may be used if dopamine is inadequate in maintaining normal blood pressure in a patient experiencing cardiogenic shock. Dobutamine is an option but is used for systemic vasodilation with stronger beta effects than the others mentioned here. Milrinone causes vasodilation and positive inotropic effects. Nitroglycerin is a potent vasodilator that would lower blood pressure rather than raise it.

44. B: Insufficient translation is not a common barrier to the application of nursing research in clinical practice. Common barriers include inadequate funding, limited access to appropriate patient populations, lack of institutional support for research initiatives, and the rapid expansion of new knowledge from multiple sources.

45. D: Mannitol is used to prevent brain herniation. It is not indicated as therapy for any of the other conditions

46. C: These are the characteristics of cauda equina syndrome, which refers to major nerve damage to a group of nerve endings that control the bowels, bladder, and legs. The other symptoms listed do not relate to this syndrome.

47. B: Third-degree burns are characterized by darkened, dead tissue (eschar) that often require debridement and skin grafts for healing. There is also reduced or absent sensations due to nerve damage and decreased blood supply. A second-degree burn is deep, but loss of sensation in the affected area doesn't occur. A first-degree burn affects only the top layer of skin, and a fourth-degree burn extends through all skin layers, and there is no pain due to the destruction of nerve endings.

48. D: An early sign of respiratory distress is agitation, along with confusion and oxygen hunger. Later signs of respiratory distress occur when the patient has become fatigued because of the respiratory effort they have put forth. These signs include decreased respiratory rate, unconsciousness, and cyanosis.

49. C: Removing the pillows from the bed is not the best option, as these are used to support the patient's limbs and reduce pressure to bony prominences. All the other interventions, including encouraging early mobility, proper nutrition, and turning and repositioning the patient every two hours will help prevent the development of pressure ulcers.

50. C: The American Hospital Association's Patient Care Partnership document mandated a decision-making partnership between the healthcare system and the patient, facilitating patients' efforts to determine their own future. This decision-making partnership highlighted the responsibilities of the healthcare system to fully communicate treatment options and the plan of care, mandating a change in care patterns and nursing practices.

51. A: Plaque buildup is a mark of atherosclerosis and is nonspecific to nicotine inhalation. The other three items listed—inflammation of the vascular endothelium, vasoconstriction, and increased blood pressure—are all effects of the toxic nature of nicotine inhalation due to cigarette smoking.

52. D: Overuse of antibiotics is what led to the mutation and uprising of drug-resistant organisms such as MRSA, VRE, and CRE. These types of "super bugs" are resistant to antibiotic treatments that used to work against them such as methicillin, amoxicillin, penicillin, and oxacillin. Stronger, broader antibiotic treatments must be used for longer periods of time to kill off drug-resistant organisms that cause infections.

53. B: The patient is in hepatic (liver) failure based on the symptomology and the presentation. Kidney failure would present with electrolyte and fluid abnormalities and their symptoms. Diseases of the stomach would present with GI symptoms such as nausea, vomiting, and abdominal pain in the left upper quadrant. Diseases of the spleen would manifest as blood disorders and would not be similar to symptoms of liver failure.

54. B: Goals of care conversations are held to keep the focus on what the dying patient wants at the end of their life.

55. D: The recurrent nightmares and flashbacks that the man is experiencing, which revisit his experiences in combat, are classic symptoms of post-traumatic stress disorder (PTSD). The man may experience panic attacks, but that disorder falls under a different category with different and specific symptoms. Bipolar disorder is another possibility, but again, it has its own specific symptoms that are not described in this scenario. Antisocial behavior involves acting aggressively and violently toward others, which is not the presentation described here.

56. D: Emphysema is a destruction of lung tissue that is characterized by the development of blebs and bullae, air trapping, and overall air space enlargement. Bronchoconstriction is a cause of asthmatic attacks and is not specifically associated with emphysema.

57. B: Diabetic ketoacidosis is an acidotic metabolic state that can be caused by poor diabetic management, leading to hyperglycemia. Diabetic management involves regular visits to the healthcare provider, taking insulin or oral anti-diabetic agents as ordered, following a healthy diet, exercising regularly, and monitoring blood glucose levels at home. Hyperglycemia can occur when the patient does not have enough insulin in the body, making Choice A an incorrect answer. Since ingesting high glucose levels leads to hyperglycemia, not reduced glucose levels, Choice C is not the correct answer. It can also occur when the oral anti-diabetic management is not sufficient to control high blood glucose levels, making Choice D an incorrect answer.

58. C: Angioplasty and stent placement often occur during routine cardiac catheterization to open up occluded blood vessels. There is no camera or scope; instead, dye is shot through the catheter and x-ray images are obtained to visualize structures. The femoral artery is the most commonly accessed blood vessel for left heart catheterization versus the brachial artery, which can be used but is not as common. The patient is not put to sleep, but rather given medicine to help them relax while keeping them awake.

59. C: A person with dark skin tones who is suspected to be anemic will show pallor in the conjunctiva of the eyes, along with the palms of the hands, bottoms of feet, buccal mucosa, and lips. Forearms, scalp, and cheeks will not show pallor, per se, but may show a gray, ashy hue if they are truly anemic.

60. A: A laparoscopic procedure is minimally invasive and makes very small incisions for the surgeon to enter the abdominal cavity and remove the gall bladder. Laparotomy involves the surgeon making a large incision to completely open up the abdominal cavity. Endoscopy is a general term referring to an interior examination of the body—usually an examination of the upper GI tract. Bronchoscopy is one type of endoscopy that nonsurgically examines the airways and lungs.

61. A: In the emergent phase, hypovolemic shock is a potential issue due to excessive fluid and/or blood loss, which will cause a drop in blood pressure. Increased urine output is unlikely unless the patient is in fluid overload. With a drop in blood pressure, heart rate will increase due to increased myocardial contractility, and vasoconstriction will occur. A person in hypovolemic shock will have pale, clammy skin due to decreased fluid or blood volume in the body.

62. B: A morning headache is a common symptom of COPD. The cough associated with COPD is usually productive. A barrel chest, not a narrowed chest, is common due to hyperinflation of the lungs. Patients with COPD will often experience weight loss and muscle wasting because of the disease.

63. B: Basophils are the white blood cells that secrete histamine, the substance that causes itching in allergic reactions. Lymphocytes are responsible for antibody creation. Neutrophils take out bacterial and fungal organisms and are quite numerous. Monocytes assist in breaking down bacterial organisms.

64. B: Sharing, supporting, and explaining the patient's point of view are activities that are consistent with advocacy. Choices *A*, *C*, and *D* contribute to good professional practice but are not specifically related to the concept of advocacy.

65. A: A patient in shock will usually exhibit oliguria, in which urine output has dramatically decreased or stopped altogether, signaling a shutting down of the kidneys due to lack of perfusion from the heart. Other signs of decreased perfusion as seen in a shock state are distant heart sounds, cyanosis, and faint and rapid pulse.

66. B: All the symptoms reported by the patient are part of severe alcohol withdrawal; however, reporting that the room is spinning points towards vestibular disturbance. Patients experiencing vestibular disturbance will feel that the room is rotating, the walls are falling, and the floor is moving. The GI symptoms, headache, and tremors relate to different systems affected by the alcohol withdrawal.

67. D: The Tennessee Classification System designates complete HELLP syndrome as having a platelet count of less than $10 \times 10^9/\mathrm{L}$, AST greater than or equal to 70 units/L, and LDH greater than 600 units/L, which account for the alterations in liver function. Additional manifestations include red cell hemolysis, elevated liver enzymes, and coagulation defects. The syndrome is associated with abnormal blood clotting that commonly creates a hematoma in the liver tissue, not in the liver vasculature; therefore, Choice *A* is incorrect. The liver function is related to the degree of severity of the syndrome; however, the liver damage may or may not improve in a liver that has been previously damaged by systemic disease, prior trauma, or infection. Irreversible damage to the liver, including rupture of hematomas and liver capsule destroying a significant part of the liver, are commonly associated with this condition; therefore, Choice *B* is incorrect. Cerebral edema and hemorrhagic stroke are among the most common complications of the HELLP syndrome due to altered coagulopathy; therefore, Choice *C* is incorrect.

68. A: Root cause is a structured examination of an incident or procedure that is focused on identifying the point at which an error occurred. The process is based on a comprehensive review of all parts of the organizational structure, which would support nurses' understanding of the systems thinking. Competency grids, process diagrams, and case studies are strategies that measure nursing competence related to the QESN patient safety criteria.

69. A: Mechanical ventilation is likely to create an acidotic state in the blood, rather than alkalotic. Neither acidotic or alkalotic states are beneficial for the patient but may be tolerated for a time with the greater good of oxygenation and perfusion being maintained until the patient is stable. Mechanical ventilation decreases the work of breathing, increases cardiac output, and creates positive end-expiratory pressure (PEEP) for a patient so they might rest until they are stabilized and can be weaned from the vent.

70. B: Phenytoin is the drug of choice when treating acute seizures. Memantine is a neurological drug used to treat dementia. Pregabalin is a drug used to treat diabetic neuropathy. Rifaximin is a drug used to treat hepatic encephalopathy.

71. C: Facilitating a patient's transition from one point on the health continuum to another requires caring practices in addition to advocacy and moral agency. Moral agency may be employed to ensure that the patient's wishes are considered, especially those wishes associated with end-of-life concerns. Developing cultural awareness is an example of a response to diversity, and the remaining two choices refer to the facilitation of learning.

72. A: Laying the head of the bed flat for extended periods of time for the patient who is on mechanical ventilation is inappropriate and may put them at risk for developing ventilator-associated pneumonia, as well as possibly causing respiratory distress. The head of the bed should be elevated to 45-90 degrees at all times. Discontinuing mechanical ventilation as soon as the patient can tolerate it is ideal. Regular oral care should be performed to keep the mouth clean and prevent infections from developing.

73. C: Antiaggregants, such as aspirin, prevent platelets from sticking together, thus preventing clotting that would lead to ischemic stroke. Antihypertensives and statins may be prescribed to control blood pressure and hyperlipidemia, respectively, but are not used for preventing coagulopathy. Beta blockers fall under the class of antihypertensives.

74. B: Bright red blood that is being vomited usually indicates an active upper GI bleed. Coffee ground blood indicates the blood has been sitting in the stomach for a while, indicating a slower bleed. The amount of blood, whether large or small, does not indicate active bleeding necessarily. For instance, a large bleed that has not fully manifested itself might result in a relatively small amount of blood vomited.

75. C: Ventricular fibrillation is the most common rhythm detected when a patient goes into cardiac arrest. This is because the fibrillation of the ventricles produces inadequate heart contraction to pump the blood to the vital organs. Without oxygen, the patient "falls out," becoming unconscious and unresponsive. Patients in ventricular fibrillation need immediate cardiopulmonary resuscitation—most importantly, defibrillation. The other rhythms mentioned—atrial fibrillation, ventricular tachycardia, and supraventricular tachycardia—may present serious complications for the patient and must be treated, but they are not the most common cause of cardiac arrest.

76. C: Acetone, a ketoacid produced during the breakdown of fatty acids during diabetic ketoacidosis, is expelled through respiration, thus giving a person in DKA a "fruity" smell to the breath. Glycerol and alanine are byproducts of fat and muscle breakdown as alternative energy sources convert to glucose. Triglycerides are broken down into free fatty acids as another alternative to glucose as energy for metabolism in the body.

77. B: Dopamine is a commonly infused drug in a mechanically ventilated patient, but not for the purpose of analgesia. Rather, it is used to maintain a normal blood pressure in a hemodynamically unstable patient. The usual drugs of choice include morphine, fentanyl, and propofol. These three are commonly used to provide analgesia to a mechanically ventilated patient.

78. C: Depression is often the first sign of the development of dementia later in life. Up to forty percent of Alzheimer's patients also have a concurrent diagnosis of depression. Panic disorder, schizophrenia, and bipolar disorder may certainly occur with dementia but are not as common.

79. D: Informed consent involves both a conversation and a signed document. All clients must provide informed consent, except in cases where their ability to consent is legally limited (e.g., minors or people with court-appointed legal guardians). In these cases, the parent or legal guardian must provide the informed consent, but nurses should still seek the patient's assent to treatment. This involves explaining all the elements of the informed consent in language the client understands, including any limitations to confidentiality and self-determination, and having the client assent, or agree, to treatment.

80. D: If a patient becomes apneic and oxygenation drops off during a spontaneous breathing trial, it is a sign that the patient should be placed back on mechanical ventilation, as they are not ready to breathe on their own. Increasing the sedation will worsen the patient's breathing function. Continuing the breathing trial will lead to organ damage due to lack of oxygenation and perfusion. An antidote is not appropriate in this scenario.

81. A: Distributive justice refers to the allocation of scarce resources, and advocacy is support for policies that protect at-risk populations. The nurse understands that scarce resource allocation may be sub-standard in certain populations. In nursing, nonmaleficence refers to the act of inflicting the least amount of harm possible in order to reach a favorable result. Fidelity refers to faithfulness but does not specifically address resources or the patient population.

82. C: A massive pulmonary embolism impairs right ventricular function as well as causing marked hypotension. Small does not affect the right ventricular function or blood pressure. Submassive affects the right ventricle without hypotension. Grand is not a category of a PE.

83. A: The central idea of the model is that synergy results when the needs and characteristics of a patient, clinical unit, or system are matched with a nurse's competencies. A patient's needs drive the nurse competencies required for patient care.

84. A: Antiplatelet therapy, commonly aspirin, is coupled with antithrombotic therapy in the postoperative period following an endarterectomy to prevent blood clotting caused by platelet aggregation, which would reocclude the blood vessels just operated on. Beta-blockers, ACE inhibitors, and ARBs are not commonly paired with antithrombotics; rather, they target blood pressure issues and heart failure.

85. D: A stroke is a potential complication of hypertension in a patient post-endarterectomy. The critical care nurse must carefully monitor and treat high blood pressure should it occur. Bleeding would be marked by low blood pressure. Infection is a noncardiac issue; thus, it is unrelated to blood pressure in this instance. Pulmonary edema can occur as a result of heart failure and is not pertinent to the monitoring for high blood pressure.

86. C: An atrial septal defect is not part of the tetralogy of Fallot. The tetralogy of Fallot includes a ventricular septal defect, an aorta arising from both ventricles, and hypertrophy of the overworked right ventricle due to pulmonary valve stenosis.

87. C: The patient is in the mania portion of the bipolar cycle, characterized by the spending spree, the promiscuous sex, and the shoplifting. The mania portion of the bipolar cycle entails a prolonged period of elation, where the patient has an inflated ego and feels that the rules no longer apply to him or her. Excessive behavior is characteristic of this portion of the bipolar cycle. Depression, panic, and anxiety are different parts of the mood disorder spectrum, with different defining characteristics.

88. B: Duloxetine may be prescribed for urinary incontinence to help increase sphincter muscle tone. Furosemide is a diuretic that would not be helpful for someone with urinary incontinence unless absolutely necessary for some other health condition. Finasteride and Doxazosin are both drugs that are prescribed for prostate enlargement and not appropriate for this particular scenario.

89. D: A viral infection is considered an immunologic cause as the immune system is weakened by the viral infection and thrombocyte levels drop as a result. Nonimmunological causes arise from a source outside of the immune system, such as sepsis and acute respiratory distress syndrome. Folate deficiency, a cause for anemia, is a nutritional deficiency, not immunological.

90. C: Research indicates that diversity in the workplace strengthens the workgroup by allowing consideration of multiple worldviews and a better understanding of the patient population served by the institution. Multiple viewpoints can also be an advantage in conflict resolution, especially when the conflict is related to diversity issues.

91. A: The novice nurse is comparing her own beliefs to the patient's beliefs and lacks the knowledge to understand the patient's point of view. This is the definition of ethnocentrism, which can adversely affect the nurse-patient relationship. The remaining observations could potentially affect the patient's refusal of the therapy; however, the patient's refusal in this example is clearly related to the religious objection.

92. D: The gastroenterologist will likely use cauterization, an application of heat, to seal the bleeding lesion. Banding is a procedure used to help stop bleeding in esophageal varices. Biopsy is where tissues are removed for histological analysis. Angioplasty is performed in cardiac catheterizations and involves balloon inflation and stent placement to open up occluded blood vessels.

93. C: Losing 1/5 or 20% percent of one's blood volume will throw a person into hypovolemic shock and is considered life-threatening. Organ failure with profound hypotension will likely follow; fluid resuscitation and blood transfusions will be needed as soon as possible.

94. D: Aseptic technique is the recommended technique to use when inserting a urinary catheter and will help in the prevention of catheter-associated urinary tract infections (CAUTIs). Sanitary and clean techniques are lower on the scale of techniques and therefore not adequate. Sterile technique is usually used in surgical procedures in which an environment without micro-organisms present is desirable.

95. D: Flail chest is not an example of an air-leak syndrome. Flail chest occurs because of rib fracture, which then causes separation of the chest wall from the rib cage. This is a medical emergency and may be associated with pneumothorax, an example of an air-leak syndrome. Emphysema and subcutaneous emphysema are both examples of air-leak syndromes.

96. A: The patient with tented T waves, widening QRS complex, and deep S waves is likely experiencing hyperkalemia. Any potassium that is being infused should be stopped, the doctor notified, and correction of the imbalance performed immediately. Hyper- and hyponatremia are not applicable here, though they are both examples of electrolyte imbalances. Hypokalemia presents differently, with weakness, polyuria, hyperexcitable cardiac cells, and muscle cramping.

97. C: Pancreatitis is the likely diagnosis based on the location of the abdominal pain and the patient's history. The hallmark symptom of pancreatitis is abdominal pain, and that is the focus of treatment. Hepatitis presents with symptoms of liver dysfunction such as jaundice, ascites, enlargement of liver, and encephalopathy. Gastritis, an inflammation of the lining of the stomach, will present with nausea and vomiting. Kidney failure will present with oliguria and fluid and electrolyte imbalances.

98. C: The institution can support diversity by providing resources that satisfy cultural practices, such as dietary rules. Institutions also may provide interpreters, information sessions for employees, and accommodations for religious observances. Under normal circumstances, requiring employees to speak a second language would severely limit the pool of eligible employees and would not be an effective strategy. Educational programs should be provided for all employees and should not be limited to supervisory staff. Offering alternative solutions to all requests for accommodation could be viewed as paternalistic and culturally insensitive. The institution is required to consider ways to satisfy all reasonable patient requests.

99. B: Stabilization of the patient's blood pressure is an excellent sign that their condition is improving. Fever, oliguria, and tachycardia (Choices *A*, *C*, and *D*) are all signs of deterioration and may point toward complications such as shock, bleeding, and/or infection, which need further investigation.

100. C: Acid reflux, along with anxiety or panic attacks, may mimic the chest pain experienced during a heart attack. The proximity of the upper sphincters of the stomach involved in acid reflux to the heart muscle are the cause of the confusion. The patient's presentation, history, and physical along with lab testing and assessment will aid in correct diagnosis. While liver cirrhosis, kidney failure, and pneumonia all involve organs close to the heart, they do not mimic the symptoms of a heart attack.

101. B: The ventricles of the brain are responsible for the production of cerebrospinal fluid. The pons are located at the end of the brain stem and are responsible for regulating breathing. The thalamus acts as a message exchange center for the cerebrum and limbic system and is located just above the brain stem. The corpus callosum is the fibrous tissue of white matter that connects the left and right brain.

102. C: Deconditioning is the term for muscle wasting and debilitation caused by bedrest. Immobility is the limited ability to move freely, which may lead to deconditioning. Decompression syndrome is a physiological condition caused by a rapid decrease in surrounding pressure and is unrelated to these symptoms. Debilitation describes a loss of strength, not necessarily muscle wasting, and thus is not the best choice to explain the described changes.

103. D: Abscesses are generally caused by bacterial infections; most commonly, they result from staphylococcal bacteria. Viruses can occasionally cause an abscess, but this is rare, so Choice *A* can be eliminated. Abscesses result from infections and are not caused by hormone shifts. Therefore, Choice *B* can be eliminated. Acne can be caused by bacteria or may lead to open wounds through which bacteria can enter. However, acne itself is not a direct precursor to the formation of an abscess, so Choice *C* can be eliminated.

104. D: Troponin is a muscle cell protein that is released when cardiac tissue is broken down during an ischemic event. Elevated levels of troponin in the bloodstream indicate cardiac muscle damage. Creatinine and BUN are waste products of the body, and higher levels of these in the bloodstream indicate kidney failure or damage, not heart damage. Creatine kinase is an enzyme found in muscle tissue. One form of the enzyme, CK-MB, is a cardiac enzyme, but its structure is similar to creatine kinase found in skeletal muscle. Therefore, it's a less specific indicator of cardiac muscle damage.

105. A: A woman may have flulike symptoms, anxiety, or jaw or back pain days to weeks before the actual cardiac event. These symptoms may be overlooked and the correct diagnosis missed if the clinician is unaware of gender differences. The other three choices listed are classic, well-known symptoms of a myocardial infarction in both men and women.

106. C: Pursed-lip breathing, breathing through a small, straw-like opening of the mouth, creates positive end-expiratory pressure (PEEP) for the patient with compromised lung function, as is the case with COPD patients. Tripod breathing is common in COPD patients but does not increase PEEP; rather, it creates more space for lung volume when they are having trouble breathing. Wide open-mouth breathing is not helpful for increasing PEEP. Frequent coughing is caused by the body's constant mucociliary response to try and clear mucus from inflamed airways.

107. A: Anemia, or a lack of red blood cells, in a patient with chronic kidney disease could indicate that erythropoietin release is decreased, meaning erythropoiesis is not being stimulated. Leukemia is a lack of white blood cells that is not affected by kidney failure. Hypovolemia is not related to a lack of erythropoietin. Hypocalcemia is an electrolyte abnormality affected by kidney failure but not by lack of erythropoietin.

108. A: While all of the steps listed are important and will likely take place at some point along the patient care pathway, controlling the airway is usually the first step in managing a maxillofacial injury. The patient needs to have enough oxygenation and ventilation to sustain him or her to care; otherwise, vital signs are likely to collapse.

109. B: An ST-segment elevation is the classic ECG reading that indicates a STEMI, in which the full thickness of the heart wall has been damaged, leading to the significant ECG changes. T-wave inversion can be linked to a number of cardiac disorders, both benign and life-threatening, but in the case of heart attacks, it is linked to NSTEMIs. The QT prolongation is part of a condition in which the patient experiences irregular, chaotic heart rhythms from time to time. The U-wave is sometimes too small to be observed on a normal ECG. It follows the T-wave and is not significant in showing heart wall damage, although it can become elevated in hypokalemia.

110. B: The four steps in systems thinking in order are react (to events), anticipate (patterns, trends, causes), design (identify the underlying structures and patterns of influence), and transform (change the beliefs and mental models).

111. C: The depth of the wound is the biggest clue as to whether the ulcer arose out of an arterial insufficiency or a venous insufficiency. Arterial ulcers are usually nonhealing and deep, eventually exposing tendons and bones if left untreated. The color of the ulcer may vary across a spectrum, regardless of the type. Cultures from the wound only tell what types of infectious agents have entered the ulcerative tissue. The size of the wound is irrelevant.

112. A: The child ate (ingested) the toxin. Breathing fumes or sniffing glue are examples of inhalation, not ingestion.

113. B: According to the systems thinking model, vulnerability refers to the presence of any stressor, actual or potential, that could adversely affect the patient's health. A history of smoking increases the patient's vulnerability to additional health alterations. Socioeconomic status and being married are related to resource availability, which refers to the availability of financial and emotional resources that are necessary to support the patient's recovery. The patient's active participation in the plan of care (Choice *D*) is considered to have a positive effect on care outcomes.

114. C: The liver is a solid organ located in the right upper quadrant of the abdomen. When a penetrating wound such as a gunshot has occurred to the abdomen, it is important to be mindful of organ damage underneath the point of penetration. The small intestine, stomach, and colon are all hollow organs located in different areas of the abdomen.

115. D: Long QT syndrome is a rare, hereditary condition found many times in healthy children and adults that may be asymptomatic until a syncopal episode or even sudden death occurs. First- and third-degree heart block occurs when there are conduction problems between the atria and ventricles, resulting in "missed" heartbeats. Bundle branch block occurs when there is an interruption in the electrical impulse across the ventricles of the heart.

116. B: Perioperative inoculation occurs around the time of surgery and happens most frequently in joint replacement surgery. Although it could be considered a post-op infection, its cause is perioperative and not postoperative. Infectious arthritis, a joint infection, is not exclusively the result of surgery.

117. D: An ankle-brachial BP index is commonly used to diagnose peripheral arterial disease by comparing the blood pressures of the two sites, thus assessing blood flow. An echocardiogram is a sonographic test used to visualize the structures of the heart, such as in heart failure. A computed tomography (CT) scan would not be useful for visualizing arterial structures of the extremities, or at least it is not commonly used. An electrocardiogram is used to measure and track electrical activity of heart muscle.

118. D: Diazepam is an anxiolytic that is not specifically used for the treatment of pulmonary hypertension. Diuretics, calcium channel blockers, and vasodilators may all be used to treat pulmonary hypertension. Sildenafil is an example of a phosphodiesterase inhibitor and is helpful in increasing blood flow in the lungs. Amlodipine is an example of a calcium channel blocker, a class of drugs that can be helpful for pulmonary hypertension. Epoprostenol is a drug specifically formulated for use in patients with pulmonary hypertension.

119. D: When the balloon inflates during diastole, blood flow back into the coronary arteries and diastolic filling are encouraged, both which improve heart function. The first two options listed, creating space in the aorta and pushing more blood out into peripheral circulation, are effects of the deflation stage of the balloon pump's actions. The function of the balloon pump is not specifically aimed at raising blood pressure, though this may be an effect of improved heart function because of the pump.

120. A: Sepsis-3 guidelines define sepsis as life threatening organ dysfunction caused by an infection. Previous definitions focused on the presence of systemic inflammatory response syndrome (SIRS) paired with a known source of infection; however, the current definition moved away from those criteria in favor of the more specific Sequential Organ Failure Assessment (SOFA) score. Hypotensive crisis and lactic acidosis typically present when sepsis has advanced to septic shock. But is not a defining factor for general sepsis.

121. D: The major premise of the Synergy Model states that synergy—optimum health—can only be achieved when agency resources and nursing competencies are congruent with the patient's needs.

122. C: Expert nurses are those who reach the point in their clinical practice where clinical reasoning and inquiry are intertwined, allowing the nurse to make clinical judgements quickly and appropriately, according to best practice standards.

123. D: An infected wound will become reddened, inflamed, and discharge pus. A surgical wound should be clean with approximated boundaries. A trauma wound may be irregularly shaped and large. A healing wound develops scabbing and possibly scar tissue but should not appear as the wound described.

124. D: The procedure described is the Roux-en-Y bypass, in which the stomach is made into a smaller gastric pouch, the rest of the stomach and duodenum are completely bypassed, and the gastric pouch then empties directly into the jejunum. This procedure makes it so the patient feels fuller faster because of the smaller gastric pouch, thus decreasing caloric intake significantly and promoting weight loss. Gastrectomy, gastric banding, and liposuction are different bariatric surgeries that do not fit the description in the scenario.

125. B: When using an artificial graft, rather than a patient's own vessel, to graft in between the femoral and popliteal arteries in the leg, narrowing and reocclusion are a concern. This is a known complication of these types of grafts. Infection is always a risk but nonspecific to this instance. Edema is associated with venous occlusion and insufficiency. Tissue graft rejection is a possibility but was not mentioned specifically in the text.

126. B: Grave's disease and Hashimoto's disease are both autoimmune disorders, but Grave's disease results in an overproduction of thyroid hormone, while Hashimoto's disease results in a deficiency of thyroid hormone. The other statements are not correct.

127. D: The pooling of blood and edematous swelling are signs of a venous insufficiency rather than an arterial one. Remember, arteries bring oxygen, so when there is a lack of oxygen, tissue cannot get oxygen, thus causing cyanosis and hair loss, and sores or wounds cannot heal. When venous blood is not returning to the heart, pooling and edema occur.

128. A: The most common complication associated with shunts is the obstruction of the proximal catheter. Over a period, the proximal tip of the catheter can become embedded in the choroid, obstructing the catheter and delaying the drainage of the CSF. The shunt valve on the proximal end can also become obstructed with blood cells and other cellular debris. Obstruction of the distal catheter is less common than proximal obstruction but occurs more frequently than infection or dislocation. Migration of the catheter tip is most commonly related to the growth of the patient, which means that this complication occurs in younger children most often. The patient referenced in this scenario was an adult at the time of insertion of the catheter; therefore, this is not a likely cause for his current problem, and Choice *B* is incorrect.

129. B: Constant clearing of the throat is a sign that a patient is silently aspirating. Integumentary symptoms such as rash are not associated with this condition. Swollen lymph nodes on the neck indicate possible upper respiratory infection. Neurological deficits such as memory and orientation loss are not associated with silent aspiration, but may occur because of stroke, which is a precursor to difficulty swallowing in some cases.

130. A: IV magnesium sulfate will be given to the pregnant woman experiencing eclampsia to prevent seizures. The other three IV medications listed are all used to correct fluid and electrolyte imbalances and may be used, but not specifically for the purpose of preventing seizures in a pregnant woman in hypertensive crisis.

131. C: Cutting her inner arms is an example of non-suicidal self-injury. NSSIs are not meant to kill oneself, but rather to relieve psychological pain by inflicting physical pain on oneself. Intentionally crashing their vehicle and ingesting the aspirin are suicidal attempts, in which taking one's life is the intention. Reporting suicidal thoughts to a friend is likely a cry for help.

132. C: Central diabetes insipidus is caused by a decreased amount of vasopressin secreted by the pituitary gland in the body. This decrease will cause massive diuresis, leading to dehydration and hypovolemia. SIADH is the opposite situation in which vasopressin is overly released, also called antidiuretic hormone, and fluid is retained, leading to hyponatremia. Diabetes type I and diabetes type II, the two types of diabetes mellitus, share the name diabetes but are slightly different. Diabetes describes a condition in which polyuria occurs, and in the case of diabetes mellitus (mellitus is Latin for "sweetened with honey," describing the sweetness of urine in diabetes mellitus), it is because of hyperglycemia that the polyuria occurs.

133. B: Hypertonic saline, in which the sodium is more concentrated, is often used to correct the dilutional hyponatremia of SIADH. Normal saline has a 0.9% concentration of sodium, which is the same as circulating blood and thus will not be helpful in correcting hyponatremia. Hypotonic saline, in which there is less than 0.9% concentration of sodium, will also not be helpful in restoring normal sodium levels to the blood. Lactated ringer's solution is generally not used for correcting hyponatremia because it is a hypotonic solution and can potentially worsen the condition.

134. C: Pain can slow thought processes and impair memory. It cannot always be controlled and does not always cause depression.

135. C: Naloxone, or Narcan, is the antidote for respiratory depression caused by an opioid overdose. Morphine and hydrocodone are examples of opioids that might cause respiratory failure if overdose occurs. Alprazolam is a benzodiazepine; it is a central nervous system depressant and can cause respiratory failure if overdosed or combined with other substances.

136. D: The patient appears to be anorexic, a psychological condition in which a patient is undernourished as a result of refusing to eat in order to meet some "ideal image" of body weight that is unrealistic. A patient with anorexia will appear pale, fatigued, underweight, and very thin. Gastritis is an inflammation of the lining of the stomach that would cause nausea, vomiting, and loss of appetite but is not applicable here. Overnutrition is a type of malnutrition associated with obesity and weight gain, not weight loss. Malabsorption is a type of nutritive disorder in which the small intestine does not absorb nutrients from food properly. Malabsorption could definitely lead to weight loss and the other symptoms but the patient's psychological issues and refusal to eat suggest a psychological condition rather than a physical disorder.

137. D: The nurse will use physical restraints to calm an agitated patient as a last resort. Verbal de-escalation should be the first intervention. If the patient continues to act out aggressively and violently, antipsychotics, both first and second generation, may be used to calm the patient down. Using restraints is a last-resort intervention, and in order to do so, the nurse must obtain a doctor's order and follow facility policy.

138. B: Vigilance refers to the ability of the nurse to recognize and respond to changes in the patient's condition. According to the Synergy Model, vigilance as a caring practice is a learned behavior that evolves with clinical experience, which means that the novice nurse will identify predictable alterations in the patient's condition, while the experienced nurse will identify and respond to more subtle changes. The most experienced nurse is capable of intervening to prevent some adverse events. Engagement refers to committing to the patient care relationship, rather than responding to changes in the patient's condition. The changes noted in the patient's condition are early, subtle indications of heart failure. The novice nurse would initially associate the changes with the surgical procedure, while the experienced nurse would assess the patient for heart failure. Although collaboration with other providers may have been an outcome of the nurse's assessment, the initial care was an independent action.

139. C: The flu vaccine should be administered every year at the beginning of the flu season. Every year a strain of flu is identified as being the likely culprit for cases of the flu for that year and used in the vaccines, thus everyone six months and older should get their flu shot each and every year. The other answers are invalid.

140. B: The risk of brain herniation is higher in patients who are immunosuppressed, over sixty years old, have a history of recent seizure activity, or have a disease of the CNS. A CT scan may be done prior to the lumbar puncture in this patient population; however, instituting antibiotic therapy to prevent morbidity remains the priority intervention. Bacterial meningitis is associated with a characteristic erythematous rash. However, depending on the causative organism, rashes may also be present with viral meningitis; therefore, the presence or absence of the rash cannot differentiate between the two conditions, which means that Choice *A* is incorrect. The protein level of the CSF is elevated, not decreased, in bacterial meningitis.

The inflammatory response resulting from the bacterial infection alters the blood-brain barrier, which allows the leakage of protein from the blood into the subarachnoid space, causing marked increase in the protein level of the CSF; therefore, Choice *C* is incorrect. The meningococcal vaccine, MCV4, is effective against meningococcal meningitis and has decreased the incidence of the disease among college students and military personnel who typically reside in close quarters. Residents of long-term care facilities are protected against pneumococcal meningitis by the PPSV; therefore, Choice *D* is incorrect.

141. B: The nurse suspects that the IV has infiltrated, meaning the catheter tip has become dislodged and IV medication and/or fluids are leaking into the surrounding tissues. The nurse should stop the infusion, remove the IV, and dress the site. An allergic reaction or infection would be warm, not cold, due to the inflammatory response present in such conditions. This is not a normal assessment of a peripheral IV.

142. D: A patient who is in renal failure with a suspected PE will likely undergo V/Q scanning, in which ventilation and perfusion of the lungs are visualized. Transesophageal echocardiography is used for visualizing the back of the heart and is not appropriate in this scenario. CT scanning with contrast is contraindicated, as the patient with renal failure cannot tolerate the dye, which is primarily metabolized by the kidneys. An MRI is not a usual scan for a PE.

143. B: Moral agency refers to decision-making that includes accountability for right and wrong decisions by the moral agent. Advocacy is an ethical principle that is not legally enforced. However, many argue that paternalism is contrary to advocacy because of the assumption that the "system" knows what is best for the patient without concern for the patient's wishes. Moral agency is not restricted to a specific population; however, the nurse will assess the ability of all patients to make informed decisions.

144. C: Nurses must acknowledge their own biases and recognize that those biases will affect their ability to provide culturally sensitive care. Standard protocols related to cultural beliefs and practices are an imperfect solution to the problem of culturally sensitive care because they are not individualized to the specific patient. Meeting the needs of the largest group in a population generally means that the cultural needs of the minority groups within the population are not met. As previously stated, culturally competent care results when caregivers first consider their own biases and the possible effect of those beliefs on patient care. If nurses base their care only on their own beliefs, the patient's beliefs and practices will be ignored.

145. D: Delirium is transient, reversible, and usually has an acute onset with an illness. Dementia, on the other hand, is a slow-developing, irreversible, and chronic condition often accompanied by another chronic diagnosis such as Parkinson's or Alzheimer's. Dementia may be slowed, but never fully reversed. Delirium usually can be treated and reversed by treating the underlying cause.

146. C: A patient with rhabdomyolysis will have a dark amber colored urine, resembling the color of cola. This is due to the myoglobin that leaked from the muscle tissue and was excreted in the urine. Yellow and clear colored urine are normal findings while blood-tinged urine is not a characteristic finding of rhabdomyolysis and may suggest another pathology.

147. C: A patient with a Behavior Activity Rating Scale (BARS) score of 1 is lethargic and difficult to rouse so immediate transfer to an ED is needed to determine cause.

148. B: Research indicates that public funds are the most common source of funding, which means that researchers are obligated to design studies that provide valid results that are applicable to some form of patient care and to disseminate the results appropriately. The remaining sources also provide funding; however, public funds are noted to be the most common source.

149. C: Immunocompromised pneumonia occurs in patients whose immune systems have been weakened. It may occur in patients who have an HIV infection or are undergoing chemotherapy or radiation regimens. Community-acquired pneumonia occurs in persons who had little to no contact with medical facilities prior to the infection. Hospital-acquired pneumonias occur in patients who have been hospitalized and as a result of immobilization. Healthcare-associated pneumonias occur in patients in long-term facilities or some other healthcare facility besides a hospital.

150. A: *Streptococcus pneumoniae* is the most common cause of bacterial pneumonia. The other three organisms listed are also bacteria and may cause pneumonia if they infect the lungs, but not as commonly as *S. pneumoniae.*

Adult CCRN Practice Test #2

1. A patient with a fever is admitted to the unit with suspected influenza. Which priority action does the nurse take?
    a. Obtain a nasal swab for analysis.
    b. Report the case to the health department.
    c. Administer the influenza vaccine.
    d. Place the patient on droplet precautions.

2. Which chronic condition listed below is most likely to lead to end-stage renal disease?
    a. Diabetes
    b. Polycystic ovary syndrome
    c. Hypertension
    d. Polycystic kidney disease

3. A nurse is providing care to a patient in hypovolemic shock due to excessive vomiting. Which pharmacological treatment does the nurse expect to administer first?
    a. Dopamine
    b. Ondansetron
    c. Lactated Ringer's
    d. Norepinephrine

4. Mickey is a 4-year-old boy who is recovering from chicken pox. His case of chicken pox was relatively mild, and his symptoms resolved after approximately ten days. Believing that he is fully recovered, his parents return Mickey to preschool after two weeks at home. After a few days back in school, Mickey's father notices that he has patches of red dots on his skin. Mickey also begins to randomly have nosebleeds, and his gums tend to bleed when he brushes his teeth. What is Mickey most likely experiencing?
    a. Shingles
    b. Continued symptoms of chicken pox, which had not fully resolved
    c. Immune thrombocytopenic purpura
    d. Guillain-Barré syndrome

5. Which of the following is NOT a right that patients and families have regarding their medical care?
    a. Accessing staffing schedules for their care team
    b. Obtaining medical records
    c. Receiving non-discriminatory care
    d. Participating in healthcare decisions

6. A nurse receives an order to wean a patient with a history of chronic obstructive pulmonary disorder (COPD) off the ventilator. The patient experiences oxygen desaturation during a breathing trial and is unable to be weaned off due to increased resistive load. Which follow up treatment does the nurse expect to implement?
    a. Decrease in sedative analgesics
    b. Replacement of the endotracheal tube (ETT)
    c. Application of supplemental oxygen
    d. Administration of bronchodilators

7. Which person is most likely to have a hemophilia diagnosis?
   a. Jake, a young boy whose mother has a mutation in her gene for factor IX
   b. David, an elderly man who has a small cancerous growth in his bone marrow
   c. Mira, an adult Asian woman
   d. Lilly, a two-year-old girl with delayed speech development

8. A patient is admitted following a traumatic fall with a spinal cord injury. Upon assessment, the patient is restless, hypotensive, diaphoretic, and has pale mucous membranes. The nurse suspects which type of hemodynamic shock?
   a. Neurogenic
   b. Cardiogenic
   c. Anaphylactic
   d. Septic

9. The nurse is receiving reports at the beginning of the shift. One of the patients has been admitted to the hospital and is awaiting transfer to the ICU with an admitting diagnosis of obstructive shock. Which of the following findings are characteristic of obstructive shock?
   a. Jugular vein distention, peripheral edema, and pulmonary congestion
   b. Decreased urine output, increased BUN, and increased creatinine
   c. Chest pain, fatigue, and lightheadedness
   d. Problems with coordination, blurred vision, and partial paralysis

10. The nurse is receiving new medication orders from the patient's medical team during rounds. Which action can help reduce medication errors?
   a. Request a verbal order.
   b. Use standard medical abbreviations when possible.
   c. Read back and verify new orders received.
   d. Rely on paper charting to double-check for error.

11. A nurse is assessing a patient diagnosed with pneumonia and atelectasis. Upon assessment, the patient is dyspneic and restless. The nurse expects to see which laboratory data to support uncompensated respiratory acidosis?
   a. pH 7.25, $PaCO_2$ 55 mmHg, HCO_3 22 mEq/L
   b. pH 7.30, $PaCO_2$ 50 mmHg, HCO_3 28 mEq/L
   c. pH 7.40, $PaCO_2$ 48 mmHg, HCO_3 30 mEq/L
   d. pH 7.38, $PaCO_2$ 38 mmHg, HCO_3 26 mEq/L

12. Which of the following, if consumed, can trigger a celiac crisis?
   a. High fructose corn syrup
   b. Gluten
   c. Nightshade vegetables
   d. Peanuts

13. Burn victims are most likely to experience renal failure as a result of which phenomenon?
   a. Sepsis
   b. Hypermetabolism
   c. Fluid creep
   d. Hypomagnesemia

14. Marcy recently had bariatric surgery. Which disorder is she most at risk of developing after the surgery?
   a. Lymphoma
   b. Anorexia
   c. Metabolic syndrome
   d. Anemia

15. A nurse is reviewing the results of arterial blood gases for a patient. The report shows the following: pH 7.36, $PaCO_2$ 46 mmHg, HCO_3 30 mEq/L. How does the nurse interpret these results?
   a. Compensated metabolic alkalosis
   b. Compensated respiratory acidosis
   c. Respiratory acidosis
   d. Metabolic alkalosis

16. A patient with a tracheostomy tube has developed tracheomalacia. The nurse knows that the major risk factor in the development of this condition is which of the following?
   a. Excessive secretions around the stoma
   b. Overinflation of the cuff
   c. Accidental decannulation
   d. Frequent suctioning

17. Upon assessment of a bariatric patient who underwent laparoscopic adjustable gastric banding (LAGB), the nurse notes a rigid abdomen, absent bowel sounds, and tenderness upon palpation. Which postoperative complication does the nurse suspect?
   a. Constipation
   b. Splenic injury
   c. Bowel perforation
   d. Aortic dissection

18. A nurse is reviewing the medication administration record of a patient post-total knee arthroplasty 24 hours ago. The nurse notes the patient has been medicated every two hours as scheduled, with breakthrough doses of more potent analgesics. The patient has no significant medical or social history and the latest physical assessment is as expected. How does the nurse interpret the patient's clinical presentation?
   a. It is considered acute pain and a normal response to surgery.
   b. The patient needs to be referred to a pain specialist.
   c. The patient is displaying drug-seeking behavior.
   d. Surgical complications are likely the cause of pain.

19. A female patient presents in the emergency room with a fever of 104°F, confusion, and tachycardia. In reviewing the patient's history, the clinical care staff notes that the patient is diabetic and regularly takes aspirin. She has also had a prescription for methimazole, but the clinical care staff cannot tell if it is an active prescription. Confirmatory lab work indicates that patient has higher than average thyroxine and triiodothyronine levels and low thyrotropin levels. What is the patient likely experiencing?
   a. An infected wound
   b. Hypoglycemia
   c. Thyroid storm
   d. A cardiovascular event

20. A patient has passed away while they have family members in the room. Which of the following is NOT an appropriate action for the nurse to take immediately after death?
   a. Continue to refer to the patient by their name after death.
   b. Assist with arrangements for funeral or burial facilities.
   c. Escort the family out of the room to begin post-mortem care.
   d. Encourage grieving and communication for the family.

21. A nurse is providing care to a patient with pulmonary hypertension. Which abnormal mechanism explains the direct progression of pulmonary hypertension to cor pulmonale?
   a. Alveolar hypoxemia
   b. Increased pulmonary vascular resistance
   c. Increased right ventricular workload
   d. Pulmonary vasoconstriction

22. The nurse is caring for a patient with fungal meningitis. Which medication would they anticipate the patient being on?
   a. Cefotaxime
   b. Gentamicin
   c. Flucytosine
   d. Intravenous immune globulin (IVIG)

23. A patient is diagnosed with cardiac tamponade following a chest CT. Which intervention does the nurse anticipate this patient receiving?
   a. Transcatheter aortic valve replacement (TAVR)
   b. Pericardiocentesis
   c. Coronary artery bypass graft (CABG)
   d. Balloon angioplasty

24. Patients with nephrotic syndrome should limit their intake of which nutrient?
   a. Carbohydrates
   b. Protein
   c. Vitamin D
   d. CoQ10

25. A patient has developed acute respiratory distress syndrome (ARDS) with pulmonary hypertension. Which medication does the nurse expect to administer to assist with improved pulmonary blood flow?
   a. Albuterol
   b. Nifedipine
   c. Nitric oxide
   d. Digoxin

26. Which of the following communication techniques represents good therapeutic communication for the nurse to use with a patient?
   a. Asking simple yes or no questions
   b. Using silence when appropriate
   c. Using clichés to establish rapport
   d. Asking patients to explain their behavior

27. A nurse is reviewing laboratory data for a patient with a history of asthma. Arterial blood gases were obtained during the initial phase of an exacerbation. Which result does the nurse expect to see in the report?
    a. $PaCO_2$ of 50 mmHg
    b. HCO_3 of 20 mEq/L
    c. $PaCO_2$ of 30 mmHg
    d. HCO_3 of 35 mEq/L

28. The nurse is caring for a patient admitted with diabetic ketoacidosis (DKA) who requests to have orange juice with their breakfast. The nurse denies this request, stating that the orange juice could raise their blood sugar to a dangerous level, and offers to get water or black coffee for the patient instead. This is an example of which ethical principle?
    a. Beneficence
    b. Autonomy
    c. Nonmaleficence
    d. This is unethical practice

29. Stage 5 of chronic kidney disease usually requires which of the following to manage the condition?
    a. Steroid and antidiuretic hormone injections
    b. Dialysis or a kidney transplant
    c. A full-time home health aide
    d. Hospice services

30. A nurse is reviewing medication orders for a patient with rheumatoid arthritis. The patient has a history of lupus with a recent renal transplant. Which medication will the nurse clarify with the healthcare provider?
    a. Acetaminophen
    b. Hydrocodone
    c. Cyclobenzaprine
    d. Ibuprofen

31. A 63-year-old male patient complains of sudden, severe upper back pain that is described as a ripping sensation. The patient has difficulty breathing, loss of vision, weakness, and a weaker pulse in their left arm. This patient is likely experiencing which medical emergency?
    a. Aortic dissection
    b. Pulmonary edema
    c. Aortic aneurysm
    d. Pulmonary embolism

32. Patients receiving hemodialysis treatments generally require a procedure every other day, with sessions lasting up to four hours. Hemodialysis complications and emergencies most commonly occur as a result of which of the following?
    a. Medical device malfunction
    b. Pathogen exposure
    c. Electrolyte imbalance
    d. Human error

33. The nurse is caring for a patient with increased intracranial pressure (ICP). Which of the following interventions would the nurse expect for the treatment of this patient?
   a. Burr holes
   b. 0.45% normal saline
   c. HOB at less than 30 degrees
   d. Mechanical hypoventilation

34. Which of the following adventitious sounds is associated with early congestive heart failure?
   a. Mediastinal crunch
   b. Late inspiratory crackles
   c. Mid-inspiratory and mid-expiratory crackles
   d. Early inspiratory crackles

35. A nurse is assessing a patient diagnosed with pneumonia who is being treated with bilevel positive airway pressure (BiPAP) therapy. Upon assessment, the patient's respiratory rate is 32 breaths/min, oxygen saturation is 84%, and the patient is unable to clear oral secretions effectively. Which intervention does the nurse expect to perform next?
   a. Prepare for intubation
   b. Switch to a CPAP machine
   c. Increase the inspiratory pressure
   d. Provide suctioning as needed

36. A nurse receives an order to initiate prone positioning for a patient on a ventilator. The nurse knows that this position produces which intended effect?
   a. Minimized risk of impaired skin integrity
   b. Reduced lung compression
   c. Improved gastric digestion
   d. Decreased systolic blood pressure

37. A 35-year-old patient is admitted to the ICU with a spinal cord injury after diving in a shallow pool. The patient has no mobility or feeling in their legs, has limited mobility with their forearms, and can breathe independently. This patient most likely has a spinal cord injury at which cervical cord?
   a. C4
   b. T9
   c. L3
   d. C8

38. A nurse is providing care to a patient on a ventilator set to assist-control (AC) mode. Which laboratory data indicates a complication of this ventilator mode?
   a. pH 7.46, HCO_3 28 mEq/L
   b. pH 7.33, $PaCO_2$ 47 mmHg
   c. pH 7.45, HCO_3 24 mmHg
   d. pH 7.47, $PaCO_2$ 32 mmHg

39. Which of the following is a complication of hypothyroidism that is often fatal?
   a. Ketoacidosis
   b. Addisonian crisis
   c. Fever
   d. Myxedema coma

40. A patient with a history of chronic obstructive pulmonary disease (COPD) is experiencing acute respiratory failure due to alveolar hypoventilation. Which clinical finding does the nurse expect to observe that best supports ventilatory failure?
   a. PaO_2 of 55 mmHg
   b. pH of 7.4
   c. Oxygen saturation of 87%
   d. $PaCO_2$ of 60 mmHg

41. Martin is a competitive high school wrestler. One day, he cuts the tip of his thumb while slicing an apple. While it bleeds heavily at first, he is able to stop the bleeding with 15 minutes of direct pressure. Unfortunately, the area is quite tender. He skips practice the next day but attends two practices later on in the week. He only experiences slight soreness at the site of his cut during these training sessions and feels that he is able to perform well. Over the weekend, he feels feverish, and his cut feels quite sore. It looks red, and he notices some white fluid within the wound which he believes is leftover antiseptic ointment. Martin takes several days off from training, but he begins to feel worse. He notices a new rash and feels like something is sitting on his chest. Martin's mother rushes him to the emergency room, where his vital signs show a faster than normal heart rate. What is Martin experiencing?
   a. A staph infection
   b. Overtraining
   c. Bacterial pneumonia
   d. A viral infection

42. The nurse is caring for a patient with a cardiomyopathy. Which type of cardiomyopathy is caused by a genetic disorder that the patient's family members should also be educated about?
   a. Hypertrophic cardiomyopathy
   b. Dilated cardiomyopathy
   c. Idiopathic cardiomyopathy
   d. Restrictive cardiomyopathy

43. Which set of laws was enacted in order to prevent healthcare facilities from turning away patients that needed life-sustaining care, regardless of ability to pay?
   a. The Patient Protection and Affordable Care Act of 2010
   b. The American Health Care Act of 2017
   c. The Emergency Medical Treatment and Labor Act of 1986
   d. The Medicare Introduction Act of 1965

44. A nurse is providing care to a patient diagnosed with a deep vein thrombosis to the right lower extremity. Upon assessment, the patient verbalizes dyspnea and has an oxygen saturation of 88%. Which other clinical finding best supports the diagnosis of a suspected pulmonary embolism?
   a. Pleuritic pain
   b. Temperature of 99.8 °F (37.6 °C)
   c. Right calf erythema
   d. Heart rate of 102 beats/min

45. The nurse is caring for a patient who has a fractured right tibia following a motor vehicle accident. Which of the following symptoms would cause the nurse greatest concern for compartment syndrome?
    a. Muscle atrophy in the affected leg
    b. Pain when stretching and pallor in the affected leg
    c. Bounding pulse in the affected leg
    d. Confusion and lethargy

46. A 75-year-old female patient who follows Orthodox Jewish traditions is admitted to the unit for pneumonia. She needs assistance cleaning up and receiving a partial bed bath. It would be appropriate for which of the following team members to participate in this care?
    a. A female nurse and female nursing student
    b. A female nurse and male nursing assistant
    c. A male nurse and female nurse
    d. A male nurse and male nursing assistant

47. A nurse is administering a blood transfusion to a patient. An hour after initiation of the transfusion, the patient experiences oxygen desaturation, fever, and hypotension. Transfusion-related acute lung injury (TRALI) is suspected. Which other clinical finding assists in the diagnosis of this condition?
    a. Hypertension on routine vital signs
    b. Sinus bradycardia on an electrocardiogram
    c. Pulmonary infiltrates on a chest x-ray
    d. Jugular venous distention upon assessment

48. A nurse is assisting a provider with a thoracentesis: removal of air or fluid from the pleural space on a patient diagnosed with empyema. Which action will the nurse take to prevent re-expansion pulmonary edema?
    a. Ensure the amount of fluid removed does not exceed 1 liter
    b. Position the patient upright with upper extremities raised and well-supported
    c. Review the patient's medical record for use of anticoagulants
    d. Instruct the patient to cough and deep breathe throughout the procedure

49. A patient who is Middle Eastern is admitted to the unit, and the nurse is informed that this patient follows typical Middle Eastern dietary restrictions. Which of the following food trays would be appropriate to give this patient?
    a. Grilled salmon with steamed vegetables and rice
    b. Cheeseburger with fries and broccoli
    c. Grilled chicken sandwich with Swiss cheese and side salad
    d. Eggs and bacon with whole wheat toast

50. The nurse is caring for a patient who is one day post-op from a lung resection and chest tube placement. The patient has been receiving acetaminophen (Ofirmev) 1000mg q6hrs and requests to have something additional for pain management. The nurse understands that recovering from this surgery with a chest tube can be extremely painful and contacts the surgeon to request an additional PRN medication for pain. This nurse is exhibiting which level of advocacy and moral agency?
    a. Level 1
    b. Level 2
    c. Level 3
    d. Level 5

51. A 65-year-old patient with unmanaged type 2 diabetes presents with an A1c of 9%. The patient's care team prescribes medication and lifestyle changes to support a reduction in the patient's A1c percentage. What is a reasonable short-term A1c goal for this patient to achieve from these interventions?

a. An A1c under 5%
b. An A1c of between 7% and 8%
c. An A1c between 5% and 6%
d. An A1c of at least 10%

52. A 45-year-old male is admitted for recent visual changes, weakness, headaches, nausea, and vomiting. The patient states that they were told five years ago that they have hypertension, but they do not like to take any medications. The nurse obtains a blood pressure of 190/125. The nurse is most concerned that the patient has developed which condition?

a. Metabolic encephalopathy
b. Bacterial meningitis
c. Hypertensive encephalopathy
d. Cerebral herniation

53. A nurse is reading a research article on new treatments for patients with COPD. In order to critically read, the nurse should actively try to determine all of the following aspects of the article EXCEPT:

a. Thesis
b. Process
c. Outcomes
d. Funding

54. A nurse is providing care to a patient who developed severe sepsis and has been in the intensive care unit for three weeks. The patient is at risk for developing post-intensive care syndrome (PICS) and having multiple deficiencies, EXCEPT in which domain?

a. Psychiatric
b. Physical
c. Cognitive
d. Emotional

55. A patient with an infected wound to the lower extremity meets criteria for systemic inflammatory response syndrome (SIRS). The nurse expects to see which conditions?

a. Respiratory rate of 22 breaths/min and oxygen saturation of 92%
b. White blood cell count of 11,000/mm^3 and serum lactate of 2 mmol/L
c. Temperature of 39 °C (102.2 °F) and heart rate of 102 beats/min
d. Blood pressure of 90/50 mmHg and urine output of 30 ml/hr

56. In a patient with moderate or severe burns who needs emergency care, what is the first intervention they should receive?

a. Wound care
b. Defibrillation
c. Fluid resuscitation
d. Airway management

57. Which is the most common source of neurological infection?
    a. Infections within the kidneys
    b. Infections within the spinal cord
    c. Infections within the bronchioles
    d. Infections within the gastrointestinal tract

58. A nurse is providing care to a patient in septic shock. The patient is receiving intensive fluid therapy. Which clinical value best reflects the expected outcome of fluid resuscitation?
    a. Mean arterial pressure (MAP) of 68 mmHg
    b. Central venous pressure (CVP) of 6 mmHg
    c. Serum lactate level of 4 mmol/L
    d. White blood cell (WBC) count of $10{,}000/\text{mm}^3$

59. A nurse is providing care to an adult patient with suspected narcotic overdose. The healthcare provider orders the administration of naloxone. How will the nurse administer the medication?
    a. 0.4 to 2 mg every two to three minutes, IV push
    b. 0.01 mg/kg every two to three minutes, IM
    c. 1 mg every two minutes, Intranasal
    d. 4 to 8 mg every two minutes, Subcutaneous

60. Which of the following is NOT a required component in informed consent?
    a. Medical team members involved in treatment or procedure
    b. Risks and benefits of alternative options
    c. Reason for the treatment or procedure
    d. Explanation of diagnosis

61. A patient arrives to the intensive care unit after being hemodynamically stabilized in the emergency department. The patient was in a motor vehicle accident at high velocity, unrestrained. Which primary complication should the nurse assess for?
    a. Ankle dislocation
    b. Traumatic brain injury
    c. Wrist fracture
    d. Lumbar compression

62. Hospital-wide decisions and committees involving client rights in a healthcare setting should include which of the following groups?
    a. Administrative heads of the hospital
    b. Doctors and nurses
    c. Medical staff, administration, patients, and family members
    d. Administration and doctors

63. Which eye complication is likely to be experienced by most patients who are diagnosed with diabetes?
    a. Non-proliferative retinopathy
    b. Proliferative retinopathy
    c. Retinal detachment
    d. Late-onset color blindness

64. A nurse is providing care to a trauma patient who is experiencing respiratory distress. Upon assessment, the nurse notes the use of accessory muscles and tracheal deviation. Which respiratory condition does the nurse suspect?
   a. Spontaneous pneumothorax
   b. Tension pneumothorax
   c. Flail chest
   d. Pulmonary embolism

65. Jonah is a 45-year-old man with a history of alcoholism. One evening, Jonah begins violently coughing to the point of vomiting. His brother helps him to the bathroom, where he notices Jonah's vomit has blood in it. Jonah looks pale, so his brother takes him to the emergency room. Which diagnosis is Jonah most likely to receive?
   a. Mallory-Weiss syndrome
   b. Crohn's disease
   c. Peptic ulcer disease
   d. Cirrhosis

66. Which of the following explanations of the fem-pop bypass is accurate information to tell a patient?
   a. A patent vessel is sewn in below the blocked vessel to restore circulation.
   b. A patent vessel is sewn in above the blocked vessel to restore circulation.
   c. The occluded vessel is removed and replaced by a patent vessel to restore circulation.
   d. A patent vessel is sewn in above and below the blocked vessel to restore circulation.

67. A nurse is providing care to a postoperative patient with a urinary catheter. The nurse knows that the most important contributing factor for the prevention of a catheter-associated urinary tract infection (CAUTI) is which of the following?
   a. Perineal care
   b. Frequent emptying of the drainage bag
   c. Hand washing
   d. Duration of catheterization

68. Which chamber of the heart is the most prone to injury from a penetrating cardiac trauma?
   a. Left ventricle
   b. Left atrium
   c. Right ventricle
   d. Right atrium

69. A nurse is providing care to a patient post-endoscopic retrograde cholangiopancreatography (ERCP). Which priority action will the nurse perform to prevent aspiration?
   a. Assess the gag reflex before feeding
   b. Position the head of the bed to at least 30 degrees
   c. Set up suction in the room post-procedure
   d. Encourage coughing and deep breathing every hour

70. When working with adult learners, it is important for the nurse to incorporate which concept into their lesson plan and teachings?
   a. Relate teachings to real-life experiences.
   b. Assume the patient has no prior knowledge of the topic.
   c. Maintain authority and control of the patient during education.
   d. Keep objectives fluid and subjective.

71. The nurse is caring for a patient with a hemorrhagic stroke. The nurse knows that which of the following is the most common cause of a hemorrhagic stroke?
   a. Hypertension
   b. Secondary brain lesions
   c. Viral neurologic infection
   d. Traumatic brain injury

72. A 35-year-old male patient with a history of heart failure is admitted for hypertensive crisis with a blood pressure of 190/135. Which intervention would be appropriate for the nurse to incorporate into the care of this patient?
   a. Administration of dobutamine
   b. Encouraging increased fluid intake
   c. Administration of nicardipine (Cardene)
   d. Maintaining bed in semi-Fowler's position

73. The nurse is working with a certified nursing assistant (CNA) to help provide care for a 55-year-old patient who is morbidly obese. Which of the following tasks would be appropriate to delegate to the CNA to perform independently?
   a. Giving an oral pain medication that has already been scanned
   b. Inserting a new peripheral IV
   c. Repositioning the patient in bed
   d. Recording output from a foley catheter

74. A nurse is caring for a patient who has an abdominal aortic aneurysm that has ruptured. Which treatment intervention does the nurse anticipate for this patient?
   a. Labetalol to control blood pressure
   b. Repeat CT scan within 24 hours
   c. Morphine 2mg IV PRN for pain
   d. Open surgical repair

75. A 27-year-old male is admitted after experiencing muscle pain, weakness, increased heart rate, and dark reddish-brown urine following a workout. An atrial blood gas (ABG) shows the patient in metabolic acidosis. The nurse is anticipating treatment for which medical condition?
   a. Diabetic ketoacidosis (DKA)
   b. Compartment syndrome
   c. Rhabdomyolysis
   d. Epicondylitis

76. A leader who discusses ideas with their group but then seldom incorporates the group's suggestions into their presented changes is said to be which kind of leader?
   a. Democratic leader
   b. Consultative leader
   c. Participatory leader
   d. Delegative leader

77. What is the most common reason a patient with sickle cell disease requires critical or emergency care?
   a. Brain bleed
   b. Losing consciousness
   c. Acute, unmanageable pain
   d. A blood clot

78. Patients who present for care as a result of intentional overdose are most commonly associated with which of the following risks?
   a. A collapsed trachea during airway management
   b. Aggression and violence upon stabilization
   c. Future suicide attempts
   d. A resulting hormone disorder

79. Which disorder is characterized by high cortisol levels and presentation of visible indicators such as a rounded face, easy bruising, and fatness on the back of the neck?
   a. Adrenal fatigue
   b. Cushing's disease
   c. Cystic fibrosis
   d. Hashimoto's disease

80. The nurse is caring for a patient who suddenly enters ventricular fibrillation. After calling a code, starting CPR, and defibrillating, what first medications should the nurse give to the patient?
   a. Epinephrine 1 mg and amiodarone 150 mg
   b. Epinephrine 1 mg and amiodarone 300 mg
   c. Adenosine 6 mg and amiodarone 300 mg
   d. Adenosine 1 mg and epinephrine 1 mg

81. The nurse is caring for a patient who has a left-sided chest tube to suction following a coronary artery bypass graft (CABG). Which finding should be reported to the provider?
   a. Serosanguinous output drainage
   b. Occasional bubbling in the water seal chamber
   c. Pain around the insertion site
   d. Chest tube output of 120 mL/hr

82. Which of the following types of bowel obstruction can resolve on its own?
   a. Intussusception
   b. Partial obstruction
   c. Complete obstruction
   d. Paralytic ileus

83. In patients diagnosed with pancytopenia, which procedure is the best option for accurately determining the underlying cause?

a. A PCR test
b. A bone marrow biopsy
c. An amniocentesis
d. A CBC panel

84. The nurse is caring for a patient with hypertensive encephalopathy. Which of the following actions is appropriate for the nurse to take during their care?

a. Maintain $PaCO_2$ between 38-40 mmHg
b. Suction secretions regularly
c. Avoid use of narcotic analgesics
d. Maintaining patient in Fowler's position and their head in neutral, midline position

85. Which of the following nursing models refers to the patient-focused care that centers around the integration of patient characteristics and nurse competencies within the healthcare environment?

a. Nursing Leadership Model
b. Professional Practice Model
c. Synergy Model
d. Modular Nursing Model

86. A 12-lead EKG shows a patient in supraventricular tachycardia with a heart rate of 180 beats per minute. Which medication would NOT be safe for this patient to take?

a. Digoxin
b. Phenylephrine
c. Verapamil
d. Adenosine

87. Billy is an ICU nurse who is taking care of a 72-year-old female patient who has experienced a complication of peripheral artery disease. Although the patient has been stable for the last six hours, Billy notices that her heart rhythm seems off. Billy checks the patient's catheter container and notices she has had very little urine output, and her lower legs and feet seem to be swelling. Which of the following might the patient be experiencing?

a. Cystitis
b. Acute kidney injury
c. Diabetic neuropathy
d. Aortic injury

88. Which of the following is a requirement to declare brain death for a patient?

a. Only primary reflexes present
b. No response to sternal rub or other stimulus
c. Respiratory rate < 6 breaths per minute without mechanical ventilation
d. Confirmation of brain death by one doctor or two RNs

89. In deep lacerations or lacerations that are older than a day, what is an important note to remember in treatment?

a. Amputation of the area may be necessary.
b. The deepest layer of skin affected should be treated first, and superficial layers of skin should be repaired in order after each deeper layer fully heals.
c. The entire wound should be closed immediately.
d. A physical therapist should provide the initial assessment to ensure that treatment aligns with the rehabilitation program.

90. Which chronic disease is most highly associated with disseminated intravascular coagulation?

a. Diabetes
b. Chronic obstructive pulmonary disorder
c. Cancer
d. Fatty liver disease

91. An untreated peptic ulcer can lead to which condition?

a. Perforation
b. Kidney stone
c. Gastric sleeve
d. Bed sores

92. A nurse is assessing a patient in status asthmaticus. Which clinical manifestation indicates rapid progression to impending cardiopulmonary arrest?

a. Patient verbalization of increased dyspnea
b. Adventitious breath sounds upon auscultation
c. Hyperventilation with accessory muscle use
d. Sudden onset of decreased wheezing

93. A patient is brought up to the unit following a diagnostic cardiac catheterization. Which task should the nurse incorporate into the care of this patient?

a. Lay patient flat in bed for at least two hours.
b. Encourage deep coughing.
c. Remove and change dressing six to eight hours after procedure.
d. Perform frequent neurovascular assessments.

94. A patient is admitted following a motor vehicle accident. Upon assessment, the nurse notes paradoxical chest wall movement, severe dyspnea, and cyanosis to the oral mucous membranes. Flail chest is diagnosed via a chest x-ray. Which treatment does the nurse expect will be ordered to stabilize this injury?

a. Positive-pressure ventilation
b. Coughing and deep breathing
c. Tracheal suctioning
d. Patient-controlled analgesia

95. A patient is admitted after facing blunt force trauma to the chest. Imaging reports that three adjacent ribs are each broken in two places on the right side. The nurse would expect which of the following findings for this patient when observing the portion of the ribs that are fractured?
   a. Skin dimpling over the affected area
   b. Expansion of the fractured segment on inspiration
   c. Edema over the affected area
   d. Retraction of the fractured segment on inspiration

96. Alexa is a competitive weightlifter. She is a training for an upcoming event and has spent most of her free time with a friend who won this event last year and has been coaching her. Alexa is highly motivated to win this event, and she spends an entire Friday evening training. She goes home and is exhausted, so she showers, drinks some water, and goes to sleep without dinner. On Saturday, she wakes up and her muscles feel extremely tender to the touch. She feels weak and slightly nauseous. When she uses the restroom, she notices her urine is a faint brown color. What diagnostic test would help Alexa most in this situation?
   a. A nasal swab for influenza
   b. A blood test for creatine kinase
   c. An electrolyte panel to check for dehydration
   d. An electromyography test to check nerve stimulation in her muscles

97. A patient with vessel occlusion of the proximal section of the right coronary artery is likely to have ECG changes in which leads?
   a. Leads V1 – V4
   b. Leads V4, V5, V6
   c. Leads I, aVL, V5, V6
   d. Leads II, III, aVF

98. The nurse is caring for a patient who is going through alcohol withdrawal. During bedside report, the patient is difficult to arouse and has difficulty telling the nurse where they are. At the end of the nurse's shift twelve hours later, the patient responds to the nurse with slowed speech and does not appear to be interested in engaging the nurse in conversation. This patient is most likely suffering from which condition?
   a. Mixed delirium
   b. Hypoactive delirium
   c. Depression
   d. PTSD

99. Which of the following is NOT one of the basic care responsibilities the nurse must practice when caring for patients?
   a. Minimizing a patient's independence
   b. Ensuring patient safety
   c. Minimizing pain and harm
   d. Decreasing medical errors

100. A nurse is preparing to discharge a patient diagnosed with tuberculosis. The nurse will provide education on the use of isoniazid, pyrazinamide, rifampin, and which other medication commonly prescribed to treat this condition?
   a. Streptomycin
   b. Penicillin G
   c. Ethambutol
   d. Gentamicin

101. A patient is admitted to the critical care unit with primary multiple organ dysfunction syndrome (MODS). To prevent progression to organ failure, which nursing care focus is most important?
   a. Infection control
   b. Maintenance of blood pressure
   c. Assessment of serum lactate
   d. Antibiotic therapy

102. A patient is diagnosed with acute pulmonary edema. Which of the following treatment orders would the nurse question?
   a. Furosemide (Lasix) 40mg IV
   b. Initiation of BiPAP
   c. Maintain head of bed less than 30 degrees
   d. Morphine 4mg IV q2-4hrs

103. A nurse is involved in a research study with 500 participants for a new vaccine that would be recommended for all people 18 years of age and older. 450 of the participants were 50 years old and older. This study would likely suffer from which kind of bias?
   a. Reporting bias
   b. Recall bias
   c. Healthy participant bias
   d. Selection bias

104. According to the DeBakey classification of aneurysms, an aneurysm that is located only in the ascending aorta is which type of aneurysm?
   a. Type I
   b. Type II
   c. Type III
   d. Type IV

105. Left-sided heart failure is most often associated with which set of symptoms?
   a. Abdominal swelling and lower extremity edema
   b. Crackles, dyspnea, and confusion
   c. Bradycardia and elevated JVD
   d. Holosystolic murmur and hepatomegaly

106. The nurse is caring for a 75-year-old patient with end-stage terminal pancreatic cancer. A family member expresses concern to the nurse that the patient has not been eating enough and wants them to receive increased supplemental nutrition. Should the nurse ethically encourage this increased nutritional intake?

a. Yes, the patient should be started on tube feeding if they cannot take in enough nutrients orally.
b. No, increased nutrition could accelerate tumor growth and lead to nausea and vomiting.
c. No, increasing their nutritional intake could lead to weight gain.
d. Yes, the increased nutrition could help extend the patient's life.

107. Which of the following is the most lethal type of skin cancer, due to its ability to quickly spread to the body's organs?

a. Squamous cell carcinoma
b. Malignant melanoma
c. Basal cell carcinoma
d. Dermatofibrosarcoma protuberans

108. A patient has received general anesthesia for a surgical procedure. After surgery is initiated, the patient develops malignant hyperthermia. Which clinical value is consistent with this complication?

a. Heart rate of 54 beats/min
b. Temperature of 38.2 °C (100.7 °F)
c. Potassium level of 3.2 mEq/L
d. CO_2 level of 47 mmHg

109. A nurse who is completely engaged in client care and can help anticipate the needs of the patient and family members is said to be at which level of caring practice?

a. Level 1
b. Level 3
c. Level 4
d. Level 5

110. A nurse is caring for a patient with a suspected myocardial infarction (MI). Which laboratory tests does the nurse anticipate being ordered?

a. Creatine kinase (CK-MB)
b. Glomerular filtration rate (GFR)
c. Prothrombin time (PT)
d. Procalcitonin (PCT)

111. The nurse is caring for a patient who is at risk of developing a deep vein thrombosis. The nurse knows that all of the following are factors that contribute to the development of a venous thrombosis EXCEPT:

a. Endothelial injury
b. Increased arterial blood flow
c. Blood stasis
d. Hypercoagulability

112. While creating an evidence-based practice and dissemination of findings guideline, a nurse is conducting research and wants to use research that has the highest level of evidence, level A. From which of the following studies should the nurse draw information?
   a. Meta-analysis
   b. Randomized-control trial
   c. Integrative interviews
   d. Cohort study

113. If the pressure in the pulmonary artery is increased above normal, which chamber of the heart will be affected first?
   a. The right atrium
   b. The left atrium
   c. The right ventricle
   d. The left ventricle

114. A nurse is providing care to a patient who is listed as an organ donor. Brain death has occurred and the nurse implements interventions to preserve organ perfusion. Which clinical parameter requires immediate action?
   a. Mean arterial pressure (MAP) of 75 mmHg
   b. pH 7.3
   c. Serum sodium 150 mEq/L
   d. Temperature of 35.1 °C (95.1 °F)

115. The nurse is caring for a patient experiencing delirium in the ICU. Which of the following medications does the nurse NOT anticipate the patient being prescribed?
   a. Trazodone
   b. Lithium
   c. Lorazepam
   d. Haloperidol

116. The nurse is caring for a patient with an emerging ischemic stroke. The nurse prepares to administer which of the following fibrinolytic agents?
   a. Urokinase
   b. Streptokinase
   c. Alteplase
   d. Tenecteplase

117. Which of the following accurately represents the population of patients that can have an advance directive?
   a. Patients with a terminal illness
   b. All patients
   c. Patients 65 years and older
   d. Patients with cancer

118. The nursing unit recently discovered a high rate of UTIs amongst post-op patients. As a result, nurses have begun removing indwelling foley catheters within 24 hours after surgery, instead of 48 hours, to try to reduce the rate of UTIs. This nursing unit is at which stage of a problem-solving strategy?

a. Evaluation of solution
b. Development of solutions
c. Identification of the problem
d. Implementation of solution

119. The nurse is caring for a patient who is recovering from a stroke. When ambulating, the patient's left arm stays down at their side and their left leg drags. The patient's right arms sways and they can properly pick up their right foot and step forward. This patient has which kind of gait disorder?

a. Hemiplegic gait
b. Diplegic gait
c. Neuropathic gait
d. Ataxic gait

120. Which of the following is NOT one of the components of effective assertive communication?

a. Look for areas of compromise.
b. Have a defined and clear message.
c. Use "you" statements.
d. Control delivery of information.

121. Which of the following are associated with an Addisonian crisis?

a. Hyperkalemia and hyponatremia
b. Hypertension and shock
c. Excessive cortisol and sweating
d. Hypokalemia and hypernatremia

122. A nurse is providing care to a patient diagnosed with pneumonia who is on a ventilator. The patient's status is declining and acute respiratory distress syndrome (ARDS) is suspected. Which PaO_2/FiO_2 ratio supports a diagnosis of moderate ARDS?

a. 85 mmHg
b. 175 mmHg
c. 250 mmHg
d. 325 mmHg

123. A patient is admitted after a head-on sports injury with slurred speech, uneven pupils, weakness, and severe headache. The nurse knows that this patient is likely suffering from which type of hemorrhage based on the cause of their injury and symptoms?

a. Subarachnoid hemorrhage
b. Intraventricular hemorrhage
c. Intracranial hemorrhage
d. Aneurysmal hemorrhage

124. A nurse is providing care to a patient with metastatic, stage IV colon cancer. The patient verbalizes they want a do not resuscitate (DNR) order. The patient's family is not in agreement. How does the nurse respond to the patient's request?

a. "You should discuss this further with your family."
b. "Let's provide you with more information on a DNR order."
c. "Are you sure you would like to sign a DNR order?"
d. "Would you like to hear about medical treatments first?"

125. In the AACN Synergy Model of nursing practice, which of the following is one of the eight types of client characteristics?

a. Medical knowledge
b. Predictability
c. Insurance coverage
d. Positivity

126. The nurse is preparing a discharge plan for a patient with risk factors for acute pancreatitis. Which of the following information should be included in this plan?

a. Endoscopic retrograde cholangiopancreatography (ERCP) imaging is required to confirm the diagnosis.
b. Ultrasonography is the most useful imaging study when significant abdominal distention is present.
c. Current research confirms the efficacy of rectal administration of indomethacin to reduce the incidence of pancreatitis due to the ERCP procedure.
d. There is no scientific rationale to explain why some individuals with chronic ETOH abuse develop acute pancreatitis, while others do not develop pancreatitis.

127. In patients who are in critical condition due to gastroenteritis, what is commonly the first intervention?

a. Highly nutritious enteral feeding
b. Airway management
c. Withholding food and beginning fluid therapy
d. Administering low-dose Zofran

128. The nurse is caring for a patient who is 36 hours post-op from a carotid endarterectomy. The patient is complaining of a severe headache that is not alleviated with administration of Tylenol. What is the most appropriate immediate action for the nurse to take?

a. Lower the head of the bed to less than 30 degrees.
b. Offer PRN opioid pain reliever.
c. Immediately notify the provider.
d. This is an expected finding; continue to monitor.

129. The nurse is caring for a patient who has just received a terminal diagnosis and was told they likely have less than a year to live. Which of the following is an appropriate response for the nurse to make?

a. Everything will turn out okay.
b. What do you think you could have done differently to prevent this?
c. This must be difficult for you; I am here to answer any questions.
d. I think you should start looking at local hospice care facilities.

130. The nurse is caring for a patient who comes from a different cultural background than themselves. The nurse respectfully asks the patient about different foods they prefer to eat in their culture so those foods can be discussed with the dietician. This nurse is at which level of responding to diversity in the Synergy Model?

a. Level 1
b. Level 2
c. Level 3
d. Level 5

131. Two nurses get into an argument during their shift about restocking the supply room and go to the charge nurse to intervene. What is the first step of conflict resolution the charge nurse should instruct them to take?

a. Present their sides of the argument.
b. Come to a compromise.
c. Discuss their disagreement in detail.
d. Dismiss their argument as non-productive.

132. Which of the following is a contraindication for thrombolytic therapy?

a. Current anticoagulant therapy
b. Over age 75
c. Severe hepatic disease
d. INR of 3.5

133. Nurses are responsible for which of the following elements of informed consent?

a. Identification of alternatives to the planned procedure
b. Description of associated risks and benefits
c. Explanation of the planned procedure or diagnostic test
d. Assessment of the patient's understanding of the information that is provided

134. A nurse is providing care to a patient who is 10 days post-right pneumonectomy. The patient has developed a low-grade fever and reports purulent sputum upon coughing. Which postoperative complication does the nurse suspect?

a. Pulmonary edema
b. Postpneumonectomy empyema
c. Chylothorax
d. Postpneumonectomy syndrome

135. Which of the following is the most common symptom of peripheral vascular disease?

a. Intermittent claudication
b. Necrotic ulcers
c. Lower extremity edema
d. Lower extremity hair loss

136. The nurse is discussing the care during rounds for a patient who has undergone a cardiac catheterization and is now having symptoms of cardiogenic shock. Which type of medication does the nurse NOT anticipate being ordered for this patient?

a. Positive inotropic medication
b. Antiplatelet medication
c. Thrombolytic medication
d. Positive chronotropic medication

137. A patient with a traumatic brain injury (TBI) is receiving a mannitol infusion. What is the correct dosing for this medication?

a. 0.5-3.5 g/kg over thirty minutes to an hour
b. 0.05-0.2 g/kg over thirty minutes to an hour
c. 0.25-2.0 g/kg over thirty minutes to an hour
d. 4.0-6.5 g/kg over thirty minutes to an hour

138. What is one way to reduce the intensity of phantom limb syndrome?

a. Cognitive-behavioral therapy focused on positive acceptance of the situation and a prosthesis
b. Updating the prosthesis each time a technological advance is made
c. Prescription antipsychotics
d. The intensity of phantom limb syndrome cannot be reduced

139. A patient is admitted after accidental ingestion of a toxic agent three hours ago. The nurse prepares for which intervention?

a. Activated charcoal
b. Gastric lavage
c. Syrup of ipecac
d. Whole-bowel irrigation

140. Which of the following inheritable diseases is characterized by widespread blisters, anemia, fused digits, and abnormal nailbeds?

a. Angelman syndrome
b. Herpes simplex 2
c. Epidermolysis bullosa
d. Familial multiple trichodiscomas

141. A 45-year-old female is admitted to the unit with vision changes, confusion, nausea, and a sudden, severe headache. This patient most likely has experienced which type of stroke?

a. Ischemic stroke
b. Transient ischemic attack (TIA)
c. Thrombotic stroke
d. Hemorrhagic stroke

142. The nurse is caring for the 25-year-old male patient with an acute spinal cord injury at the C3 to C4 level. Which of the following manifestations is consistent with this injury?

a. Vital capacity 45 percent of normal, hemoglobin 10.4 g/dL, heart rate 96 beats per minute
b. Loss of somatic and reflex function, BP 160/90, effective cough effort
c. Coarse and fine crackles bilaterally, heart rate 56 beats per minute, core temperature 96.7 °F
d. BP 104/60, urinary output 18 mL over the last 60 minutes, heart rate 120 beats per minute

143. A nurse is providing care to a patient who is 24 weeks pregnant. The patient suddenly reports excruciating localized uterine pain and has dark red vaginal bleeding. The nurse suspects abruptio placentae. Which subsequent complication is the nurse most concerned with?
   a. Idiopathic thrombocytopenic purpura
   b. Disseminated intravascular coagulation
   c. Uterine atony
   d. Pulmonary embolism

144. Which of the following is NOT one of the eight indicators of nursing competencies?
   a. Systems thinking
   b. Facilitation of learning
   c. Clinical inquiry
   d. Adherence to discharge plans

145. Problems with the kidneys can first manifest as referred pain in which region?
   a. Lower torso and flank
   b. Upper torso and neck
   c. Popliteal area
   d. Shoulder tips

146. Robbie was in a motorcycle accident that caused moderate road rash across his right arm. In addition, he experienced a severe cervical injury that was the primary focus of treatment when he was taken to the emergency department. His arm was cleaned, irrigated, disinfected, and bandaged. However, as he recovers, he notices two thick bumps under the surface of the skin on his forearm. They feel uncomfortable to touch. What do these bumps indicate?
   a. Robbie may have serious nerve damage in his wrist.
   b. Robbie may have skin cancer.
   c. Robbie is healing normally; the bumps will slough off soon.
   d. Robbie's arm is presenting granulomas.

147. The nurse is providing discharge education for a 66-year-old patient with type 2 diabetes who has had a TIA. Which of the following patient statements indicates that the teaching has been effective?
   a. "There is nothing I can do to change my risk for another episode."
   b. "The best thing I can do is to keep my A1C level below 6.5 like my doctor said."
   c. "I only have type 2 diabetes, so that doesn't affect my blood vessels."
   d. "I'm glad I don't have to take insulin to fix this."

148. Which defect is considered an acquired structural heart defect?
   a. Myocarditis
   b. Tetralogy of Fallot
   c. Atrial septal defect
   d. Patent ductus arteriosus

149. A nurse is performing a primary survey on a pregnant patient who sustained a traumatic fall. The patient is supine, the airway has been cleared, and intravenous access has been established. The patient suddenly verbalizes lightheadedness, heart palpitations, and the blood pressure is 84/48 mmHg. Which initial action does the nurse take?

a. Infuse a fluid bolus.
b. Reassess the patient's airway.
c. Turn the patient to the left lateral position.
d. Contact the healthcare provider.

150. Which of the following findings would the nurse NOT expect in a patient with bacterial meningitis?

a. WBC count 20,000/mL
b. Blood glucose 30 mg/dL
c. Nuchal rigidity
d. Hand tremors

Answer Explanations #2

1. D: Choice *D* is the priority action for this patient. The nurse should ensure infection control measures are taken to prevent the virus from spreading to others. Choice *A* should occur after infection control measures are in place. Choice *B* is performed when there are influenza outbreaks or a novel influenza A virus has been confirmed. Choice *C* is not a priority action at this time. The influenza vaccine should be administered after the patient's symptoms have subsided and the diagnosis is confirmed.

2. A: Diabetes is strongly linked with developed kidney disease and is the leading cause of end-stage renal disease, in which the kidneys fail. Almost half of end-stage renal disease cases result from diabetes. In diabetic patients, the kidneys are constantly exposed to high blood glucose levels. This is highly taxing for the kidneys and ultimately causes kidney dysfunction and damage. Choice *B* is incorrect because polycystic ovary syndrome, an endocrine disorder in which cysts develop on the ovaries, is not highly associated with end-stage renal disease. Choice *C* is incorrect because hypertension is only the second-leading cause of end-stage renal disease; diabetes has a stronger association. Choice *D* is incorrect because, while the genetic disorder known as polycystic kidney disease can increase a person's chances of ultimately developing end-stage kidney disease, it is not the leading cause.

3. C: Choice *C* is correct because Lactated Ringer's is an isotonic crystalloid solution used in fluid resuscitation. The patient's fluid volume should be corrected first before other pharmacological treatment. Choices *A* and *D* are not correct because dopamine and norepinephrine are vasopressors that should be administered only if fluid replacement does not correct hypotension associated with hypovolemic shock. Choice *B* is not correct because although ondansetron will help with nausea and vomiting, the patient is already in hypovolemic shock. Fluid resuscitation is the priority.

4. C: Immune thrombocytopenic purpura (ITP) can suddenly occur in small children after viral infections. It is especially common after chicken pox. It is characterized by bleeding easily due to decreased platelet counts in the body. In most children, it resolves normally within a few weeks. In some children, it can take six months for the condition to resolve. The patches of dots on Mickey's skin are bleeds known as petechia, and he is also showing other symptoms of ITP such as nosebleeds and gum bleeds. Choice *A* is incorrect because shingles would not normally be seen a child immediately after recovery from chicken pox. Instead, shingles is a painful condition that affects adults who had chicken pox in childhood when the previously dormant virus becomes active. Choice *B* is incorrect because chicken pox symptoms tend to clear within 10 days and the patient is considered recovered at that point. Choice *D* is incorrect because Guillain-Barré syndrome is a rare condition that occurs after viral infections but is characterized by paralysis and muscle weakness.

5. A: Patients and families do not have the right to access staffing schedules; however, they should be kept informed regarding who is actively participating in their care. Choices *B, C,* and *D* are incorrect because these are all rights that patients and families have in the healthcare setting. They have the right to obtain and review their medical records, receive capable and non-discriminatory care, and actively join in medical care decisions.

6. D: Choice *D* is correct because bronchodilation is the expected treatment for a patient with history of chronic obstructive pulmonary disorder. Increased resistive load is primarily due to bronchoconstriction and decreased airflow. Choice *A* is incorrect because a decrease in sedative analgesics is indicated for excessive sedation, which can lead to a decreased ventilatory drive. Choice *B* is incorrect because replacement of the endotracheal tube (ETT) is not indicated unless there is luminal narrowing or the ETT is small for the patient's size. Choice *C* is incorrect because application of supplemental oxygen is indicated for hypoxemia, which causes an increase in ventilator demand.

7. A: Hemophilia is blood disorder that prevents adequate clotting and can result in heavy bleeding due to low levels of blood proteins, called clotting factors, that work with platelets to form blood clots. The condition is commonly inherited from the mother when the mother has a mutation in the genes that are responsible for clotting factors 8 and 9. Consequently, the offspring with the inherited trait is unable to make the proteins that are responsible for clotting wounds. Most cases of symptomatic hemophilia are passed on by women to male offspring; women only show symptoms in very rare cases.

Choice *B* is incorrect because, while some cancers can result in acute hemophilia, most bone marrow cancers disrupt the production and function of white blood cells rather than clotting factors. Choice *C* is incorrect because, as previously stated, women often do not show symptoms of hemophilia and primarily serve as carriers. Unless they are specifically tested for it or know they have family history, they tend to be undiagnosed. Additionally, people of Asian descent are less likely to have hemophilia than those of other races. Choice *D* is incorrect even though hemophilia could result in brain bleeds that delay speech development. Speech delays can be caused by many other factors and there is not enough information about the toddler to know the cause. Additionally, because Lilly is female, she is more likely to be a carrier for hemophilia rather than showing symptoms herself.

8. A: Choice *A* is correct because neurogenic is a type of distributive shock that causes massive vasodilation due to loss of sympathetic tone. Spinal cord injuries and head trauma are the main risk factors for the development of neurogenic shock. Choice *B* is not correct because cardiogenic shock is due to cardiac complications such as an infarction, dysrhythmia, or stenosis. Choice *C* is not correct because anaphylactic shock occurs as a result of an allergic reaction. Choice *D* is not correct because septic shock develops as a result of a bacterial infection.

9. A: Jugular vein distention, peripheral edema, and pulmonary congestion are characteristics of blood volume backing up due to an obstruction. Decreased urine output, increased BUN, and increased creatinine are signs of renal failure. Chest pain, fatigue, and lightheadedness are signs of an MI. Problems with coordination, blurred vision, and paralysis are symptomatic of a stroke.

10. C: Any new orders should be read back to the provider to verify they are correct, and any additional questions or concerns should be addressed at this time. Choice *A* is incorrect because verbal orders should be avoided when possible, as there is a higher possibility of error. Instead, electronic orders or clearly legible handwritten orders should be used first. Choice *B* is incorrect because medical abbreviations should be avoided to help reduce the likelihood of medication errors. Choice *D* is incorrect because the nurse should utilize the electronic medical record to double-check orders and reduce incidences of medication error. Using electronic methods allows for medication barcodes and scanning, which is an additional check to decrease error.

11. A: Choice *A* is indicative of uncompensated respiratory acidosis. The pH level is abnormal, with an abnormal $PaCO_2$ value and a normal bicarbonate level. Choice *B* is expected in partially compensated respiratory acidosis. The pH level is abnormal with both the $PaCO_2$ and HCO_3 levels out of normal range. Choice *C* is indicative of compensated respiratory acidosis. The pH level is normal with both the $PaCO_2$ and HCO_3 levels being abnormal. Choice *D* is a normal acid-base balance, indicative of no acute condition or a corrected acid-base imbalance.

12. B: Celiac disease is an inherited autoimmune disorder that affects the small intestine. People with celiac disease cannot digest gluten, a protein found in many grains. Consuming gluten can cause severe pain, diarrhea, vomiting, weight loss, irreparable damage to the small intestine, and general gastrointestinal distress in these patients. If the reaction is extremely severe and results in metabolic disruption, it is known as a celiac crisis and requires hospitalization. Choices *A*, *C*, and *D* are incorrect because high fructose corn syrup, nightshade vegetables, and peanuts do not contain gluten and do not tend to trigger a celiac crisis.

13. C: Fluid creep occurs when victims with large burns receive excess amounts of fluid during initial treatment. Due to shock and other complications from burns, these patients may not necessarily be able to circulate fluid well and can experience edema throughout their body, ultimately resulting in renal failure. Some studies indicate that fluid creep results in renal failure in up to one-third of burn victims. The Parkland formula is a concentration of fluid and colloid treatments that attempt to manage fluid creeps in patients who have large burns. Choice *A* is incorrect because, although burn patients are vulnerable to infections and any infection can progress to sepsis and, ultimately, renal failure, this is not the primary cause of renal failure in burn victims. Choice *B* is incorrect because burn victims may experience hypermetabolism due to hormone disruption after renal failure occurs; however, burn victims do not typically experience hypermetabolism preceding renal failure. Choice *D* is incorrect because hypomagnesemia, a condition in which the body does not have enough magnesium, can occur in burn victims but is not the primary factor in their renal failure.

14. D: People who undergo bariatric surgery, or surgeries that influence the gastrointestinal system to ultimately support weight loss, are at risk of developing anemia for the rest of their lives because they tend to have a harder time absorbing nutrients, including iron. Choice *A* is incorrect because bariatric surgeries are not associated with a higher incidence of lymphoma, a type of cancer originating in the lymph nodes. Choice *B* is incorrect despite patients tending to have smaller appetites and being physically unable to tolerate large quantities of food after bariatric surgery. While some patients may develop anorexia or other eating disorders after such a surgery, the odds of doing so are lower than developing anemia. Choice *C* is incorrect because patients often seek bariatric surgery to address weight-related health issues such as metabolic syndrome. Bariatric surgery may resolve metabolic syndrome in up to 90% of patients.

15. B: Choice *B* is correct because the provided values demonstrate compensated respiratory acidosis. The pH level is normal, the $PaCO_2$ (partial pressure of carbon dioxide) is elevated (indicating acidosis was previously present), and the HCO_3 (bicarbonate) level is elevated (indicating compensation occurred). Choice *A* is incorrect because a pH level of 7.36 does not support compensated metabolic alkalosis. The expected pH would be between 7.41 and 7.45. Choice *C* is not correct because respiratory acidosis would be characterized by a high $PaCO_2$ level and a decreased pH level. Choice *D* is incorrect because metabolic alkalosis would be characterized by elevated HCO_3 and pH levels.

16. B: Choice *B* is correct because tracheomalacia is characterized by erosion of the tracheal cartilage. Overinflation of the cuff causes pressure and damage to the tracheal tissue wall. Choice *A* is incorrect because excessive secretions cause skin excoriation and erosion of the tracheal stoma. Choice *C* is incorrect because accidental decannulation is considered a medical emergency. The cannula must be reinserted to maintain airway patency. Choice *D* is incorrect because frequent suctioning can lead to the formation of granulation tissue, a complication that can cause airflow obstruction.

17. C: Choice *C* is among the most common laparoscopic complications in a bariatric patient. The patient's symptoms are indicative of bowel perforation and peritonitis. Choice *A* is a common postoperative condition due to manipulation of the bowel during the procedure. However, constipation does not cause a rigid abdomen. Choice *B* is a possible complication of LAGB. However, characteristic signs of splenic injury include bruising to the abdomen and left shoulder radiating pain. Choice *D* is a possible complication of bariatric surgery. However, symptoms of an aortic dissection are emergent, including chest pain, respiratory distress, and loss of consciousness.

18. A: Choice *A* is the best interpretation of the patient's clinical presentation. Acute pain is a defense mechanism, particularly after an acute event such as surgery. The patient's lack of medical or social history do not indicate substance use. Choice *B* is not correct because postoperative pain is expected. Pain that does not decrease over the course of days or weeks may require further intervention. Choice *C* is not correct because there is no indication that the patient has a history of substance use. Acute pain after a surgical procedure is expected. Choice *D* is not correct because the latest physical assessment is as expected. There is no indication of surgical complications.

19. C: Thyroid storm is a rare but critical complication in patients with hyperthyroidism. Most presentations are clinical and confirmed with lab work that shows elevated thyroxine and triiodothyronine levels and low thyrotropin levels (thyroid hormones). Clues that the patient may be experiencing this include the prescription for methimazole, a medication used to treat hyperthyroidism. Thyroid storm also most commonly affects women, and compounds found in aspirin have been shown to trigger thyroid storms. Choice *A* is incorrect because, although an infected wound can lead to a fever, this does not account for all the presenting symptoms and medical history; considered holistically, these indicate a thyroid storm. Choice *B* is incorrect because, although diabetic patients can experience hypoglycemia, this does not account for all the presenting symptoms and medical history; considered holistically, these indicate a thyroid storm. Choice *D is* incorrect because, although tachycardia is a cardiovascular condition, this does not account for all the presenting symptoms and medical history; considered holistically, these indicate a thyroid storm.

20. C: Following a patient's death, the family members should not be immediately asked to leave the room. The family should be allowed to stay in the room with the patient to grieve, process their emotions, and participate in care if safe and appropriate. Choices *A, B,* and *D* are incorrect because these are appropriate actions for the nurse to take to help provide support to the family and remain respectful to the patient.

21. C: Choice *C* is correct because cor pulmonale is characterized by adaptation of the right ventricle in response to increased workload, dilation, and hypertrophy. Choices *A*, *B*, and *D* are precursors to pulmonary hypertension. All of these mechanisms are caused by chronic pulmonary disease and occur before the right ventricular workload is increased.

22. C: A patient with fungal meningitis is likely to be placed on an anti-fungal medication such as flucytosine, fluconazole, or amphotericin B. Choice *A* is incorrect because cefotaxamine (Claforan) is a cephalosporin antibiotic that is more likely to be used for the treatment of bacterial meningitis. Choice *B* is incorrect because gentamicin is an aminoglycoside antibiotic that could also be used in the treatment of bacterial meningitis. Choice *D* is incorrect because intravenous immune globulin (IVIG) is a therapy made of antibodies that is often used in autoimmune disorders or treatment of viral meningitis.

23. B: A patient found to have cardiac tamponade must undergo a pericardiocentesis to quickly drain the excess fluid in the pericardial sac. Without this procedure, the fluid puts pressure on the heart, causing it to inadequately pump blood, which can lead to shock, organ failure, and death. Choice *A* is incorrect because transcatheter aortic valve replacement (TAVR) is used in the treatment of severe aortic stenosis. Choice *C* is incorrect because a coronary artery bypass graft (CABG) is used to treat severe cardiovascular occlusion and is most often utilized in the presence of severe coronary heart disease. Choice *D* is incorrect because a balloon angioplasty is a type of peripheral stent used to treat peripheral vascular insufficiency.

24. B: Patients with nephrotic syndrome have damaged kidneys that allow excessive protein in the urine. Based on the severity of their disease, patients are advised to eat a low-protein diet, as consuming more protein can strain the kidneys further and cause more damage. Choice *A* is incorrect because patients with nephrotic syndrome are encouraged to eat low-sodium grains, beans, fruits, and vegetables—all sources of carbohydrates. Choice *C* is incorrect because patients with nephrotic syndrome tend to be deficient in Vitamin D and some studies indicate that supplementing with Vitamin D can help manage symptoms of nephrotic syndrome. Choice *D* is incorrect because CoQ10 may support cardiovascular function, but there is no evidence that it helps or harms patients with nephrotic syndrome. Therefore, it is not known whether or not patients with nephrotic syndrome should limit this nutrient.

25. C: Choice *C* is correct because nitric oxide is a potent vasodilator used in the treatment of pulmonary vasoconstriction and subsequent pulmonary hypertension. Nitric oxide improves oxygenation and blood flow to functioning alveoli. Choice *A* is incorrect because albuterol is primarily used to treat bronchospasms in patients with asthma or chronic obstructive pulmonary disease. Choice *B* is incorrect because nifedipine is an anti-hypertensive medication primarily used to produce coronary vasodilation. Choice *D* is incorrect because digoxin is an antiarrhythmic medication that increases cardiac output. This medication does not specifically improve pulmonary blood flow.

26. B: When indicated and appropriate, using silence allows time for the patient to reflect on how they are feeling, process their thoughts, and come up with their own solutions. Choice *A* is incorrect because yes or no questions can be limiting; instead, open-ended questions should be used to garner more information from the patient and allow for better communication. Choice *C* is incorrect because clichés can come across as insincere and may add little meaning to the conversation. Choice *D* is incorrect because asking patients to explain their behavior may come across as accusatory and cause a patient to close off their communication.

27. C: Choice *C* is correct because a $PaCO_2$ (partial pressure of carbon dioxide) of 30 mmHg indicates hypocarbia, which is an expected finding during the initial phase of an asthma exacerbation. Hypocarbia is due to hyperventilation. Choice *A* is incorrect because a $PaCO_2$ of 50 mmHg indicates hypercarbia, which is evident during the late states of an asthma exacerbation. Hypercarbia results from inadequate ventilation. Choices *B* and *D* are incorrect because an abnormal bicarbonate (HCO_3) level is associated with metabolic, not acute, respiratory conditions.

28. C: A patient requesting drink or food that may dangerously raise their blood glucose level and increase mortality and morbidity with diabetic ketoacidosis (DKA) should be denied; this is defined within the ethical principle of nonmaleficence, which means to cause no harm to a patient. Choice *A* is incorrect because beneficence is the ethical principle to promote welfare and actively help the patient. Choice *B* is incorrect because autonomy refers to the ethical principle and right for patients to make informed, independent decisions about their care. The patient in this scenario is not being denied their autonomy; instead, they are being redirected to make a safer decision. Choice *D* is incorrect because this is not unethical practice. The nurse made a decision in the best interest of the health of the patient and offered them appropriate alternative choices.

29. B: Stage 5 chronic kidney disease is the last stage of progression for this condition. By this time, it is serious enough to require constant dialysis (a process that filters the blood for the kidneys) or a kidney transplant because the kidneys have failed.

30. D: Choice *D* should be clarified with the provider. Ibuprofen is a non-steroidal anti-inflammatory drug (NSAID) that can cause nephrotoxicity if combined with immunosuppressant (transplant anti-rejection) medications. Choice *A* is not contraindicated in a patient with a kidney transplant. Renal failure is possible only with chronic use or high doses. Choice *B* is an opioid that contains acetaminophen. It is not contraindicated in patients with renal transplants. Choice *C* is a muscle relaxant and is not contraindicated in patients with a renal transplant.

31. A: An aortic dissection is the tearing through of some layers of the aortic wall, causing blood to leak into the layers of the aorta. Common symptoms associated with an aortic dissection include a sudden and severe tearing or ripping feeling, difficulty breathing, stroke-like symptoms, weaker pulse in one arm or thigh, loss of consciousness, and paralysis. Choice *B* is incorrect because common symptoms of pulmonary edema include difficulty breathing; a suffocating feeling that worsens when lying down; a cough with pink, frothy sputum; and wheezing. Choice *C* is incorrect because an aortic aneurysm is the bulging or weakening of the aortic wall without tearing and may have an asymptomatic presentation. Symptoms of an aortic aneurysm are often not present unless a dissection or rupture of the vessel occurs. Choice *D* is incorrect because common symptoms of pulmonary embolism include shortness of breath, cough, chest pain, cyanosis, irregular heartbeat, sweating, and back pain.

32. D: Although hemodialysis is an intensive procedure in patients who are considerably more vulnerable than the general population, emergency situations are rare. When they do occur, they are usually the result of human error. This may include communication breakdowns between a clinical provider and a home caregiver, indirect medication errors, patients missing appointments, or other mismanaged health issues that complicate treatment. Choice *A* is incorrect because modern dialysis machines are high-tech, manufactured under rigorous standards, and have numerous safety mechanisms; it is rare for them to malfunction. Choice *B* is incorrect because hemodialysis machines incorporate cleaning solutions that virtually eliminate exposure to harmful pathogens. Choice *C* is incorrect because, although hemodialysis patients are vulnerable to electrolyte imbalances, this not the most common cause of emergency situations in this patient population.

33. A: A patient with increased intracranial pressure (ICP) is at risk of seizure, coma, and death due to increased fluid in the brain, called hydrocephalus. Burr holes, or decompressive craniectomy, can be used to relieve this pressure and may done on these patients. They may also have ventricular drains placed to help remove fluid. Choice *B* is incorrect because 0.45% normal saline is hypotonic and could cause an increase of fluid and therefore pressure in the brain. Typically, 3% normal saline, which is hypertonic, or mannitol is used to help pull fluid off of the brain back into the vascular space to help reduce pressure. Choice *C* is incorrect because the head of the bed should be maintained at 30 degrees or higher to help promote fluid drainage from the brain. Choice *D* is incorrect because, although these patients often require mechanical ventilation, they should be hyperventilated because it can cause arterial vasoconstriction which would lower cerebral blood flow and decrease ICP.

34. B: Early congestive heart failure is associated with crackles that are fine, profuse, and persistent. The sounds are originally audible at the bases but may progress upward as the failure becomes more severe.

These crackles are also heard in interstitial lung disease that is characterized by fibrosis. A mediastinal crunch is defined as the presence of precordial crackles that are associated with the heart rate, not the inspiratory rate. They are also best heard in the left lateral position. However, these sounds are due to mediastinal emphysema; therefore, Choice *A* is incorrect. Mid-inspiratory expiratory crackles may be due to bronchiectasis, but they have not been demonstrated in patients with heart failure; therefore, Choice *C* is incorrect. Early inspiratory crackles occurring in patients with chronic bronchitis and asthma are of short duration and number and may be associated with expiratory crackles; therefore, Choice *D* is incorrect.

35. A: Choice *A* is correct because the patient's symptoms are indicative of respiratory distress. Bilevel positive airway pressure (BiPAP) therapy is contraindicated in patients who are unable to clear their own secretions or maintain airway patency. Choice *B* is incorrect because a continuous positive airway pressure (CPAP) machine is typically used to treat obstructive sleep apnea. This therapy is not indicated for the patient's symptoms. Choice *C* is incorrect because increasing the inspiratory pressure will not resolve the patient's inability to clear their own oral secretions. Choice *D* is incorrect because providing suctioning as needed is a short-term solution to clearing the oral secretions. The patient's symptoms indicate a deterioration in respiratory status.

36. B: Choice *B* is correct because prone positioning reduces lung compression, which improves ventilation and oxygenation in the ventilated patient. Choice *A* is incorrect because the prone position can still cause pressure on various surfaces of the skin (e.g., face, ears, cheek, forehead). Choice *C* is incorrect because the prone position increases gastric volume and can produce emesis. Choice *D* is incorrect because a decrease in the systolic blood pressure is not an intended effect. Hypotension is a complication of prone positioning.

37. D: A patient with a spinal cord injury at C8 will have paralysis that affects their legs and the trunk of their body; however, because it is below C5, the patient's nerves that innervate their diaphragm are still functional and they can breathe on their own. Injuries that are from C4 through T1 can have an effect on the use of arms and hands, but to varying degrees. Choice *A* is incorrect because an injury at C3 through C5 would cause paralysis in the diaphragm, requiring the patient to be on mechanical ventilation. Choices *B* and *C* are incorrect because injuries in the lumbar and lower thoracic region are less likely to have an effect on the ability of a patient to use their forearms.

38. D: Choice *D* is correct because a pH of 7.47 and a $PaCO_2$ (partial pressure of carbon dioxide) of 32 mmHg indicates respiratory alkalosis. Respiratory alkalosis is a potential complication of an assist-control (AC) mode ventilator setting due to the patient's effort to breathe above the set respiratory rate. Choice *A* is incorrect because a pH of 7.46 and a HCO_3 (bicarbonate) level of 28 mEq/L indicates metabolic alkalosis, a complication not expected for an AC ventilator setting. Choice *B* is incorrect because a pH of 7.33 and a $PaCO_2$ level of 47 mmHg indicates respiratory acidosis. Retention of CO_2 is not expected. Choice *C* is incorrect because a pH of 7.45 and a $PaCO_2$ level of 42 mmHg is a normal finding.

39. D: Myxedema coma can occur when hypothyroidism goes untreated and can be fatal in up to 60% of patients. It is characterized by hypothermia, confusion, and respiratory muscle weakness. Choice *A* is incorrect because ketoacidosis is typically a critical complication of diabetes. Choice *B* is incorrect because Addisonian crisis is a critical complication of adrenal insufficiency. Choice *C* is incorrect although it is true that fever is a symptom of many critical diseases. However, patients with hypothyroidism who experience critical events are more likely to experience hypothermia and other drops in temperature rather than fever.

40. D: Choice *D* is correct because a $PaCO_2$ (partial pressure of carbon dioxide) level of 60 mmHg is indicative of respiratory acidosis, primarily caused by the inability to adequately move air in and out of the lungs. Choice *A* is incorrect because although a PaO_2 (arterial oxygen partial pressure) of 55 mmHg is characteristic of acute respiratory failure (ARF), the value supports oxygenation, not ventilatory failure. Choice *B* is incorrect because a pH of 7.4 does not support ARF. ARF is characterized by a pH level of less than 7.3. Choice *C* is incorrect because an oxygen saturation of 87% is expected in a patient with history of chronic obstructive pulmonary disease.

41. A: Staph infections are bacterial infections that begin on the skin or in the nose. They can enter open cuts and enter the bloodstream. This allows the bacteria to proliferate in the blood and/or reach other organs, such as the heart. Staph is especially common in wrestlers, placing Martin at higher odds of experiencing this type of infection. He is also exhibiting common staph symptoms such as fever, pus in the wound, a new rash, and chest pain (which can occur from endocarditis caused by the infection). Choice *B* is incorrect because overtraining is typified by flu-like feelings that can occur when someone exercises heavily without allowing adequate time for their body to recover. It is more common in athletes, but the question indicates that Martin spent several days resting and recovering. He is also not showing classic signs of overtraining, such as muscle soreness, poor performance, poor sleep, and loss of interest in the activity. Choice *C* is incorrect because it does not fit all the symptoms, even though Martin's infection could progress to bacterial pneumonia if the bacteria spreads to his lungs. Bacterial pneumonia is characterized by chest pain upon coughing or breathing, extremely high fevers, and coughs that result in thick discharge. Fortunately, Martin is not showing any of these symptoms. Choice *D* is incorrect because it does not fit all the indications in Martin's case. Viral infections do have some similar symptoms to bacterial infections, such as fever and rash. However, Martin's other indications, such as the open wound with white discharge and wrestling history, are more likely to be signs of a bacterial infection than a viral infection.

42. A: Hypertrophic cardiomyopathy is caused by a genetic disorder that is most often diagnosed in middle or late adulthood once symptoms become more present. This causes thickening of the heart muscle, which makes it more difficult for blood to be pumped through the body. Since this is a genetic disease, it is important to educate both the patient and their family members on symptoms and treatments. Choices *B, C,* and *D* are incorrect because these cardiomyopathies are not caused by genetic factors. Dilated cardiomyopathy is often caused by coronary artery disease, drug and alcohol use, and metabolic disorders. There is no certain cause of idiopathic cardiomyopathy, but it is theorized it may be caused from immune responses, metabolic injuries, viruses, or tachycardia. Restrictive cardiomyopathy is often caused by a buildup of fibroelastic tissue that may be secondary to a multitude of external causes.

43. C: The Emergency Medical Treatment and Labor Act of 1986 (EMTALA) was a direct response to healthcare facilities turning away patients that were unable to pay for treatment, even in life-or-death situations. However, facilities are not reimbursed for losses by this law, and this has had an effect on overall healthcare costs.

44. A: Choice *A* is correct because pleuritic pain is one of the most common symptoms associated with a pulmonary embolism. Pleuritic pain is characterized by severe pain in the chest that worsens upon inspiration and expiration. Choice *B* is incorrect because a temperature of 99.8 °F (37.6 °C) is slightly above normal range. Low grade fever is a *non-specific* sign associated with pulmonary embolism. Choice *C* is incorrect because right calf erythema is an expected finding for deep vein thrombosis. This finding does not directly support a diagnosis of pulmonary embolism. Choice *D* is incorrect because a heart rate of 102 beats/min is slightly above normal. Tachycardia is associated with pulmonary embolism. However, it is not as specific to the respiratory system as pleuritic pain.

45. B: A patient can experience compartment syndrome from a crush injury, fracture, or frequent athletic exertion. Having pallor on or pain in the affected limb, especially when stretching or moving, can be a sign of compartment syndrome. Other common signs of compartment syndrome include paresthesia, poikilothermia, and weak or absent pulse. Choice *A* is incorrect because building or wasting of muscle is not a sign of compartment syndrome. Choice *C* is incorrect because a bounding pulse would not be expected in the affected limb; a weak, thready, or absent pulse would be expected. Choice *D* is incorrect because confusion and lethargy are not symptoms associated with compartment syndrome; however, any changes in level of consciousness should be monitored and reported.

46. A: Patients who practice Orthodox Judaism often follow practices where unnecessary touching from non-family members and any physical contact from members of the opposite sex is not allowed. A female nurse and female nursing student would be an appropriate care team to handle this patient's care. Choices *B, C,* and *D* are incorrect because each of these care teams includes at least one male team member, which would not be appropriate for this patient's care based on their religious beliefs. In medical emergencies, these practices may have exceptions, but it is important that cultural and religious preferences be respectfully discussed and honored with patients throughout their care.

47. C: Choice *C* is correct because chest imaging is one of the diagnostic tests used to identify lung injury. All suspected transfusion-related acute lung injuries (TRALIs) will show pulmonary infiltrates on a chest x-ray. Choice *A* is incorrect because hypotension, not hypertension, is suspected in TRALI. Choice *B* is incorrect because sinus bradycardia is not a clinical finding used to diagnose TRALI. Choice *D* is incorrect because jugular venous distention is expected with fluid volume overload, seen in conditions such as transfusion-associated circulatory overload.

48. A: Choice *A* is correct because the removal of large amounts of fluid or exudate may cause pulmonary edema due to a rapid re-expansion of the affected lung. The nurse should monitor the amount of fluid being removed, with 1 liter being the recommended limit. Choice *B* is incorrect; although sitting upright with the upper extremities raised and well-supported is the preferred position, this action primarily prevents accidental needle injury of internal structures. Choice *C* is incorrect because this action prevents excessive bleeding, a possible complication of the procedure. Choice *D* is incorrect because the patient should remain completely still during the procedure to prevent needle injury.

49. A: A patient who follows traditional Middle Eastern practices may follow certain dietary restrictions, such as not eating pork or mixing meat and dairy products. Grilled fish with vegetables and a grain would be in-line with this culture's dietary restrictions. Culture and traditions should never be automatically assumed; the nurse should always respectfully discuss with the patient what their dietary preferences and restrictions are. Choices *B* and C are incorrect because they mix meat and dairy on the same plate. Choice *D* is incorrect because bacon is pork, which is often not allowed in Middle Eastern diets.

50. A: There are three levels of nurse advocacy and moral agency: Levels 1, 3, and 5. The nurse who is easily able to advocate for a patient and agrees morally with the decision the patient is making is exhibiting Level 1 advocacy and moral agency, the most basic level that emphasizes the work of the nurse. Choice *B* is incorrect because Level 2 is not a level of advocacy and moral agency. Choice *C* is incorrect because Level 3 advocacy and moral agency has the nurse advocate for the patient even if what they are advocating for does not directly align with their own personal values. Choice *D* is incorrect because Level 5 advocacy and moral agency is when the nurse uses their position and power to empower clients to request the care and resources that are within their best interests, even if it goes against their personal values.

51. B: A1c percentages indicate what percentage of oxygen-transporting proteins in the blood are glycated; the higher someone's A1c, the higher their risk of complications from diabetes. In an older patient with diagnosed type 2 diabetes, an A1c reading between 7% and 8% indicates that the patient's blood sugar is managed well enough to avoid significant complications. Choice *A* is incorrect because patients without diabetes have A1c percentages below 5.7%; therefore, anything below 6% would be considered difficult to achieve in the short-term for a patient who has been diagnosed with type 2 diabetes. Choice *C* is incorrect for the same reason; it is much too low a goal for a person with diagnosed type 2 diabetes. Choice *D* is incorrect because an A1c of 10% or higher is exceptionally high, and significant complications such as diabetic neuropathy and retinopathy begin to occur at that level. Therefore, it is not a reasonable goal for the patient.

52. C: A patient with a systolic blood pressure greater than 180 and diastolic pressure greater than 120 is said to be in hypertensive crisis. A patient with untreated hypertension who is now in hypertensive crisis in addition to weakness, headache, visual changes, nausea, and vomiting is likely to have hypertensive encephalopathy that causes cerebral edema. These patients can have a sudden onset of symptoms and the increased pressure should be treated immediately. Choices *A*, *B*, and *D* are not correct because the symptoms of these diseases do not align with the patient's presentation.

53. D: When critically reading a new research article, it is not imperative that the nurse sees where funding comes from for the research. While funding can have some influence over research and should be examined when appraising research, it is not necessary when trying to critically read and understand new research information. Choices *A, B,* and *C* are incorrect because the nurse should determine the thesis, process, and outcomes when critically reading research.

54. D: Choice *D* is correct because emotional is not a defined domain for post-intensive care syndrome (PICS). Choice *A* is not correct because severe sepsis can lead to the development of psychiatric disorders such as anxiety, depression, and post-traumatic stress disorder (PTSD). Choice *B* is not correct because a patient with severe sepsis can have lasting physical effects due to cardiovascular and respiratory compromise. Choice *C* is not correct because severe sepsis is a major risk factor for the development of cognitive impairment in patients who show signs of PICS.

55. C: Choice *C* is correct because systemic inflammatory response syndrome (SIRS) is characterized by the presence of two or more conditions that indicate sepsis. A temperature of 39 °C (102.2 °F) and a heart rate of 102 beats/min meets criteria for SIRS. Choice *A* is not correct because oxygen saturation is not one of the criteria used to define SIRS or sepsis. Additionally, an oxygen saturation of 92% is normal. Choice *B* is not correct because a white blood cell (WBC) count of 11,000/mm^3 does not meet SIRS criteria. Serum lactate levels are used to evaluate septic shock. Choice *D* is not correct because urine output is used to evaluate hypoperfusion in severe sepsis. Additionally, 30 ml/hr is the minimum normal limit for urine output.

56. D: Almost three fourths of people who experience moderate to severe burns also experience inhalation injuries, meaning their airway has been damaged. They likely are not receiving enough oxygen. Inhalation injuries are highly associated with deaths of burn victims. Burn victims with moderate to severe burns may experience unpredictable air obstruction events; therefore, stabilizing the airway should be the primary intervention. At the minimum, this requires supplemental oxygen; however, some patients may require mechanical ventilation. Choice *A* is incorrect because, although wound care is an important component of burn treatment to prevent infection, the patient must be stabilized first.

Choice *B* is incorrect even though some patients may be in shock after a burn and experience dangerously low blood pressure. A defibrillator is an aggressive intervention and can cause more harm to the burn patient, so airway management should still be the primary intervention. If blood pressure or shock is an issue, medications that support vascular function are typically a better intervention. Choice *C* is incorrect because fluid resuscitation is generally done after airway management in burn patients. Immediate and aggressive fluid resuscitation while the patient is not stable can lead to over-resuscitation, which is harmful for burn victims and leads to fluid creep.

57. B: The most common source of neurological infections is from infections in the spinal cord and meninges around the brain. Often, neurological infections are secondary to another infection somewhere else in the body. Neurologic infectious diseases can be viral, bacterial, or fungal. Although neurologic infections can start from an infection anywhere in the body, the spinal cord and meninges are most common, therefore Choices *A, C,* and *D* are incorrect.

58. A: Choice *A* is correct because the expected mean arterial pressure (MAP) is 65 mmHg. A MAP greater than 65 mmHg indicates resolution of hypotension and adequate fluid volume. Choice *B* is not correct because the central venous pressure (CVP) goal during fluid resuscitation is above 8 mmHg. Choice *C* is not correct because a serum lactate level of 4 mmol/L indicates hypoperfusion and persistent septic shock. Choice *D* is not correct because although a white blood cell (WBC) count of 10,000/mm^3 is considered normal, this value is not the expected outcome of fluid resuscitation.

59. A: Choice *A* is correct because 0.4 to 2 mg every two to three minutes, IV push is the recommended dose for an opiate overdose. The maximum dose is 10 mg. Choice *B* is not correct because 0.01 mg/kg every two to three minutes, IM is the recommended dose for neonates experiencing post-operative respiratory depression due to opioids. Choice *C* is not correct because the recommended intranasal dose is 4 to 8 mg every two to three minutes. Choice *D* is not correct because 4 to 8 mg every two minutes is a usual dose for an intranasal administration, not a subcutaneous administration. The usual route for a subcutaneous administration is 0.4 mg every two to three minutes.

60. A: It is not a requirement for the informed consent to list all members of the team involved in the treatment or procedure. However, the patient should still have a general understanding of the care they will be receiving from team members. Choices *B, C,* and *D* are incorrect because these are required components in informed consent. Other required components include risks and benefits of not having the procedure.

61. B: Choice *B* is an expected injury for a patient who is unrestrained in a motor vehicle accident. The lack of seat belt propels the body forward and causes head injuries against the windshield. Choices *A, C,* and *D* are not predictable injury patterns for a motor vehicle accident. Ankle dislocations, wrist fractures, and lumbar compression fractures are primarily seen with traumatic falls.

62. C: When committees are being constructed to make hospital-wide changes regarding client rights, it is best to involve not only administrative and medical staff, but also patients and their family members, since these matters directly concern them. Additional feedback can be gained from patients and family members through surveys, feedback cards, and follow-up appointments. Choices *A, B,* and *D* are incorrect because they do not include all groups of people that should be involved in decisions regarding client rights.

63. A: Non-proliferative retinopathy affects capillaries in the eyes. In this condition, the capillaries become inflated and less efficient at transporting blood and nutrients. Almost all patients with diabetes, whether type 1 or type 2, will experience some degree of non-proliferative retinopathy. When caught early, this condition can be easily managed. Choice *B* is incorrect because, although non-proliferative retinopathy can become proliferative, it usually does not, in part because most patients with diabetes are encouraged to maintain comprehensive eye care with frequent exams. For the same reason, Choice *C* is incorrect; most cases of non-proliferative retinopathy will not progress to retinal detachment. Choice *D* is incorrect because diabetes is not associated with or a general risk factor for color blindness, a hereditary condition that is normally present from birth.

64. B: Choice *B* is correct because a distinctive sign of a tension pneumothorax is tracheal deviation. Tension pneumothorax results from trapped air in the pleural space, which causes pressure on the heart and lung and displaces the trachea to the unaffected side. Choice *A* is incorrect because a spontaneous pneumothorax is due to a bleb rupture on the lung that is not associated with trauma. Choice *C* is incorrect because a flail chest is characterized by an unstable chest wall and paradoxical chest wall movement. Choice *D* is incorrect because a pulmonary embolism is a blood clot that restricts blood flow within the lung. Tracheal deviation is not a characteristic sign of a pulmonary embolism.

65. A: Mallory-Weiss syndrome refers to esophageal tears that occur from violent coughing or vomiting and are most commonly seen in patients with a history of alcoholism, although occasionally can be seen in pregnant women or patients experiencing a hernia. Alcoholics tend to have a history of more frequent vomiting than other people, as well as chronic gut inflammation. This makes them more vulnerable to Mallory-Weiss syndrome as well. Choice *B* is incorrect because Crohn's disease is characterized by inflammation of the digestive tract and symptoms such as severe diarrhea and weight loss. Alcoholism may exacerbate the issue but does not generally contribute to the onset of the disease. Additionally, vomiting is typically not present in Crohn's disease. Choice *C* is incorrect because peptic ulcer disease, which results from sores that develop along the digestive tract, is characterized by pain and acid reflux, but not typically by vomiting unless the patient significantly overeats. There is no indication that Jonah has recently overeaten, or that he is showing other symptoms of peptic ulcer disease. Finally, Choice *D* is incorrect because Jonah is not showing typical symptoms of cirrhosis complications, which include hypertension, jaundice, swelling, and itchy skin.

66. D: In fem-pop, or femoral-popliteal bypass surgery, a patent vessel, either from a transplanted or synthetic graft, is sewn in above and below the occluded vessel to bypass the blockage and restore circulation. The occluded vessel remains in the leg with the new patent vessel implanted around it. Choices *A, B,* and *C* are incorrect because these are not accurate or complete descriptions of the fem-pop bypass surgery.

67. D: Choice *D* is the most contributive risk factor for the development of catheter-associated urinary tract infections. The catheter should be removed as soon as possible to prevent bacteria from entering the urinary tract. Choice *A* is important. However, perineal care alone does not prevent bacterial colonization in other areas of the catheter, such as the drainage bag. Choice *B* helps prevent stagnant urine. However, this factor alone does not prevent CAUTIs. Choice *C* protects the healthcare providers from contamination but does not protect the patient from developing a CAUTI.

68. C: The chamber of the heart that is most prone to penetrative cardiac trauma is the right ventricle. This is due to the anatomical position of the right ventricle being the most anterior on a person's body. Choices *A, B,* and *D* are incorrect because the left ventricle, left atrium, and right atrium are not the chambers most prone to cardiac traumas caused by penetrative forces, due to their more lateral or posterior positioning in the body. Other chambers of the heart can still experience penetrative injuries, especially secondary to medical procedures, but they are not the most afflicted chamber.

69. A: Choice *A* is correct because the gag reflex is often affected during moderate sedation and/or topical anesthesia used to perform an endoscopic procedure. Assessing the gag reflex before feeding ensures the patient can swallow adequately. Choice *B* is incorrect because, although positioning the head of the bed to at least 30 degrees facilitates the passage of oral secretions, this is not a priority action to prevent aspiration in a patient who underwent an endoscopic procedure. Choice *C* is incorrect because setting up suction is a safety precaution in case the patient's airway is compromised. However, this intervention does not specifically prevent aspiration. Choice *D* is incorrect because coughing and deep breathing promote removal of oral secretions, but this is a standard intervention for every patient receiving anesthesia.

70. A: When working with adult learners, it is important for the nurse to relate the teachings to real-world experiences. This acknowledges patients' prior knowledge and experience and helps provide a more robust teaching and understanding that adult learners can utilize. Choice *B* is incorrect because the nurse should not assume the patient has no prior knowledge, as this can come off as belittling and limit the extent to which the nurse can teach. Instead, the nurse should assess the prior knowledge the patient has and tailor the teaching level and material accordingly. Choice *C* is incorrect because by maintaining authority and control, the nurse does not allow the patient to be involved in learning and may invalidate concerns they have. This approach may also come off as disrespectful when trying to educate adult learners. Instead, the nurse should have a professional and collaborative approach. Choice *D* is incorrect because keeping objectives fluid and subjective may make it more difficult for patients to understand the goals they are trying to reach and more difficult for the nurse to assess their learning. Objectives should be clear, measurable, and goal focused.

71. A: The most common cause of a hemorrhagic stroke is untreated and uncontrolled hypertension. Other major risk factors for a hemorrhagic stroke can be cerebral cavernous malfunctions, arteriovenous malformations, anticoagulation medications, head trauma, cerebral aneurysm, and bleeding disorders. Choices *B, C,* and *D* can cause many complications in the brain; however, they are not the most common or likely causes of a hemorrhagic stroke and are therefore incorrect.

72. C: In the treatment of hypertensive crisis, patients are often started on vasodilators, such as nifedipine (Cardene), to help lower and control blood pressure. Other medications that are commonly used in the treatment of hypertensive crisis include alpha-adrenergic blockers, labetalol, and calcium channel blockers like diltiazem and verapamil. Choice *A* is incorrect because dobutamine is contraindicated in patients with hypertensive crisis because it causes vasoconstriction which can further raise blood pressure. Choice *B* is incorrect because increased fluid intake could further raise blood pressure. In addition, this patient has a history of heart failure, and the excess fluid could increase the work on their heart and cause further cardiac and systemic damage. Choice *D* is incorrect because the head of the bed in patients with hypertensive crisis should be maintained at 90 degrees, and semi-Fowler's position has the head of the bed between 30 and 45 degrees. Keeping the patient in an upright position decreases the amount of blood returning to the heart and can help lower blood pressure.

73. D: It is appropriate for the nurse to delegate the task of recording output to a certified nursing assistant (CNA). Certified nursing assistants can also be delegated other routine care such as recording intake/output, vital signs, and activities of daily living as appropriate. The nurse should be able to assess if each task is necessary, appropriate, and within the CNA's scope of practice. Choice *A* is incorrect because passing medication is outside of the regular scope of a CNA's practice. The nurse should pass this medication if it was scanned and charted under their name and license. Choice *B* is incorrect because inserting a new IV is outside of the regular scope of practice for a CNA. Some facilities may allow training for CNAs for additional skills, so the nurse should be familiar with the policies at their facility. Choice *C* is incorrect because, although it is within the scope of practice for a CNA to reposition a patient, it is not appropriate to ask a CNA to independently reposition an obese patient. This task can cause injury to the CNA and patient; instead, the nurse should either assist the CNA or ensure the CNA has additional help.

74. D: When an abdominal aortic aneurysm ruptures, it has torn through all layers of the aorta and the patient is at risk for massive blood loss and death. This is a medical emergency that requires immediate surgical repair. An open repair is a surgical intervention that is used if the vessel has completely ruptured. Choice *A* is incorrect because beta-blockers, such as labetalol, are used to help prevent aortic aneurysms from progressing further but would not be able to treat a ruptured aneurysm alone without surgical intervention. Choice *B* is incorrect because repeat imaging scans, such as CT, MRI, or X-ray, would be used to monitor an aneurysm before it is ruptured. It would still be a priority to surgically repair the aneurysm to prevent morbidity or mortality. Choice *C* is incorrect because although morphine may be used to help manage pain associated with an aneurysm, it would not be the immediate action that should be taken for this patient to help minimize damage and maximize likelihood of survival.

75. C: Muscle pain, weakness, elevated HR, dark reddish-brown urine, and metabolic acidosis are all signs of rhabdomyolysis. Rhabdomyolysis is a rapid breakdown of muscle tissue that releases protein into the blood and can cause severe kidney damage. This can be caused by overexertion in workouts, infection, trauma, immobility, and certain medications. Choice *A* is incorrect because, although patients with DKA may have metabolic acidosis, the other described symptoms more closely reflect a diagnosis of rhabdomyolysis. Choice *B* is incorrect because compartment syndrome would present with symptoms such as pallor, pulselessness, paresthesia, poikilothermia, and pain. Choice *D* is incorrect because epicondylitis (also called tennis elbow) may cause pain, but it will not commonly present with other clinical manifestations as described here.

76. B: Someone who allows their group to present ideas and solutions, but does not use these group ideas, is said to be a consultative leader. In this leadership style, staff may feel that their input is being heard, even if it is not taken seriously into consideration. Choice *A* is incorrect because a democratic leader collaborates with their staff to hear ideas and solutions and will take those ideas into account when making their decision. Choice *C* is incorrect because participatory leadership is another name for democratic leadership and has the same meaning. Choice *D* is incorrect because in delegative leadership, similar to laissez-faire leadership, the leader is hands-off and assigns tasks and problems to their group to complete without the leader's instruction or input.

77. C: People with sickle cell disease have red blood cells that are crescent-shaped rather than round and less flexible than healthy red blood cells. These cells are prone to getting stuck in blood vessels due to their curved shape and tough walls, and this can result in extreme pain that can last up to several weeks. It typically happens multiple times a year and is the most common reason for hospitalization in these patients. Choice *A* is incorrect because patients with sickle cell disease are not prone to internal bleeding; rather, they often do not have adequate blood flow or enough red blood cells. Choice *B* is incorrect because people with sickle cell disease do not commonly lose consciousness even though they are often fatigued due to having decreased red blood cells. Choice *D* is incorrect because, while people with sickle cell disease are more prone to clots than other people, it is not the most common reason for these patients to seek emergency care.

78. C: Patients who have intentionally overdosed have likely done so as an attempted suicide; therefore, they are at a much higher risk for suicide within the year following admittance to the emergency room. Researchers have indicated the need for ongoing intervention and follow-up after stabilizing a patient who has been admitted for intentional drug overdose to address the root cause of the patient's suicidal ideations and any other mental health comorbidities. While all patients who overdose require initial airway management, collapsed tracheas are generally not a risk during the intake and stabilization process. Patients who are stabilized following a drug overdose are not likely to become immediately violent or aggressive, as they may be too weak or sedated. Hormone disorders typically do not result from an overdose incident.

79. B: Cushing's disease is a disorder affecting the pituitary gland, causing the body to produce too much cortisol over time. This results in considerable swelling and fat deposits around the torso, face, and upper back. Choice *A* is incorrect because adrenal fatigue is not a disorder, but rather a collection of symptoms that may be caused by the body irregularly producing cortisol. These symptoms may include irregular wake-sleep times and fatigue. Choice *C* is incorrect because cystic fibrosis is a genetic disorder that affects the lungs. Choice *D* is incorrect because Hashimoto's disease is an autoimmune disorder that affects the thyroid gland and thyroid hormones related to metabolism.

80. B: In the event that a code is called due to a patient having ventricular fibrillation, after starting CPR and defibrillating, the nurse should first administer epinephrine 1 mg via IV push, followed by amiodarone 300 mg. Choice *A* is incorrect because an amiodarone dose of 150 mg is only given if a second dose of amiodarone is needed and is not used as the initial dose. Choice *C* is incorrect because adenosine 6mg is used to treat supraventricular tachycardia or narrow complex tachycardias. Choice *D* is incorrect because adenosine is not used to treat ventricular fibrillation and is more commonly used as a 6 mg dose, not a 1 mg dose.

81. D: Chest tube output of greater than 100mL/hr following a coronary artery bypass graft (CABG) is abnormal and should be reported to the provider. Increased chest tube output could be a sign of bleeding or complications from the surgery. Choice *A* is incorrect because the drainage from the chest tube is expected to be serosanguinous. Choice *B* is incorrect because occasional bubbling, especially during exhalation and coughing, is an expected finding for a chest tube that is to suction. Choice *C* is incorrect because pain at and around the insertion site of the chest tube is common and should be managed with prescribed pain medication.

82. D: Paralytic ileus, also known as a pseudo-obstruction, has symptoms similar to a partial or complete bowel obstruction but, upon examination, there is often no visible blockage. Instead, the muscles may be paralyzed and unable to contract in order to move food and nutrients through the digestive tract.

This can occur due to some medications, hormone disorders, neurological disorders, and general stress. While patients may remain in the hospital for monitoring, this condition can resolve on its own or through minimally invasive mechanisms, such as changing the patient's diet. Surgery is almost never involved. Choice *A* is incorrect because intussusception, which occurs when one part of the intestinal tract telescopes into another part, is a true obstruction that will require either a radiologic or surgical procedure. Choice *B* is incorrect because a partial bowel obstruction will require one or more surgical procedures to resolve. Choice *C* is incorrect because a complete bowel obstruction will also require surgery.

83. B: Pancytopenia refers to an abnormally low blood cell count. It can result from a variety of causes including, but not limited to, viral infections, complications of pregnancy, pharmaceutical drugs, autoimmune disorders, and congenital issues. A biopsy of the patient's bone marrow quickly eliminates many of the possible causes, saving time and unnecessary testing for the patient and allowing for more prompt care. Choice *A* is incorrect because a PCR test detects the presence of specific viral particles, which may or may not relate to the pancytopenia diagnosis. Choice *C* is incorrect because an amniocentesis is a procedure performed during pregnancy to detect specific congenital diseases in the fetus. It is generally not used to detect pancytopenia in the mother or the fetus. Choice *D* is incorrect because, although a complete blood count (CBC) panel is often the first indicator that a patient is experiencing pancytopenia, this test does not provide helpful information to determine the underlying cause.

84. D: A patient with hypertensive encephalopathy has fluid leaking into their brain, which can cause increased intracranial pressure (ICP) and make cranial cerebral drainage difficult. The patient's body and head should be positioned to not restrict blood flow and allow for easier fluid drainage. Choice *A* is incorrect because $PaCO_2$ should be maintained between 33-37 mmHg to prevent an increase in ICP. Choice *B* is incorrect because suctioning should be avoided as it can cause an increase in ICP and blood pressure. Choice *C* is incorrect because helping to control a patient's pain can help reduce increase in pressure. Additionally, narcotic pain medications are often used in the treatment of hypertensive encephalopathy.

85. C: The model of nursing that shows the interactions and interconnectivity of a patient's health, the nurses' knowledge and clinical expertise, and the healthcare environment describes the Synergy Model of nursing practice. The Synergy Model encompasses eight client characteristics, eight nursing competencies, and six indicators of quality outcomes in the healthcare environment. Choice A is incorrect because the Nursing Leadership Model describes collaborative nursing environments that encourage teamwork and motivation. Choice *B* is incorrect because the Professional Practice Model refers to the overarching model of nursing practice that describes general values and beliefs in the nursing profession. Choice *D* is incorrect because the Modular Nursing Model describes the hierarchy and separate care units involved in patient care.

86. B: Phenylephrine is commonly used as a decongestant but can also trigger a fast heartbeat and supraventricular tachycardia (SVT). Other common medications that may cause SVT include antihistamines, asthma medications, and other decongestants. Choices *A, C,* and *D* are incorrect because digoxin, verapamil, and adenosine are all commonly prescribed medications in the treatment of SVT. Other treatment options for SVT include vagal maneuvers, cardiac ablation, and cardioversion.

87. B: The patient has several risk factors and symptoms for acute kidney injury. ICU admittance and age older than 65 years are both risk factors for acute kidney injuries. Additionally, this patient has peripheral artery disease. This increases the risk for acute kidney injuries because they may not get enough blood. The patient is also showing other kidney-related problems, such as minimal urine outflow and swelling in the legs and feet. Choice *A* is incorrect because cystitis is an infection of the bladder; symptoms include pain, the need to urinate, fever, and passing blood through the urine. The patient is not showing these symptoms. Choice *C* is incorrect because diabetic neuropathy is nerve damage that can occur in diabetic patients. It is characterized by irregular sensitivity to the sensations of touch, pressure, and temperature. It can also cause pain and weakness in various parts of the body. The patient is not showing these symptoms. Choice *D* is incorrect because the patient does not have symptoms of aortic injury, which often results in unbearable pain in the chest, neck, back, and stomach and can lead to loss of consciousness.

88. B: One finding to declare brain death for a patient is unresponsiveness to any stimuli. Choice *A* is incorrect because to declare brain death, primary reflexes should be absent in a patient. Choice *C* is incorrect because a patient needs to be apneic to declare brain death. Choice *D* is incorrect because two nurses alone cannot declare brain death. Additionally, in some areas, two physicians are required to declare brain death at separate times.

89. B: In order to prevent infection and needing to reopen the wound, the deepest layer of the wound should be repaired and allowed to heal fully before treating the next layers of skin. The superficial layers of skin should be kept sterile and covered during recovery. The other options listed are not relevant to the process.

90. C: Disseminated intravascular coagulation (DIC) is a critical condition in which a patient's blood begins abnormally clotting, eventually leading to vascular blockages and internal bleeding. While most cases of DIC are acute and occur after infections and/or traumatic injuries, they can occur more gradually in the presence of blood cancers. Choice *A* is incorrect because diabetes is a chronic disease and, apart from cancer, DIC events are generally not associated with chronic diseases. Choice *B* is incorrect for the same reason; chronic obstructive pulmonary disorder is a chronic disease. Choice *D* is also incorrect for the same reason; fatty liver disease is a chronic disease.

91. A: A perforation can occur when an untreated ulcer ultimately creates a tear in the stomach wall. This can cause related complications such as peritonitis, which typically requires emergency hospitalization. Choice *B* is incorrect because kidney stones are not related to peptic ulcers. Kidney stones are generally caused by diet, obesity, and some medications; they also have a family history component. Choice *C* is incorrect because gastric sleeves are used in bariatric procedures. They can make a patient more susceptible to developing peptic ulcers in the future; however, they are not a complication of peptic ulcers. Choice *D* is incorrect because bed sores are not related to gastrointestinal disorders. Instead, they are irritated, tender areas on the body that form when a patient remains in a single position for too long.

92. D: Choice *D* is correct because a sudden onset of decreased wheezing indicates the airway is completely obstructed. The healthcare team must intervene rapidly (intubation) to prevent cardiopulmonary arrest. Choice *A* is incorrect because increased dyspnea is characteristic of status asthmaticus. The patient's ability to verbalize their condition indicates their airway is still open. Choice *B* is incorrect because adventitious (wheezing) breath sounds are expected in respiratory conditions where the respiratory airways are narrowed. Impending cardiopulmonary arrest is characterized by diminished or absent breath sounds. Choice *C* is incorrect because hyperventilation is an expected finding during an asthma exacerbation. Hyperventilation indicates the airway is still open.

93. D: A patient who has undergone cardiac catheterization is at higher risk of neurovascular dysfunction and injury and should be assessed frequently. The nurse should assess for extremity circulation, signs of cardiogenic shock, and other common signs of bleeding. Choice *A* is incorrect because following a diagnostic cardiac catheterization, patients should be instructed to lay flat, with the head of the bed less than 30 degrees for at least four hours following the procedure. For an interventional cardiac catheterization, a patient should stay in this position for at least six hours. Choice *B* is incorrect because deep coughing or vomiting can cause clot dislodgment from the surgical site and put the patient at higher risk of internal bleeding. Choice *C* is incorrect because the dressing on the procedure site should not be removed until 24 hours after the procedure to reduce risk of clot dislodgement and bleeding.

94. A: Choice *A* is correct because a severe flail chest injury is stabilized with the use of positive-pressure ventilation. The goal of therapy is to establish adequate gas exchange via mechanical ventilation. Choice *B* is incorrect because coughing and deep breathing are not enough to stabilize a severe chest injury. The patient's symptoms indicate inadequate gas exchange. Choice *C* is incorrect because tracheal suctioning is indicated when the patient cannot clear their own oral secretions. The patient's immediate need is to stabilize the injury and promote adequate gas exchange. Choice *D* is incorrect; although patient-controlled analgesia is likely to be ordered for pain management, this therapy does not stabilize the injury.

95. D: Fractures on at least two adjacent ribs in two places each can cause a flail chest. This results in parodical chest movement with breathing, meaning the fractured segment of ribs will retract during inspiration and expand on expiration. Choices *A* and *C* are incorrect because they are not typical findings associated with this specific type of fracture. Choice *B* is incorrect because chest expansion during inspiration represents normal chest movement in an uninjured body, not flail chest movement.

96. B: Alexa is showing clear signs of rhabdomyolysis, including muscle pain, weakness, and dark urine. Rhabdomyolysis occurs when muscle tissue is severely damaged and releases macronutrients into the blood stream. The muscle damage that leads to rhabdomyolysis can be the result of either overuse or trauma; Alexa's activities indicate overuse. The only way to confirm the condition and begin targeted treatment is with blood tests that detect creatine kinase (released by the damaged muscles). Choice *A* is incorrect because Alexa is not showing comprehensive flu symptoms, nor do her daily activities indicate that she may be coming down with the flu. Choice *C* is incorrect because, while an electrolyte panel may provide additional information to help Alexa's healthcare provider, she does not need to be treated for dehydration; rather, she needs treatment for the severe muscle injury. Choice *D* is incorrect because electromyography tests are performed for abnormal, chronic muscle weakness. This does not apply to Alexa.

97. B: A patient experiencing an MI with vessel occlusion in the proximal section of the right coronary artery is likely to have ECG changes in leads V4, V5, and V6. This can result in right ventricular ischemia. Choice *A* is incorrect because ECG changes in leads V1 – V4 are associated with vessel occlusion in the right coronary artery or circumflex artery and can indicate a posterior infarct. Choice *C* is incorrect because ECG changes in leads I, aVL, V5, and V6 are associated with vessel occlusion in the circumflex coronary artery or the branch of the left coronary artery and indicate a lateral infarct. Choice *D* is incorrect because ECG changes in leads II, III, and aVF are associated with vessel occlusion in the right coronary artery and can indicate an inferior infarct.

98. B: A patient who is going through active alcohol withdrawal is at higher chance of suffering some type of delirium. Patients with a sudden onset of confusion and who are difficult to arouse, listless, have decreased awareness of surroundings, and have decreased activity, action speed, and speech speed are said to have hypoactive delirium. Hyperactive delirium is new onset of confusion accompanied with increased activity, restlessness, and loss of control of activity. Choice *A* is incorrect because mixed delirium is when patients exhibit signs of both hypoactive and hyperactive delirium in a twenty-four-hour period. Choice *C* is incorrect because, although patients with depression may have hypoactive features, a patient with confusion, active alcohol withdrawal, and prominent hypoactive actions is more likely to be suffering from hypoactive delirium. Choice *D* is incorrect because these symptoms do not describe common features of a patient with PTSD. A patient with PTSD may present with irritability, trouble sleeping, be easily frightened, and have a fixation on memories of trauma.

99. A: Since it is important to help promote a patient's independence to assist them with recovery, discouragement of this goal would be counter to the basic care responsibilities of the nurse. Choices *B, C,* and *D* are incorrect because these are the basic care responsibilities the nurse must provide. The nurse should provide safe care, minimize harm and pain, and reduce or eliminate any occurrence of medical errors.

100. C: Choice *C* is correct because ethambutol is part of a typical four-medication regimen to treat tuberculosis. Ethambutol works by suppressing bacterial RNA synthesis. Choice *A* is incorrect because streptomycin is only prescribed when patients have a multidrug-resistant strain of tuberculosis. Streptomycin has a high level of toxicity. Choice *B* is incorrect because penicillin G is an anti-infective used primarily in the treatment of pneumococcal pneumonia. Choice *D* is incorrect because gentamicin is an aminoglycoside antibiotic used to treat gram-negative bacterial infections. Gentamicin is not typically prescribed to treat tuberculosis.

101. A: Choice *A* is the major focus of nursing care for a patient with multiple organ dysfunction syndrome (MODS). Infection increases the mortality risk of a patient with MODS. Hand hygiene and universal precautions should be strictly adhered to when providing patient care. Choice *B* maintains adequate cardiac output and organ perfusion. However, this intervention alone does not prevent progression of MODS. Choice *C* is a vigilant strategy to detect early signs of sepsis. However, assessing laboratory data is not sufficient to prevent progression of MODS. Choice *D* helps to treat concurrent infections that can affect the recovery from MODS. However, infection control is the preferred preventative strategy.

102. C: Keeping the head of the bed in a lower position than 30 degrees is often contraindicated in a patient with acute pulmonary edema, and the nurse should question and verify this order with the provider. This positioning can make it more difficult for the patient to breathe, move oxygen, and remove fluid from their lungs. Patients with acute pulmonary edema should be maintained in an upright, high Fowler's position. This helps with ease of breathing, oxygenation, and fluid draining from the lungs. Choice *A* is incorrect because IV diuretics, such as furosemide (Lasix), are commonly given to help promote removal of fluid. Choice *B* is incorrect because BiPAP provides positive end-expiratory pressure (PEEP) that helps oxygenate patients and push excess fluid out of their lungs. Choice *D* is incorrect because morphine is often given to these patients to help alleviate pain and anxiety as well as decrease preload in the body.

103. D: Since most of the participants are over 50 years old and the treatment is for all adults over 18 years old, these participants do not accurately reflect the population for which the vaccine is intended.

This can lead to skewed results due to a selection bias, a bias that comes from study participants not being reflective of the true population. Choice *A* is incorrect because reporting bias comes from under-reporting or over-reporting certain characteristics or variables to skew results. Choice *B* is incorrect because recall bias is when participants are not able to accurately or completely remember information that is asked in a study. Choice *C* is incorrect because healthy participant bias is when someone is more likely to participate in a medical study if they are already careful and considerate about their health.

104. B: An aneurysm that is in the thoracic region of the body, specifically in only the ascending aorta, is a Type II aneurysm according to the DeBakey classification. The DeBakey classification is used to categorize an aneurysm based off the location in the body that it occurs. Choice *A* is incorrect because a Type I aneurysm is located in the thoracic region that starts in the ascending aorta but extends through to the descending aorta. Choice *C* is incorrect because a Type III aneurysm, also called an abdominal aneurysm, is located only in the descending aorta. Choice *D* is incorrect because Type IV is not a classification of aneurysm in the DeBakey classification. Aneurysms in the DeBakey classification system can only be Type I, Type II, or Type III.

105. B: Crackles in the lungs, dyspnea, and confusion are all symptoms associated with left-sided heart failure. Left-sided heart failure backs up to the lungs, where it causes the presentation of symptoms. Other symptoms with left-sided heart failure include a wet cough and wheezing. Choices *A, C,* and *D* are incorrect because these are all symptoms of right-sided heart failure. Right-sided heart failure backs up to the rest of the body and can cause more systemic problems. As left-sided heart failure persists and progresses, it can eventually cause right-sided heart failure and its associated symptoms.

106. B: A patient who is terminally ill may not physiologically need as much nutritional intake due to the dying process. The nurse should understand ethically that even though this nutrition may extend life for the patient, it can cause a great deal of discomfort, increase nausea and vomiting, and even cause increased tumor growth. The nurse should always explain their reasoning to the patient and family members and encourage open discussion. Choice *A* is incorrect because starting supplemental tube feeding can cause the aforementioned side effects and may not be within the wishes of the patient. Choice *C* is incorrect because weight gain is not a strong concern during the dying process and does not present an ethical dilemma for the nurse. Choice *D* is incorrect because although nutrition can extend life, it can result in a lower quality of life that the patient may not wish to endure.

107. B: Compared to other types of cancers, skin cancers have a fairly good prognosis if caught in their early stages. However, malignant melanoma is the most serious and aggressive form of skin cancer; it can spread rapidly and advance to late-stage cancer in under two months. Choice *A* is incorrect because squamous cell carcinoma is a common skin cancer with a very high survival rate. Choice *C* is incorrect because basal cell carcinoma is the most common type of skin cancer. Patients tend to notice and treat this type of cancer before it spreads; when removed from a local site, it has a 100% survival rate. Choice *D* is incorrect because dermatofibrosarcoma protuberans is a rare type of skin cancer that spreads slowly; it almost never spreads beyond the skin, which makes its relatively easy to treat.

108. D: Choice *D* is correct because one of the primary manifestations of malignant hyperthermia is hypercarbia. A carbon dioxide level of 47 mmHg is above normal. The normal CO_2 level is 35-45 mmHg. Choice *A* is not correct because a heart rate of 54 beats/min is not expected with hyperthermia. Tachycardia, or increased heart rate, is expected. Choice *B* is not correct because a temperature of 38.2 °C (100.7 °F) is on the higher end of normal. Choice *C* is not correct because a potassium level of 3.2

mEq/L is not expected in malignant hyperthermia. Hyperkalemia, an elevated potassium level, is consistent with the complication.

109. D: There are three levels of caring practice for the nurse: level 1, level 3, and level 5. A nurse who is completely involved in a patient's care and able to anticipate needs to provide safe, dignified, and comfortable care is considered to be at the highest level of caring practice, level 5. Choice *A* is incorrect because level 1 care provides the most basic care of creating a safe environment for a patient. Choice *B* is incorrect because level 3 care involves kind and compassionate care from a nurse, but the nurse may not be as fully engaged in managing and anticipating a patient's needs. Choice *C* is incorrect because level 4 is not one of the levels of caring practice for the nurse.

110. A: A common laboratory test in a patient with a suspected myocardial infarction (MI) is creatine kinase (CK-MB). CK-MB will show increased levels four to eight hours after myocardial injury. Other common lab values that are measured in a suspected MI are troponin levels, ischemia-modified albumin (IMA), and myoglobin. Choices *B, C,* and *D* are incorrect because these are not laboratory values that would be ordered for diagnosis or monitoring of an MI.

111. B: Increased arterial blood flow is not a factor that contributes to development of a venous thrombosis. Increased blood flow and perfusion may help decrease the likelihood of venous thrombosis. Choices *A, C,* and *D* are incorrect because endothelial injury, blood stasis, and hypercoagulability are all part of Virchow's Triad describing the three factors that can lead to venous thrombus formation.

112. A: Evidence is usually graded on a letter scale, with A being the highest level of evidence. The type of research with the highest level of evidence is a meta-analysis. Choice *B* is incorrect because a randomized-control trial is the second highest level of evidence, level B. Choices *C* and *D* are incorrect because integrative interviews and cohort studies have a moderate level of evidence and are both level C.

113. C: The blood leaves the right ventricle through a semi-lunar valve and goes through the pulmonary artery to the lungs. Any increase in pressure in the artery will eventually affect the contractibility of the right ventricle. Blood enters the right atrium from the superior and inferior venae cavae veins, and blood leaves the right atrium through the tricuspid valve to the right ventricle. Blood enters the left atrium from the pulmonary veins carrying oxygenated blood from the lungs. Blood flows from the left atrium to the left ventricle through the mitral valve and leaves the left ventricle through a semi-lunar valve to enter the aorta.

114. D: Choice *D* is correct because thermoregulation is lost after brain death. A temperature of 35.1 °C (95.1 °F) indicates hypothermia and can compromise organ perfusion. Choice *A* is not correct because a mean arterial pressure (MAP) of 75 mmHg is ideal for maintaining cardiac output and organ perfusion. The acceptable MAP parameter is 60-110 mmHg. Choice *B* is not correct because a pH level of 7.3 is an acceptable parameter after brain death. The pH should be kept between 7.3 and 7.5. Choice *C* is not correct because serum sodium should be kept less than or equal to 155 mEq/L after brain death.

115. B: Lithium is a mood stabilizer that is often used in the treatment of hypermania and hypomania. Lithium, however, is not often used to treat delirium because lithium toxicity can cause delirium. Choices *A, C,* and *D* are incorrect because trazodone, lorazepam, and haloperidol are commonly used medications in the treatment of delirium to relax patients. The nurse should be cautious using these medications because they can worsen confusion in elderly patients.

116. C: Alteplase is the single fibrinolytic agent approved for the treatment of ischemic stroke because it is associated with fewer adverse effects than the remaining agents. Streptokinase and tenecteplase have been used effectively to treat patients with acute myocardial infarction; however, in patients with ischemic stroke, streptokinase has been associated with an increased risk of intracranial hemorrhage and death. Current evidence for the efficacy and safety of urokinase and tenecteplase does not support their use for the treatment of ischemic stroke. Therefore, Choices *A, B,* and *D* are incorrect.

117. B: Advance directives can be made available to any and all patients that are admitted. This allows for the protection of the patient's legal right to self-determination in their care. Advance directives can also include types of do-not-resuscitate (DNR) orders that may be more commonly seen in terminally ill or elderly patients. Choices *A, C,* and *D* are incorrect because they do not include the entire patient population that is eligible to receive an advance directive as part of their medical care.

118. D: This team is now at the implementation stage of problem-solving because their team is actively using their possible solution by removing catheters within 24 hours of surgery. Choice *A* is incorrect because evaluation would be the next step in this process and would include the team seeing if this is an effective strategy in reducing UTIs. In this scenario, the nursing team has already identified a problem, in this case high UTI rates, and developed a possible solution of removing catheters earlier in the post-op period; therefore, Choices *B* and *C* are also incorrect.

119. A: Gait that is characterized by one-sided weakness resulting in the affected arm staying at a person's side and not swinging and the affected foot dragging while walking is considered to be hemiplegic gait. The unaffected side allows for normal movement of the limbs with ambulation. This gait is often caused by stroke. Choice *B* is incorrect because diplegic gait is when hips, knees, and ankles are turned in on both sides of the body, affecting ambulation. This is often caused by stroke, cerebral palsy, or head trauma. Choice *C* is incorrect because neuropathic gait is when the foot drops down when lifting the leg and stepping, causing the patient to have to lift their knee higher with each step. This is a common gait in patients with ALS, MS, and peripheral neuropathy. Choice *D* is incorrect because ataxic gait is considered to be a staggering or uncoordinated walk that is often caused by alcohol intoxication.

120. C: Using "you" statements may place needless blame and pressure on the patient or learner. In the case of disagreement and communication, it is better for the nurse to use "I" statements to help them take responsibility for both ideas and feelings to help move a conversation forward. Choices *A, B,* and *D* are incorrect because these are encouraged communication tactics in successful assertive communication.

121. A: Addisonian crises occur from acute adrenal insufficiency in which the adrenal glands fail. Hyperkalemia (high potassium) and hyponatremia (low sodium) are electrolyte imbalances that occur during Addisonian crises in which the patient's potassium levels are too high and their sodium levels are too low. This imbalance has a domino effect on the patient's overall cardiovascular health and stress response. Choice *B* is incorrect because, while Addisonian crisis is associated a high risk of shock, it is associated with low blood pressure (hypotension) rather than high blood pressure (hypertension). Choice *C* is incorrect because excessive cortisol and sweating indicate excessive activity, while patients in Addisonian crisis tend to lose alertness, become severely weak and confused, and lose consciousness from shock-like symptoms. Choice *D* is incorrect because a hypokalemia (low potassium) and hypernatremia (high sodium) are the opposite effects of those caused by an Addisonian crisis.

122. B: Choice *B* is correct because a $\mathrm{PaO_2/FIO_2}$ (arterial oxygen partial pressure/fraction of inspired oxygen) ratio of 175 mmHg is classified as moderate acute respiratory failure syndrome (ARDS) per the

Berlin Definition of ARDS. Choice *A* is incorrect because a PaO_2/FIO_2 ratio of 85 mmHg is considered severe ARDS. Choice *C* is incorrect because a PaO_2/FIO_2 ratio of 250 mmHg is considered mild ARDS. Choice *D* is incorrect because a PaO_2/FIO_2 ratio of 325 mmHg is not a value that supports a diagnosis of ARDS.

123. C: A traumatic injury in combination with unequal pupils, weakness, headache, and slurred speech are symptomatic of an intracranial hemorrhage, or bleeding around the brain, that can lead to a hemorrhagic stroke. Choice *A* is incorrect because subarachnoid hemorrhage often results in hemodynamic instability, respiratory changes, and decreased level of consciousness. Subarachnoid stroke can also be caused by traumatic injuries. Choice *B* is incorrect because intraventricular hemorrhage can cause decreased level of consciousness and elevated heart rate and blood pressure. Intraventricular hemorrhages can be chronic or due to traumatic injury. Choice *D* is incorrect because aneurysmal hemorrhage is another name for subarachnoid hemorrhage and has the same causes and symptoms.

124. B: Choice *B* honors the patient's wishes while providing more information on end-of-life care. The nurse should respect the patient's autonomy and ensure the patient and family are educated on end-of-life decisions. Choice *A* does not respect the patient's autonomy. While it is important to take the family's thoughts into consideration, the patient makes the ultimate decision on their end-of-life care. Choice *C* does not provide sensitive care. The nurse's duty is to provide information and respect the patient's wishes. Choice *D* is not the best response. The patient's illness is advanced and medical treatments are likely to be futile.

125. B: Predictability is one of the eight types of client characteristics in the AACN Synergy Model. The other client characteristics are resiliency, stability, vulnerability, complexity, resource availability, participation in care, and decision-making ability. Choices *A, C,* and *D* are incorrect because these are not characteristics or factors that affect the patient aspect of the Synergy Model.

126. D: Chronic alcohol abuse and biliary tract dysfunction are the most frequent causes of acute pancreatitis; however, there are no identified criteria that explain why some individuals will experience pancreatitis while others do not. Acute pancreatitis is most often diagnosed by the presenting history and physical examination. ECRP is only indicated in patients with acute pancreatitis and concomitant biliary disease; therefore, Choice *A* is incorrect. Ultrasonography is generally less useful than CT imaging for pancreatitis, and its efficacy is significantly decreased in the presence of abdominal distention, which distorts the images; therefore, Choice *B* is incorrect. Although rectal indomethacin is used commonly to treat acute pancreatitis resulting from ERCP imaging, controversy remains regarding the efficacy of the therapy; therefore, Choice *C* is incorrect.

127. C: Gastroenteritis, or inflammation in the stomach lining, is typically caused by a virus, bacteria, parasite, or other pathogenic microbe. Patients may present with vomiting, diarrhea, gastrointestinal distress, and fever. Patients typically progress to needing critical care due to dehydration, and they often are unable to digest food initially. Therefore, withholding food and providing fluid therapy is generally the first line of care to stabilize the patient. Choice *A* is incorrect because the patient may not be able to manage enteral nutrition initially. Choice *B* is incorrect because patients with gastroenteritis usually do not have respiratory concerns, and while airway vitals may be checked, airway management would not be the first intervention. Choice *D* is incorrect because the use of anti-emetic drugs such as Zofran is not currently the primary intervention used to treat gastroenteritis, although it may support primary interventions such as fluid therapy, especially in pediatric patients.

128. C: A patient who is experiencing a severe, unrelieved headache after a carotid endarterectomy may be hemorrhaging. This is a medical emergency, and the nurse should immediately notify the provider before additional measures are taken. Carotid endarterectomy is a surgical procedure used to treat carotid artery stenosis that opens an occluded artery and removes the plaque. Choice *A* is incorrect because lowering the head of the bed may cause an increase in pressure in the brain and could cause more complications for the post-op patient. Choice *B* is incorrect because although the patient may need additional pain medication, the provider should be notified first, since this could indicate a medical emergency. Choice *D* is incorrect because a headache that is not relieved by Tylenol is not an expected finding.

129. C: Nurses should always try to use therapeutic communication, but they should take special care when speaking with patients and family members who have received difficult news. The nurse is letting the patient know in this response that they are available to care for the patient's needs and recognize the stressful situation they are in. This communication helps put the focus on the patient and allows for an open line of communication. Choice *A* is incorrect because this gives false reassurance to the patient and may make it more difficult for the patient to accept their prognosis. Choice *B* is incorrect because this question is accusatory and places blame on the patient, which is not comforting or productive. Choice *D* is incorrect because the nurse is offering advice when it may not be the patient's wish to begin looking at hospice. This also does not put the patient as the focus of the nurse's response and does not allow them time to properly process the new information they received.

130. C: There are three levels of responding to diversity in the Synergy Model: levels 1, 3, and 5. According to the Synergy Model of responding to diversity, a nurse who is seeking information about the cultural background of a patient and beginning to incorporate some of this diversity into the patient's care is said to be at a level 3 of diversity response. Choice *A* is incorrect because at level 1, the nurse is just beginning to assess different cultural backgrounds with basic questions but may not be incorporating these findings into diverse care. Choice *B* is incorrect because level 2 is not one of the levels of responding to diversity in the Synergy Model. Choice *D* is incorrect because level 5 is when the nurse is actively incorporating diverse cultural knowledge into the patient's care and is able to help think of alternative or preferred models for delivery of care that are aligned with the patient's diverse cultural beliefs.

131. A: The first step of conflict resolution should be for both sides to present their side of the disagreement calmly and professionally. This allows whoever is mediating the conflict to understand the opinions of both sides. Choices *B* and *C* are incorrect because these steps come later in conflict resolution. After presenting the sides of the argument, the disagreement should be discussed in detail, eventually coming to a compromise or some negotiation or re-evaluation. Choice *D* is incorrect because disagreements should not be dismissed. Using conflict resolution can help teams grow and build better communication.

132. D: An INR of 3.5 is elevated and will cause bleeding complications if thrombolytic therapy is initiated before the INR returns to the normal level of less than or equal to 1.1.

133. D: While the physician is legally responsible for satisfying all elements of informed consent, nurses are ethically responsible for assessing the patient's ability to process and understand the implications of informed consent. Nurses protect the patient's autonomy by raising these questions and concerns. The remaining elements of informed consent are required of the physician, rather than the nurses.

134. B: Choice *B* is correct because postpneumonectomy empyema is a collection of pus in the postpneumonectomy space. Signs and symptoms reflect an infection, such as fever and purulent drainage. Choice *A* is incorrect because pulmonary edema is a postoperative complication characterized by respiratory distress and hypoxemia. It typically occurs within 72 hours post procedure. Choice *C* is incorrect because a chylothorax is characterized by an abnormal accumulation of chyle in the postpneumonectomy space. Clinical manifestations include an elevated central venous pressure, dyspnea, and tachycardia. Choice *D* is incorrect because postpneumonectomy syndrome occurs when the mediastinum shifts due to hyperinflation of the remaining lung and compression of the trachea and mainstem bronchus.

135. A: The most common symptom of peripheral vascular disease is intermittent claudication, or pain in the leg caused by obstructed blood flow in arteries. Necrotic ulcers, as well as lower extremity edema and hair loss, may be symptoms in patients with peripheral vascular disease but none are the most common symptom; therefore, Choices *B, C,* and *D* are incorrect.

136. D: Positive chronotropic medications increase heart rate and can increase the workload on the heart following a cardiac catheterization. If a patient is experiencing cardiogenic shock, the patient may also have tachycardia, and a medication that further increases the heart rate would be dangerous. Choice *A* is incorrect because positive inotropic agents, such as norepinephrine and dopamine, are medications commonly used in the treatment of cardiogenic shock following a cardiac catheterization to increase contractility. Choices *B* and *C* are incorrect because antiplatelet medication, such as clopidogrel, and thrombolytics, such as alteplase, are used to help reduce risk of clotting with cardiac catheterization or cardiogenic shock.

137. C: The correct dose for mannitol is 0.25-2.0 g/kg infused over thirty minutes to an hour for a patient with a TBI. Mannitol causes osmotic diuresis and helps draw fluid off the brain, lowering ICP. Hypertonic saline is also infused and used for the same purposes. Choices *A*, *B*, and *D* are incorrect because they are not the correct dose to run a mannitol infusion for a patient with a TBI.

138. A: Phantom limb syndrome is most likely to diminish if the patient mentally feels comfortable with the prosthesis and accepts it as an artificial limb, therefore allowing the brain to perceive that area of the body as missing. This changes the brain's neural processing for the area over time.

139. D: Choice *D* is correct because whole-bowel irrigation is administered to patients who have ingested a toxic agent more than two hours before seeking treatment. Whole bowel irrigation is performed orally or through a nasogastric tube using polyethylene glycol electrolyte solution. Choices *A* and *B* are not correct because although activated charcoal and gastric lavage are commonly used to absorb and excrete toxic agents, they are most effective when administered within one to two hours of the ingested toxin. Choice *C* is not correct because syrup of ipecac is no longer recommended as treatment for toxic ingestions.

140. C: Epidermolysis bullosa is an inheritable disorder that affects a person's connective tissues. People with this disorder have fragile tissues, and routine tactile exposure (such as getting dressed) can result in skin irritation and blistering. Blisters can also occur across or inside the body without any external cause. This can be extremely painful and even fatal in cases where vital organs are affected. Patients also experience abnormalities in their hands and feet including thick, calloused skin and calcified, disfigured nailbeds. Choice *A* is incorrect because Angelman syndrome is an inherited disorder that affects a person's nervous system and development. Symptoms include musculoskeletal delays and developmental delays. Choice *B* is incorrect because the question is about an inheritable disease, and herpes simplex 2 is most commonly sexually transmitted or is spread in ways other than inheriting. Choice *D* is incorrect because the rare, inherited disease known as familial multiple trichodiscomas results in hair and skin lesions, but it does not cause blistering, anemia, or issues with the hands and feet.

141. D: Symptoms of vision changes, confusion, nausea, vomiting, difficulty speaking or walking, and paralysis can all be general signs of any type of stroke. However, a sudden and severe headache, along with the other described symptoms, is a hallmark sign of a hemorrhagic stroke. Choices *A, B,* and *C* are incorrect because, although patients with these kinds of stroke may experience many of these symptoms, a patient with a sudden and severe headache is likely to have a hemorrhagic stroke.

142. C: Injuries above the T6 level are associated with neurogenic shock, due to alterations of the autonomic nervous system, resulting in the loss of vagal tone. This manifests as decreased vascular resistance and vasodilation. Injury at this level is also associated with alterations in respiratory function, which results in symptoms such as decreased vital capacity and the presence of adventitious breath sounds. In addition, hypothermia is common; therefore, Choice *C* is correct. A vital capacity level that equals 45 percent of normal is associated with injuries at the T1 level or below and is an indication of hemorrhagic shock rather than neurogenic shock.

143. B: Choice *B* is the most common complication after abruptio placentae. Disseminated intravascular coagulation is a serious complication characterized by internal and external bleeding. Choice *A* is a genetic autoimmune disorder that can result in postpartum hemorrhage. Choice *C* occurs after birth and is the inability of the uterine muscle to contract adequately. Choice *D* is a complication that can occur with any pregnancy. Pregnancy increases the risk of developing deep vein thrombosis with subsequent embolus.

144. D: Adherence to discharge plans is not one of the eight indicators of nursing competencies; however, it is one of the six indicators of quality outcomes in the healthcare setting. Choices *A, B,* and *C* are incorrect because they are all indicators of nursing competencies. The other nursing competencies are clinical judgement, advocacy, caring practices, collaboration, and diversity response.

145. A: Most patients who are experiencing renal issues first present to the emergency department with pain in the flank or lower torso (including lower abdomen, lower back, and groin). Choice *B* is incorrect because referred pain to the upper torso and neck is more indicative of heart and lung issues. Choice *C* is incorrect because pain in the popliteal area is usually a result of muscle strains or sprains in the hamstrings, calves, or quadriceps. Choice *D* is incorrect because referred pain in the tips of the shoulders is often caused by gall bladder or spleen issues.

146. D: Granulomas are inflamed or infected tissues that look like thick bumps under the surface of the skin. They develop around microscopic foreign bodies. Patients who are in emergency situations tend to have higher rates of experiencing foreign body complications, as these can get overlooked when emergency teams are focused on life-sustaining measures instead. The presence of bumps on Robbie's arm are not indicative of the other options.

147. B: The elevated glucose levels associated with both type 1 and type 2 diabetes result in atherosclerosis, or wall thickening of the small arterioles and capillaries, which alters the circulation in the brain, retina, peripheral nerves, and kidneys. These changes are cumulative and irreversible; however, long-term control of the serum glucose level as measured by the A1C can limit the progression of this process. Current research indicates that the optimum A1C level is patient specific. In this discussion, the patient knows his personal A1C target and understands the association between the elevated glucose levels and the occurrence of the TIA; therefore, Choice *B* is correct. Two of the $ABCD^2$ score categories are modifiable risk factors. Maintaining the systolic and diastolic blood pressure and blood glucose level as defined by the A1C within normal limits may lower the risk of a repeated attack.

148. A: Myocarditis is a structural heart defect that is acquired through bacterial and viral infections or other conditions that cause inflammation. Other acquired structural heart defects include those caused by valvular disease, cardiomyopathy, and cardiac hypertrophy. Treatment for acquired heart defects usually includes medication therapy and surgical repair. Choices *B, C,* and *D* are incorrect because these are all structural heart changes that are caused by congenital defects. These defects are diagnosed either at birth and infancy or later in childhood once symptoms start presenting. The most common treatment for congenital defects is surgical repair.

149. C: Choice *C* is the appropriate intervention for this patient. During pregnancy, the enlarged uterus applies pressure to the vena cava when in the supine position and causes decreased venous return. Turning the patient to the left lateral position will relieve compression. Choice *A* should occur after non-pharmacological interventions have been attempted. Choice *B* is not indicated. The patient's airway has already been cleared and the symptoms are not indicative of respiratory complications. Choice *D* is indicated only if the patient's symptoms persist after performing initial interventions.

150. D: Hand tremors are not an expected finding in patients with a bacterial infection in their nervous system. These patients, however, are at risk for seizures and should be monitored closely. Patients with bacterial meningitis have toxins that are released into the body that can cause brain cell damage quickly. Since damage and infection can start so rapidly, the nurse should be able to recognize common signs of bacterial infection and anticipate treatment measures. Choices *A* and *B* are incorrect because an elevated WBC and low blood glucose levels are a common laboratory finding in patients with bacterial meningitis. Choice *C* is incorrect because nuchal rigidity, or neck stiffness, is a common sign of bacterial meningitis.

Adult CCRN Practice Tests #3 - #15

To keep the size of this book manageable, save paper, and provide a digital test-taking experience, the 3rd – 15th practice tests can be found online. Scan the QR code or go to this link to access it:

testprepbooks.com/bonus/ccrn

The first time you access the tests, you will need to register as a "new user" and verify your email address.

If you have any issues, please email support@testprepbooks.com.

Dear Adult CCRN Test Taker,

Thank you for purchasing this study guide for your Adult CCRN exam. We hope that we exceeded your expectations.

Our goal in creating this study guide was to cover all of the topics that you will see on the test. We also strove to make our practice questions as similar as possible to what you will encounter on test day. With that being said, if you found something that you feel was not up to your standards, please send us an email and let us know.

We would also like to let you know about other books in our catalog that may interest you.

CNOR

This can be found on Amazon: amazon.com/dp/1637753004

CEN

amazon.com/dp/1637757891

DTR Flashcards

amazon.com/dp/1637754078

We have study guides in a wide variety of fields. If the one you are looking for isn't listed above, then try searching for it on Amazon or send us an email.

Thanks Again and Happy Testing!
Product Development Team
support@testprepbooks.com

Online Resources

Included with your purchase are multiple online resources. This includes the practice tests in an interactive format and a convenient study timer to help you manage your time.

Scan the QR code or go to this link to access this content:

testprepbooks.com/online387/ccrn

SCAN ME

The first time you access the page, you will need to register as a "new user" and verify your email address.

If you have any issues, please email support@testprepbooks.com.

Thank you for letting us be a part of your studying journey!

Made in the USA
Monee, IL
15 September 2026

63182434R00153